Nutritional Grail

ANCESTRAL WISDOM, BREAKTHROUGH SCIENCE,
and the DAWNING NUTRITIONAL RENAISSANCE

Christopher James Clark

EXTROPY PUBLISHING

Copyright © 2014 by Christopher James Clark

All rights reserved. No part of this publication may be reproduced, distributed, or transmitted in any form or by any means, including photocopying, recording, or by other electronic or mechanical methods, without the prior written permission of the publisher, except brief quotations embodied in critical reviews, editorials, and certain noncommercial uses permitted by copyright law. For permission requests, write to the email address below, "Attention: Permissions Coordinator."

Extropy Publishing
www.extropypublishing.com
info@extropypublishing.com

Cover Artwork: Manvee Singh – manveesingh@gmail.com
Graphic Design: Ben Hopfer – benhopfer.4ormat.com
Copyediting: Ruth Goodman – ruthgoodman.com

Ordering Information:
Special discounts are available on quantity purchases by corporations, associations, institutions, and others. For details, write to the email address above, "Attention: Special Sales Department."

Nutritional Grail/Christopher James Clark—1st edition
ISBN 978-0-9912595-0-2

Table of Contents

Dedicated to all my teachers

May you live as long as you wish and love as long as you live.

—Robert A. Heinlein

Foreword

In a jungle of dietary advice, food choices, and eating habits, it's hard to know which foods are best. In past eras, food choices were much more restricted. People ate what was available. Today, our food choices are seemingly limitless. So how can we determine the best diet for the twenty-first century?

- Should we formulate our meals based on "conventional knowledge," with four parts carbs, two parts protein, and one part fat?
- Should our diets center around grains and starches?
- Are vegan and vegetarian diets healthy?
- Is dairy healthy? What about red meat?
- Should we avoid gluten?
- Should we eat soy or avoid it like the plague?
- Should we eat mostly raw foods?
- Should we eat like chimpanzees, like Okinawans, or perhaps like people from the Caucasus?

The list of questions is very long. To gain a better perspective, we should step back, momentarily, from the details and intricacies of dietary theory. In doing so, two things become apparent:

1. There are some established dietary principles, which the vast majority of scientists, practitioners, and health advocates agree upon.

2. These principles are consistently seen in the diets and eating habits of indigenous populations, as well as those of ancient man.

In this book, Christopher Clark explores the forgotten nutritional principles and practices of the past, including those of traditional cultures and Paleolithic man. In my opinion, we have strayed very far from this ancestral wisdom. Embracing this wisdom represents the first and most logical step towards living healthier.

But Clark goes far beyond this. He takes a scientific approach, explaining in great detail, according the latest nutritional research, which foods are most healthy and which are most problematic. He has done a remarkable job with his research and has thoroughly documented, in a scholarly manner, all the information he presents. Clark offers fascinating insights regarding:

- Our dietary misdirection and mistakes
- The deterioration of our food quality
- Effective detoxification through natural foods
- The importance of reducing chronic inflammation and oxidative stress, both of which underlie many degenerative diseases

To those who will listen, modern science is increasingly saying that contemporary Western diets are damaging our health significantly. We can best avoid the diseases of modernity by merging ancestral dietary wisdom with modern nutritional science, and adjusting our diets accordingly.

But establishing a healthy diet requires a basic understanding of the reasons for choosing certain foods and avoiding others. This book helps because it clearly and coherently explains the most essential information regarding each food group and each macronutrient category.

Clark does not ask us to accept any doctrine or dogma. He simply informs us about many foods and food preparation techniques, based on science and tradition, which can greatly improve our health and increase our longevity.

We now know a lot about ancient man, including details about his lifestyle and diet. According to paleontologists, our distant ancestors hunted and gathered their food for every meal. They ate when food was available, which was not necessarily every day. Our ancestors certainly derived satisfaction from their food, but probably not the same satisfaction we derive from sophisticated gastronomy.

Things are much different today. We have a plethora of food constantly at hand. So readily accessible is food that sometimes it becomes mundane. Consequently, we continually look for ways to stimulate our senses. Additionally, we must compensate for the constant stresses of modern life, which include our heavy workloads, social commitments, insecurities about the future, and the physiological stress caused by eating denatured food and living in polluted environments. We can alleviate stress through meditation, yoga, and sports, but the most effective approach is returning to wholesome, nourishing food, which, as Clark demonstrates, can also deeply satisfy our senses.

For many people today, diet has become mechanical. We quickly scarf down our morning bread with butter and jam. We hurriedly drink our coffee so as not to be late for work. We watch television while eating, giving little attention to our food. And, for lack of time and motivation, we frequently opt for fast food or readymade meals. We establish bad habits, which are difficult to overturn.

Clark proposes that eating healthy can and should be pleasurable, never a struggle or a burden. He gives us the keys for implementing his dietary advice, which include simple, straightforward recipes requiring very little time to prepare. From both a health perspective and an implementation perspective, this book begs the question, "Why would anyone choose to eat differently?"

Christopher Clark brilliantly showed me that eating healthy must not mean eating sadly. To the contrary, he showed me that sitting down for our meals should be a double pleasure: the pleasure for our taste buds and the pleasure of feeling healthy. What could be better?

Jean-Luc Morel, MD

- President of the French Association of Morpho-Aesthetic Medicine and Anti-Aging (Président de l'Association Française de Médecine morpho-Esthétique et anti-âge)
- Former Education Director at multiple French Universities (Ancien Directeur d'enseignement à l'Université)

Introduction

started thinking about it when I was quite young, maybe 9 or 10 years old. Most of my peers probably never gave it any thought. I attribute this disparity mostly to my grandmother. After my immediate family, she was my closest and most influential relative. She died when I was 18 after an arduous, 15-year battle with heart disease. I spent a good chunk of my childhood at Akron General, the hospital in Akron, Ohio, where she routinely was a patient. I grew to despise hospitals and heart disease, and resolved to avoid both throughout my life. That's why from such a young age I was thinking about the relationship between diet and health.

Like many Americans during the 1980s and 90s, I was convinced that saturated fat and cholesterol were the primary drivers of heart disease. This conventional wisdom was echoed ad nauseam by the US government, the food industry, prominent health institutions, and my grandmother's cardiovascular specialists. I had no reason to question such an unshakable consensus of experts. Moreover, I had firsthand proof that fat and cholesterol were the culprits—my grandmother's fatty cuisine. Danish meatballs, known as frickadeller in my family, were her specialty. To make them, she would combine ground beef, onions, breadcrumbs, and eggs, form the mixture into balls, then pan-fry them in bacon grease. What could be more artery-clogging? At least the breadcrumbs were healthy, or so I thought. As I explain throughout this book, however, the breadcrumbs are the most objectionable ingredient while the other ingredients are actually quite healthy.

I loved those meatballs, but increasingly avoided them during my pre-teen years and beyond. During those same years, I began choosing low-fat yogurt, low-fat snack foods, and "heart-healthy" breakfast cereals. Wheat and sugar featured prominently in my childhood diet, both of which I fully believed were healthy. According to the health experts of those days, whole wheat prevents heart disease and sugar is benign. I wouldn't succumb to heart disease by drinking sodas and eating crackers, as I often did. I would avoid that fate by carefully restricting my saturated fat and cholesterol consumption. That's why I frequently lobbied for Wendy's.

My family regularly drove the four hours from my suburban Detroit hometown to Akron, where my grandparents lived. We didn't eat fast food often—only a few times per week like every freedom-loving American family. McDonald's and Burger King were my family's preferred choices, but both were on my B-list. McDonald's was too fattening and Burger King's burgers, according to a persistent rumor that nobody really believed, caused cancer. I decided to play it safe. By my calculations, Wendy's was the healthiest option. First of all, Wendy's had thicker fries, which to my mind meant proportionally more potato and less fat. Second, Wendy's offered a grilled chicken sandwich whereas McDonald's and Burger King only had fried chicken sandwiches. Furthermore, I absolutely loved Wendy's Frosty desserts, which were low fat—or at least low fat enough for me.

I was outnumbered four to one by my parents and two brothers. Accordingly, I used persuasion, guilt tactics, and statistics to undermine the democratic process. During those long drives to Ohio, I usually convinced my family to opt for Wendy's. Since our destination was often the Cardiovascular Intensive Care Unit at Akron General, "heart-healthy" Wendy's seemed like the sensible choice. Cruising along the Ohio Turnpike, washing down my grilled chicken sandwich and fries with an icy Coke (followed, of course, by a Frosty), I enjoyed the feeling of proactively cheating my genetic predisposition to heart disease. I was winning.

I went to college in Ann Arbor at the University of Michigan, where I considered studying medicine. All those years of visiting hospitals, however, made me rather squeamish. I couldn't even watch surgery videos without feeling nauseous. The sight of a scalpel cutting flesh made me lightheaded. One sunny spring day during my first year of college, my biology professor played a video for our class, which featured some surgery scenes. I decided to test my mind-over-matter skills, convincing myself I could watch it without incident. This was not a good decision. After several minutes, I hastily collected my belongings and staggered from the class, blurry-eyed and desperately seeking the nearest exit and a breath of fresh air. Lying on a patch of grass for the next half hour, I decided to forget about medicine and instead focus on getting into Michigan's prestigious business school.

I graduated from Michigan with my bachelor of business administration degree before moving to Chicago to work for United Airlines, then a Fortune-100 company. The most important thing I learned in school was how to learn—how to analyze problems and situations while objectively finding solutions and drawing conclusions. I worked as a pricing and market analyst for United, eventually developing strategic pricing initiatives and managing markets worth $350 million annually. Although I became a very good analyst, I felt unfulfilled. I had bigger goals and a better purpose. The corporate business world taught me much, but my heart was elsewhere.

I thought a lot about health and nutrition during those years. I had my own apartment and, for the first time, was regularly cooking most of my meals. I was shopping at organic supermarkets and reconsidering my warped childhood ideas about food. Sugar, I finally realized, is completely unhealthy, as are processed foods and fast foods, even my beloved Wendy's. I wanted to go deeper into nutrition, but I didn't know how or where to start. By this time, I was rather weary of allopathic medicine, invasive surgery, and pharmaceutical drugs, all of which failed to heal my grandmother's heart. I started looking into traditional Chinese medicine. Gradually, I realized that food is our most effective, most fundamental form of medicine. I again began contemplating studying medicine. This time, however, I wasn't thinking about medical school. I was thinking about culinary school.

I started searching for healthy cooking schools in 2001. Both the Internet and the holistic health movement were much less developed then. Consequently, I didn't find many options. Eventually, I decided to attend a macrobiotic school in Austin, Texas. Macrobiotics is a philosophy that borrows from traditional Chinese medicine and advocates a mostly vegetarian, grain-based diet, including vegetables, legumes, and various fermented foods. Although my dietary philosophy today looks nothing like macrobiotics, my macrobiotic experience was invaluable. Most importantly, I met hundreds of wonderful people who were passionate about health and dedicated to promoting health-conscious lifestyles. After completing my macrobiotic studies, I managed the kitchen of a yoga resort in Greece for five years. I also taught cooking workshops throughout Europe, and worked with scores of individuals, restaurants, and spas, advising them on recipes, menus, and diet plans.

During my entire career as a chef and health food advocate, two questions nagged me continually: 1) What is really the healthiest way to eat, and 2) How can I be sure? I never stopped being a student and never stopped asking such probing, fundamental questions. After studying macrobiotics, I started branching out, deeply exploring many other dietary philosophies and traditions. By embracing the scientific aspects of established diets and sifting out the unscientific aspects, I gradually pieced together a working philosophy. From macrobiotics, for example, I embraced miso and other fermented foods while rejecting its heavy reliance on grains. From raw vegan diets, I embraced certain raw vegetables and herbs while rejecting the wholesale exclusion of animal foods. Eventually, I realized that answering those nagging questions would require starting from square one. I would have to approach nutrition as a scholar— objectively, critically, and scientifically. Thus began an intensive, two-year writing and research project, finally culminating in this book.

This brings me to an important question that many readers will undoubtedly ask: What qualifies you, Christopher Clark, to write a book on nutrition? To answer this question, I'll first pose a more general question: What qualifies anyone to write about nutrition? I suggest there are four general categories of qualified people. The first category includes doctors and practitioners with professional experience guiding people to improved health through diet and nutrition. These professionals have seen firsthand what does and doesn't work. The second category consists of people who have overcome diseases or chronic conditions by changing how they eat. Some have overcome cancer, others autoimmune diseases such as Crohn's disease. People from categories one and two have stories to tell. Their recommendations may not always be scientifically sound, but nevertheless, for certain people with certain conditions, they have been effective.

The third category consists of scientists doing original research. These people are the backbone of the entire field. Without their invaluable work, nutrition would be little more than folklore. Unprincipled corporations and opportunistic individuals would make every nutritional claim that suits them. Snake oil would be the cure for everything that heals nothing. Nutritional scientists deserve tremendous respect for conducting original research, which can potentially benefit the entire world.

The fourth category consists of people who carefully study the work of those from category three, and to a lesser extent those from categories one and two. Nutritional research is either primary, including experimental and epidemiological studies, or secondary. Primary research generates new data, whereas secondary research gathers, analyzes, and interprets data from numerous primary sources. In general, primary research attempts to answer very focused questions, whereas secondary research asks broader questions. Primary research normally requires a scientific degree, whereas secondary research benefits from a scientific degree, but does not require one.

My qualifications come via category four. Although my analytical background prepared me to conduct secondary research, I have neither the medical degree nor the nutritional science degree that would perhaps reassure some readers. With this in mind, I have worked tirelessly to thoroughly and precisely document this entire book. Every important statement, assertion, and conclusion is footnoted and linked to post-chapter notes. I don't expect readers to simply accept my ideas at face value. Writers should provide references so readers can better draw their own conclusions. Many nutrition books are only partially documented. Others are poorly documented or not documented at all. There is a logical reason for this—thoroughly documenting a book requires great time and perseverance. I know this because I have done it.

Despite the lengthy time commitment, I suggest that meticulous documentation is essential for scholarly writing. Why should readers presume that an author knows his subject? Of course some authors, based on past experience, command a certain amount of authority and can justifiably publish undocumented content. Less-known authors like myself, however, should provide extensive documentation if they wish to create high-quality books. Students of nutrition, practitioners, and anyone interested in improving his or her health can easily examine and access my original sources. Throughout this book, you will find over 500 citations from peer-reviewed, scientific journals and other highly credible sources. The book speaks for itself. Your author makes no pretense to being an authority. The studies I show you and the scientists who conducted them are the authorities. Your humble author is simply a diligent, hard-working researcher with a thirst for knowledge and a passion for health.

From Dark Ages to Renaissance

The quest for the Holy Grail ranks among Western civilization's most important and most enduring mythological tales. The original version was written near the end of the twelfth century, a tumultuous era characterized by dangerous consolidations of power, violent Middle East Crusades, and heightened awareness regarding the need for change. Although modern life is considerably different from life during the twelfth and thirteenth centuries, from a big-picture perspective, there are striking parallels. Corporations and governments, for example, are increasingly integrating, thus broadening their collective spheres of influence. War, occupation, and general meddling are commonplace in many Middle East countries. And most significantly, ordinary people on every continent are yearning for change. The grail story and its historical context, as we will see, offer remarkable insights regarding our current health and nutritional crises and how we can resolve them practically.

The Roman Empire crumbled during the fifth century, leaving a power vacuum, which the Catholic Church gradually filled. The church maintained power during the ensuing Dark Ages by scorning individuality and championing conformity. Those who questioned Catholic doctrine or simply thought creatively were punished or killed for heresy. Through fear and superstition, the church prevented alternative perspectives on religious and societal issues. By the thirteenth century, however, many people were becoming disillusioned by the corruption and power abuses they saw emanating from the church. Catharism, an evangelical Christian movement, started flourishing in many regions of southern Europe, particularly southern France. This enraged Pope Innocent III, who ruled from 1198 until his death in 1216. One of the most powerful and most influential popes, Innocent III was a vigorous opponent of heresy. In 1209, he initiated the Albigensian Crusade, an aggressive, twenty-year campaign to decimate the Cathars and stamp out heresy. Like the Crusades the church was waging throughout the Middle East, this crusade was an affront to free thought, humanism, and individualism.

The European Renaissance was characterized by great advancements in science, the arts, intellectual thought, and humanism. The Renaissance began in Florence during the fourteenth century, but its roots extend back to the twelfth century. The church was rampantly corrupt and, consequently, new ideas were emerging and spreading through society. The twelfth century brought increased awareness about the natural laws governing man and the cosmos, increased confidence in the power of reason, and greater emphasis on human dignity and virtue.[1] Religious writings and the literature of the day frequently explored such themes as the self, the inner man, the inner mystery, and the inner landscape. Also, the concept of choosing one's path gained acceptance, although choices were limited to certain preapproved social roles, as opposed to forging one's own path. Nevertheless, many of our contemporary ideas on individuality, self-expression, autonomy, identity, and self-realization are rooted in twelfth-century thought. Robert A. Johnson, a world-renowned Jungian analyst, once observed,

> *"The twelfth century began so many of the issues that we struggle with today. It has been said that the winds of the twelfth century have become the whirlwinds of the twentieth century."*[2]

Against this cultural-historical backdrop, sometime between 1181 and 1190, a French poet named Chrétien de Troyes wrote *Perceval: The Story of the Grail*, which has since become one of Western civilization's most important stories. The grail is an archetype symbolizing the individual's journey towards self-realization and higher planes of consciousness. The grail story reveals much about the human psyche and the human condition. Among its most significant themes are:

1. The importance of asking questions
2. The transformative power of serving others (and serving one's higher Self)

To heal the Fisher King, the young knight, Perceval, must ask the pivotal question, "Whom does the grail serve?" Simply by asking this question, the king will be healed and Perceval will learn a fundamental truth: that life is about serving something greater than oneself.

The grail story has much to teach us about health and nutrition. During the past century, our relationship with food became greatly imbalanced. Cancer, heart disease, and diabetes rates skyrocketed. How did this happen? How can we heal ourselves? Simply by asking questions, the nutritional grail quest begins. Like Perceval, we must ask several critical questions: Whom does my food serve? Does my food serve me physically, mentally, and spiritually? Does my food serve my higher Self? Does the knowledge of what to eat, why to eat it, and how to prepare it help me serve others? The nutritional grail overflows with nourishing, healing food. Obtaining the grail physically, however, would only feed you for a day. Instead, you must obtain the grail intellectually and spiritually. For its essence is knowledge—to learn why it contains what it contains—and the magnificent possibilities implied by that knowledge.

Perceval and the Fisher King

The Story of the Grail follows a young knight, Perceval, and his lifelong quest to find a mysterious grail with healing properties.[*] Perceval's father is a valiant knight who fights honorably during the Crusades but eventually dies in battle before the birth of his son. Perceval's mother is the queen of Wales. Dejected by the knighthood and mourning her husband's death, she abandons her noble home to raise Perceval in isolation, in a faraway forest. She raises him to be ignorant of both his name and his heritage. Growing up in the forest, Perceval learns nothing about chivalry and the knighthood. Accordingly, his mother reasons, he will avoid his father's fate. Perceval grows up happy, adventurous, and strong, but naïve and hopelessly innocent. One

---

[*] Chrétien died before finishing the original grail story. Other writers added various endings and alterations. This summary encapsulates several different versions of the story.

day, while playing in the forest, he encounters a group of knights. They speak with him about the knighthood and Perceval becomes enthralled, immediately setting his heart on becoming a knight. His mother cries and protests, but finally accepts her son's destiny. With his mother's blessing, Perceval leaves the forest and eventually makes his way to King Arthur's court.

Upon accepting Perceval for knight training, the court assigns him a mentor. Though he learns combat skills quickly, Perceval asks too many innocent questions. His mentor sternly informs him, "A knight takes orders. He does not ask questions. He simply does what he is told." This lesson has severe repercussions when Perceval later enters Grail Castle. Although he struggles to understand this rigid mentality, Perceval learns that asking questions always leads to embarrassment and discipline.

After several years, Perceval completes his knight training and starts receiving some minor missions. On one such mission, we find Perceval patrolling a remote wooded area. Dusk falls as he begins wondering where he will sleep. Approaching a small lake, Perceval sees an old man fishing. He asks the man if there is a nearby inn. "No inns for thirty miles," the old man replies, "but you can stay at my place. It's just down the road." Perceval happily accepts the man's generous offer and continues along the road. No houses are around. The road is barren and desolate. Perceval wonders if he has missed the house. Then, as if from nowhere, a large castle suddenly appears. Intrigued and perplexed, Perceval crosses the drawbridge. A girl, who seems to be expecting him, welcomes him and escorts him to his room.

Some hours later, the girl invites Perceval to the castle's magnificent main hall where an elaborate ceremony is about to begin. Perceval witnesses a long procession of men and women, many of whom are carrying mysterious objects. As Perceval later finds out, he is staying at Grail Castle, the home and protectorate of an illustrious grail with healing powers. Every night, the castle hosts the same ceremony. Near the end of the ceremony, a woman carries the brilliantly glowing grail into the main hall. Each person from the procession drinks from the grail, instantly receiving its healing grace. The only person who does not drink is the king of the castle, also known as the Fisher King, the same man who invited Perceval to stay there.

The Fisher King grew up as the prince of Grail Castle. When his father died, he took over as king, assuming the honor and privilege of protecting the grail. For many years, he ruled graciously and effectively. The kingdom enjoyed great prosperity. But over time, a combination of greed, corruption, and negligence threw the kingdom out of balance. Certain knights used trickery, deception, and temptation to weaken the Fisher King. Consequently, he developed a severe illness, which causes him chronic pain and immense suffering. He has become too sick to live yet not sick enough to die. Only when he goes fishing does he gain some temporary relief. As his health declines, his kingdom becomes a barren wasteland. The land becomes infertile, the vegetables stop growing, and the cattle stop grazing.

The health of the king, and hence the entire kingdom, depends on a young knight, an innocent fool, who according to prophecy, will come to Grail Castle and witness the ceremony. This knight will have the opportunity to ask one simple question: "Whom does the grail serve?" With this question, the king's health will be restored and the kingdom will become prosperous once again. Perceval, the innocent fool, finds himself in precisely this situation. The grail has been revealed. The members of the procession are drinking. Everyone drinks except the king. All eyes turn towards Perceval, as if cueing him to ask the question. But he simply cannot ask. His sheltered upbringing and his knight training prevent him from doing so. He wants to ask but he chooses silence instead, which he thinks is proper and knightly.

The next morning Perceval finds himself alone. The castle has vanished and the Fisher King is nowhere to be seen. Perceval saddles his horse and continues along the road, knowing he has failed. He goes on to fight many battles and complete many missions, but eventually grows tired of the knighthood. He wonders if perhaps he has been fighting not for the forces of light, but for the forces of darkness. He becomes introspective, trying to understand his life and his purpose. He informs King Arthur of his decision to retire, but Arthur insists on one more mission. Dutifully, Perceval begins his final quest.

After riding all day, dusk falls and Perceval looks for an inn. He approaches a man fishing by the lake, instantly recognizing him as the Fisher King, who again invites him to Grail Castle. As always, there is an elaborate ceremony that night, featuring a grand procession. This time, Perceval is ready. He watches while men and women drink from the grail, each receiving its healing grace. He looks empathetically at the Fisher King, stretched out on a mattress, consumed by pain and unable to drink. In a loud, confident voice, Perceval asks, "Whom does the grail serve?" The procession stops. All eyes turn towards Perceval. A mysterious, faceless voice answers, "The grail serves the king." Energy pulsates through the king's body, restoring his health and that of his entire kingdom. The land once again becomes fertile. Water flows, the vegetables grow, and the cattle graze. The people rejoice and three days later, the king dies peacefully. Perceval then assumes the kingship of Grail Castle.

Nutritional Grail

The characters of Perceval and the Fisher King offer great insight concerning our current nutritional crisis. The Fisher King becomes ill when his kingdom becomes imbalanced, primarily due to his own negligence and complacency. We, too, have become imbalanced, both societally and individually, regarding the foods we eat. The past century can be thought of as the Dark Ages of nutrition, a time when synthetic foods and nontraditional foods started replacing wholesome, nourishing, traditional foods. Like the Fisher King, we became sick with chronic, degenerative diseases like cancer, heart disease, and diabetes. This outcome could have been avoided if, like Perceval, we would have asked a critical question: "Whom does this food serve?"

In Western nations, many people are raised to be innocent and somewhat naïve, like Perceval. We are raised, for example, to trust experts and rarely doubt them. But what happens when the experts are wrong? As detailed throughout this book, during the twentieth century, the Dark Ages of nutrition, the health experts were wrong time after time. Consequently, food consumption patterns shifted dramatically. Healthy, traditional foods like butter, eggs, and red meat were wrongly shunned while sugar, soy, refined wheat, and various artificial foods were whole-heartedly embraced. If we were more aware of our ancestors' dietary wisdom, and less trusting of governments, institutions, and corporations, perhaps more people would have scrutinized this shift. More people would have asked obvious questions such as, "Whom does hydrogenated corn oil serve?" But like Perceval, we kept quiet, trusting the experts were correct. Grail Castle disappeared and we carried on with our battles.

During the past several decades, people have been asking critical questions about food, health, and nutrition. By asking these questions, collectively, we are gradually correcting past mistakes. Modern nutritional science has overturned many misguided theories, including the theories that sugar is benign, that wheat- and corn-heavy diets are healthy, and that saturated fat causes heart disease. Ancestral wisdom is gaining more and more respect. Our ancestors, as many people now realize, enjoyed much healthier diets than do most modern humans, especially our distant ancestors, before the advent of agriculture. Ancestral wisdom and breakthrough science are guiding us towards a nutritional renaissance, but as during the twelfth century, the renaissance hasn't yet arrived—it's only now dawning. We have turned the corner on the Dark Ages of nutrition, but are still burdened by rigid bureaucracies and institutions, which are still fighting various crusades while resisting the inevitable—change. Now is truly the time for seeking the nutritional grail.

By seeking the grail—by asking the pertinent questions—we raise the collective consciousness of humanity regarding food and health. In this way we serve others. We serve the entire Grail Kingdom, which has become a desolate wasteland, and all its inhabitants. We serve the Fisher King, restoring his health while giving him the chance to die peacefully. We serve our own inner Perceval, giving him wisdom, strength, courage, compassion, and humility while he ascends to the kingship of Grail Castle, assuming the honor of protecting the nutritional grail for future generations. This ascent symbolizes self-realization, or what Carl Jung described as moving the center of gravity of the personality from the ego to the Self.

This book is the result of asking questions. I wish to share with you the answers that I found. You will learn, for example, how certain incorrect theories—like the fat and cholesterol theories that shaped my childhood eating choices—evolved and why they still persist. You will learn why grain-based diets like macrobiotics, which are certainly better than typical Western diets, are ultimately flawed. You will learn about breakthrough nutritional research, which is overturning many core theories established during the past century. As a compendium of research, this book can help anyone working towards revising outdated governmental and institutional dietary recommendations. More importantly, however, this book can benefit you directly by helping you improve your own health.

Besides explaining the *what* and *why* of healthy eating, I also explain the *how*. I'm neither a medical doctor nor a nutritional scientist, but I am an expert on healthy cooking. That's why I have included over one hundred simple, delicious recipes, plus an entire Implementation chapter. I am truly honored that you have decided to read my book. Accordingly, I have gone to great efforts to make your reading experience enjoyable, rewarding, and potentially life-changing.

Notes

[1] Caroline Bynum, "Did the Twelfth Century Discover the Individual?" *Journal of Ecclesiastical History*, January 1980, vol. 31, no. 1, pg. 1–17

[2] Robert A. Johnson, *The Fisher King and the Handless Maiden: Understanding the Wounded Feeling Function in Masculine and Feminine Psychology*, published by Harper One, 1995, pg. 10

CHAPTER ONE

The Seven Pillars

Nutrition and health are processes of discovery and deepening awareness. While we can generalize nutritional advice, we must allow for individual adjustments based on multiple factors, including lifestyle, activity level, age, sex, and physiological uniqueness. There has never been, nor will there ever be, a standardized diet that is best for everyone. In other words, what works for some may not work for others. This fundamental reality opens the door to many nutritional philosophies, some based on religion, ethics, and popular culture, others based on personal experience, observational data, and scientific inquiry. To understand and evaluate any nutritional philosophy, one should first examine the pillars upon which it stands. The research project that evolved into *Nutritional Grail* began with three simple motivations:

- To learn which foods and which nutritional strategies best promote vitality, strength, longevity, clarity, and harmony
- To identify weaknesses in my own diet and implement appropriate changes
- To make my research and advice available to others

I commenced by suspending everything I thought I knew about nutrition. I didn't have an agenda. I wasn't writing to prove or disprove the efficacy of any particular diet. Instead, I set out to carefully and objectively examine the scientific literature on nutrition, to explore ancestral dietary wisdom, and finally, to consolidate my findings into this book. Briefly put, my philosophy rejects rigidity while embracing flexibility. I accept what is. In the spirit of progress, I strongly support evidence and results over presumption and beliefs. My nutritional philosophy rests upon the following seven foundational attributes.

No Dogma

Nutrition, like religion, has many established institutions. These institutions sometimes use their clout to promote certain ideas, concepts, and beliefs. When an institution has enough prominence, people generally accept its assertions uncritically. In time, unchallenged ideas become dogma. Should science later disprove dogmatic ideas, the institutions championing those ideas rarely correct themselves. In many cases, they ignore, harass, or slander those who challenge such ideas scientifically. From the institution's perspective, reversing its stance on important issues could mean compromising its reputation and thus undermining its authority.

In some circles, admitting error is commendable. The progression of science, after all, depends on such intellectual honesty. Nevertheless, we have seen far too many scientific organizations become far too politicized. Take, for example, the issue of water fluoridation. While topical fluoride can indeed prevent dental caries, ingested fluoride provides no such protection. Even the American Dental Association (ADA) and Centers for Disease Control (CDC), the two most outspoken advocates of water fluoridation, have acknowledged that only topical fluoride prevent caries.[1] Ingested fluoride is a carcinogen, neurotoxin, and endocrine disruptor (see Chapter 7). So why is fluoride still added to drinking water and why does the CDC still rank fluoridation as "one of the ten greatest public health achievements of the twentieth century?"[2]

We have seen similar conduct from the American Heart Association (AHA), which decades ago fingered saturated fat and cholesterol as primary drivers of heart disease. The AHA began discouraging traditional fats while recommending industrial seed oils, particularly those rich in polyunsaturated omega-6, an inflammation-promoting fat with many detrimental side effects. The AHA's position on fat became dogma and remains so today. Modern science has completely vindicated saturated fat while exhaustively demonstrating how excessive omega-6, far from preventing heart disease, actually promotes it. Nevertheless, the AHA and other related institutions remain steadfast supporters of industrial seed oils (see Chapter 3).

To be clear, I am not against institutions. I am against dogma. All knowledge, all theories, and all positions must remain open to scrutiny, inquiry, and investigation. Institutions are not exempt. Mistakes and setbacks are inevitable, but refusing to acknowledge them contradicts the spirit of science. So how do scientific institutions become dogmatic in the first place? There are many possibilities. Cozy relationships with large, influential corporations, for example, are highly suspicious, especially when those corporations manufacture patently unhealthy foods.

The Academy of Nutrition and Dietetics (AND) is the world's largest organization of nutrition professionals, with more than 71,000 members. The AND works closely with the US Department of Agriculture (USDA) and the US Department of Health & Human Services to establish US dietary guidelines. The AND describes itself as "an evidence-based organization" that "extensively analyzes relevant scientific studies before taking a position on any issue."[3] According to their professional Code of Ethics:

- "The dietetics practitioner practices dietetics based on evidence-based principles and current information."

- "The dietetics practitioner is alert to the occurrence of a real or potential conflict of interest and takes appropriate action whenever a conflict arises."[4]

While the AND does not define conflicts of interest, their policy apparently does not preclude corporate sponsorship relationships with the world's largest food and beverage companies. Coca-Cola, ConAgra, General Mills, Kellogg's, Mars, PepsiCo, and the National Dairy Council are just some of the academy's publically disclosed sponsors.[5] Their trade group and corporate sponsors swelled from just ten in 2001 to thirty-eight in 2011.[6] Some sponsors become "Academy Partners," which entitles them to co-sponsor events, educate registered dieticians (RDs) about their products, and use the academy's logo in marketing campaigns. During the 2012 AND annual meeting, for example, the Corn Refiners Association (lobbyists for high fructose corn syrup) sponsored three educational sessions for RDs, including "High Fructose Corn Syrup: Myth vs. Science" and "High Fructose Corn Syrup: Danger or Distraction?" Meanwhile, Kellogg's sponsored a "Kids Eat Right" symposium aimed at promoting the whole grain goodness of their sugary breakfast cereals, which they aggressively market towards children.[7]

The AND requires all RDs to regularly accrue Continuing Professional Education (CPE) credits. The AND authorizes "accredited providers," including Coca-Cola, ConAgra, General Mills, Kellogg's, Kraft, Nestlé, and PepsiCo, to directly educate RDs through webinars, seminars, and symposiums.[8] Although the AND promotes the CPE program as educational, their Commission on Dietetics Registration (CDR) openly touts the "marketing opportunities" available to CPE corporate participants, including "exposure to a market of over 90,000 CDR Credentialed Practitioners."[9] Special relationships between large corporations and ostensibly objective scientific organizations are raising many eyebrows. For example, a commentary published in the *Journal of the American Medical Association* in 2010 astutely observed,

> *"The food industry has sought credibility by teaming with respected partners (e.g., a beverage company partnering with a medical professional association). This tarnishes the partner and is seen as a cynical way of buying influence and goodwill."* [10]

Not surprisingly, through its position papers and dietary guidelines, the AND overwhelmingly supports its partners' products while downplaying associated health risks. For example, Coca-Cola and PepsiCo are among the world's biggest purveyors of aspartame-containing products. The AND conveniently overlooks studies showing that aspartame impairs memory performance, increases brain oxidative stress, and is especially agitating for people suffering from mood disorders and depression (see Chapter 4). According to the AND, "Studies have found no evidence of a wide range of adverse effects of aspartame."[11] They even permit Coca-Cola to educate registered dieticians about aspartame safety via various CPE programs.[12]

Coca-Cola and PepsiCo are also massive sugar peddlers. The AND says sugar is safe when consumed according to US Dietary Reference Intakes (DRI) or Dietary Guidelines for Americans (DGA).[13] The DRI allows for "a maximal intake level of 25 percent or less of energy from added sugars."[14] The DGA groups "solid fats" with added sugars and limits the bundle to no more than 15 percent of calories.[15] The DGA says, "Added sugars are no more likely to contribute to weight gain than any other source of calories." But the research presented in Chapter 4 suggests otherwise. Excessive sugar consumption is the common thread connecting most degenerative diseases. To be fair, the AND acknowledges that higher intakes of sugar can promote obesity, diabetes, and heart disease, but for an organization dedicated to nutrition, their sugar allowances seem unreasonably high. Perhaps their relationships with some of the world's largest sugar players have influenced their recommendations.

And what about genetically modified foods? Coca-Cola, PepsiCo, General Mills, and Kellogg's are huge manufacturers of GMO-containing foods. To educate RDs about GMO safety, the AND permitted Coca-Cola to sponsor a CPE taught by the director of international biotechnology of the University of California, Davis.[16] The AND is officially neutral on GMOs, having promised a position paper by the end of 2013.[17] Their now-expired position paper from 2006, however, strongly endorsed GMOs. "Food biotechnology techniques can enhance the quality, safety, nutritional value, and variety of food available for human consumption," wrote Christine Bruhn, the paper's lead author.[18] Bruhn, a University of California professor, is an outspoken opponent of GMO labeling and longtime advocate of GMO technology. To write its purportedly unbiased 2013 position paper, the AND again commissioned Bruhn.

Carole Bartolotto, an AND dietician working on the organization's GMO review panel, was concerned that Bruhn's participation might violate the AND's conflicts of interest policy. Bartolotto had similar concerns about two other panel members with ties to biotech companies, including Monsanto. Bartolotto was also troubled by the AND's decision to exclude all animal studies from the review process. Only a few short-term human GMO studies would be assessed.[†] In a letter to senior employees, Bartolotto voiced her concerns. Shortly thereafter, she was dismissed.[19] Dogma and conflicts of interest are antithetical to science and the pursuit of knowledge. They are nevertheless all-too-common problems for scientific organizations and associations. My nutritional philosophy rejects dogma while embracing revision and refinement, always based on sound evidence.

Holism

Holistic medicine acknowledges the importance not only of the physical, but also the nutritional, environmental, emotional, social, and spiritual dimensions of health. The interplay between these dimensions determines a person's overall health and wellness, or disease and distress. Changes in one dimension typically ripple through the others, creating a multiplying effect capable of dramatically altering the whole. Toxicity within one's physical environment, for example, can interfere with nutrient absorption and metabolism, disrupt emotional wellbeing, increase stress levels, and even cloud one's spiritual perspective. For better or for worse, our dietary choices have profound ripple effects.

Holistic nutrition involves more than just counting calories and analyzing protein, carbohydrates, and fat. Such analyses, while certainly useful, are severely limited. No two foods are exactly alike. Every food contains unique, synergistic combinations of macronutrients and micronutrients. Each metabolizes differently. The digestion and metabolism of broccoli, for example, is much different from that of ice cream. Also, certain dietary fats digest and metabolize much more efficiently than others.

Nutritional analysis provides useful information, but doesn't tell the whole story. A truly holistic perspective must also consider how foods are grown, how they are processed, how they are cooked, and how they combine with other foods. In other words, we must consider the big picture, including both the macro perspective and the fine details.

[†] As this book was going to print the AND had not yet published its updated GMO position paper.

Dynamism

Both nutritional science and nutritional cooking are dynamic, constantly evolving disciplines. New discoveries, fresh insights, and progressive technologies continually expand and refine the collective nutritional and culinary knowledge gleaned by many cultures during many millennia. By confirming, quantifying, and advancing ancient nutritional wisdom, modern nutritional science is helping us to live quantitatively longer and qualitatively better lives.

But nutritional science is not immune from the wayward hands of politics and corporate influence. During the twentieth century, the Dark Ages of nutrition, a combination of carelessness, naiveté and greed misdirected nutritional science, thus prompting untold millions to embrace dangerously unprecedented diets. Processed foods, synthetic ingredients, low-fat diets, wrong-fat diets, excessive sugar, and many other radical departures from traditional dietary wisdom became the norm.

Nevertheless, science has certain self-correcting mechanisms, which eventually overturn and correct its errors. I feel grateful to have lived (and survived) through the latter stages of the twentieth century, experiencing firsthand the cultural and physiological effects of widespread nutritional myopia. I am even more grateful for the opportunity to write this book now, during a significant correction period, with the full benefit of hindsight. Decades of scientific studies now soundly refute the past century's misguided nutritional adventurism. This book represents the cutting edge of nutritional science, fourteen years into the twenty-first century. The future will surely bring new insights, new perspectives, and greater refinement. My nutritional philosophy welcomes these adjustments as scientific progress depends on humility, transparency, and nonattachment.

Science

Nobel Prize-winning physicist Richard Feynman once observed, "It doesn't matter how beautiful your theory is, it doesn't matter how smart you are. If it doesn't agree with experiment, it's wrong."[20] There are plenty of dietary and nutritional theories, some based on empirical data, others based on historical precedent, epidemiology, conjecture, pseudoscience, ethics, idealism, or novelty. Adherents of most theories, at least to some degree, characterize their positions as scientific. But do most nutritional theories actually withstand rigorous scientific scrutiny?

Nutritional science is limited by several factors. First, controlled human studies are not always feasible, especially long-term studies. Second, each person has his own unique metabolism. What's good for some may not be good for others. Third, many nutritional studies are poorly designed, and fourth, the results of many studies are wrongly interpreted. Based on these limitations, different studies sometimes yield contradictory conclusions. Many people are justifiably confused and frustrated when, for example, some studies claim red meat is healthy, while others conclude it causes cancer, or when some studies claim saturated fat causes heart disease, while others declare it wholesome and healthy. How and why do such contradictions arise?

Most published nutritional research studies are either a) controlled experimental studies, or b) epidemiological studies. Most experimental studies are conducted on animals, not humans. Indeed, animal testing has contributed greatly to the current state of nutritional knowledge. David Baker, in a 2006 *Journal of Nutrition* article on animal testing for nutritional research, commented, "The last 50 years could be thought of as the quantitative era, a time when nutrient requirements, nutrient-nutrient interactions, and pharmacologic aspects of nutrients were the focus."[21] The bulk of this knowledge came from animal studies, primarily because:

- Larger groups can be studied more economically.
- Dietary consumption and living conditions can be carefully controlled.
- Shorter life spans improve the feasibility and efficiency of studies.
- Invasive tissue sampling allows for accurate nutrient status assessment.

But as nutrition becomes more holistic, the limitations of animal studies become more evident. As Baker points out, animals cannot explain how different foods make them "feel." And while humans can provide this qualitative feedback, human studies are inherently difficult to organize and monitor. At some point, the most practical, informative, and relevant nutritional studies are those you conduct independently, within the laboratory that is your own body-mind.

Poorly designed or wrongly interpreted experimental studies sometimes lead to contradictory conclusions. This happens, for example, when physiological differences between humans and animals are overlooked. Other reasons experimental studies sometimes fail include:

- The effects of single nutrients cannot be isolated.
- The synergistic effects of certain nutrients are sometimes not accounted for.

- Each person has unique genetics, which can skew study results.

- Metabolism is individualistic, partly due to unique gut bacterial composition.

- Nutritional studies cannot control for all lifestyle factors, including exercise, sleep quality and duration, stress, exercise, meditation, drug interactions, etc.

- Most nutritional studies lack randomized control groups.

- Data can be severely flawed due to inaccurate food reporting by subjects.

The limitations of experimental studies are many, but those of epidemiological studies are far greater. Also known as observational studies, epidemiological studies involve establishing cohorts of subjects, administering questionnaires, and following these subjects for years or even decades. With this data, which costs thousands or even millions of dollars to collect, researchers can construct databases showing foods consumed, diseases, and deaths. Thereafter, they can interpret associations before formulating hypotheses.

The primary problem with epidemiological studies is they only show associations, not causality. For many reasons, journalists and certain vested interests sometimes portray associations as causal relationships. In 2012, for example, Harvard School of Public Health researchers published an epidemiological study associating red meat consumption with increased heart disease. Senior author Frank Hu declared, "This study provides clear evidence that regular consumption of red meat, especially pro-cessed meat, contributes substantially to premature death."[22] Hu failed to mention, however, that his results were merely *associative*, not causal. *The New York Times* at least mentioned this key descriptive word: "Eating red meat is associated with a sharply increased risk of death from cancer and heart disease, according to a new study, and the more of it you eat, the greater the risk."[23]

Broadly speaking, there are three potential problems with definitive conclusions drawn from associations:

1. Miniscule associations are oftentimes blown out of proportion.

2. Associations are sometimes merely coexistent, not causal, phenomena.

3. Hypotheses drawn from associations are not always tested experimentally.

The Harvard study found increased mortality rates of 13 and 20 percent associated with increased consumption of unprocessed and processed red meat, respectively. While these rates may seem significant, for epidemiological studies, they are not. Contrast these rates, for example, with those from the first epidemiological study linking smoking to lung cancer. Published in 1950 in the *British Journal of Medicine*, this landmark study observed increased lung cancer rates of 2,600 percent associated with fifteen to twenty-four daily cigarettes.[24]

Ideally, good epidemiological studies inspire hypotheses. These hypotheses can later be confirmed or rejected through experimental studies. Without a follow-up experimental study, an epidemiological study can only infer causality, and only when observed associations are relatively large, as per the smoking study. Only 20 years ago, most scientific journals typically rejected epidemiological studies demonstrating associative relationships less than 300 or 400 percent.[25] During the 1990s, however, journals started becoming less restrictive. More and more weak-association studies began creeping into the scientific literature. In 1995, award-winning science writer Gary Taubes called attention to this trend with a seminal article penned for *Science* exploring the limits of epidemiology. Taubes observed,

> *"The search for subtle links between diet, lifestyle, or environmental factors and disease is an unending source of fear—but often yields little certainty."* [26]

In epidemiology, associations are sometimes simply coexistent phenomena. The Harvard study failed to consider, for example, that increased red meat consumption can correlate positively with smoking, alcohol consumption, and sedentary lifestyles. Was red meat causing the premature deaths or were cigarettes or some other factors? The Harvard study does not prove that red meat consumption increases mortality. It simply shows that people who eat higher amounts of red meat generally die earlier than those who don't. The causes of these deaths could be many different factors or many factors combined. At best, the Harvard study could inspire a series of follow-up experimental studies, controlling for various risk factors to test the hypothesis that red meat consumption increases mortality.

According to Karl Popper, a prominent philosopher of science, "The method of science is the method of bold conjectures and ingenious and severe attempts to refute them."[27] A theory that withstands such attempts *might* be true—possibly, maybe. But science always allows for new evidence, fresh insight, and further experimentation. I have organized my approach to nutrition around this principle. I create menus based on modern nutritional research and ancient dietary wisdom. Then, through personal experimentation, observation, and further research, I refine my menus, gradually homing in on my personal, optimized diet. I also create generalized menus for others, which of course are always subject to person-specific adjustments and modifications.

Science is sometimes criticized, but pure science is simply an open-minded, logical approach to learning. Every nutritional theory worth its salt should embrace, not shy away from, pure scientific inquiry.

Reverence

Traditional Chinese medicine, Ayurveda, and other ancient wisdom traditions have contributed immensely to modern nutritional understanding. Many traditional cultures developed invaluable culinary insights and technologies based on the foods, tools, and resources available to them. These cultures had certain advantages over modern science. Specifically, they could understand the health properties of different foods by observing patterns over vast spans of time. Some foods promoted harmony; others promoted disharmony.

Knowledge accumulated over centuries or millennia is generally functional and highly refined. Traditional dietary wisdom therefore tends to be highly credible. Of course traditional concepts, processes, techniques, and recipes must also withstand critical thinking, rational analysis, and scientific scrutiny. Nevertheless, if something worked before, it probably still works today. Therefore these traditions are excellent starting points and excellent sources of inspiration.

Regarding tradition, I refer to genuine, authentic, longstanding tradition. As a regular world traveler, I often sample traditional foods from around the world. Never will I forget the answer I received in Colombia upon asking my local guides about the traditional recipe for coconut rice. I was told that Coca-Cola is an essential ingredient of the "traditional" recipe. I have also seen countless "traditional" recipes calling for industrial seed oils for frying. Coca-Cola and industrial seed oils are modern synthetic creations, not traditional foods. Contrast these products, for example, with miso.

From a nutritional perspective, soybeans are highly problematic. To nullify some of soy's inherently unhealthy properties, traditional Asian cultures developed various fermentation techniques. Miso, for example, originated between China and Japan as a preservation and nutrient-improvement technique. Miso involves a fermentation process, which gradually transforms soy into an easily digestible food with potent medicinal properties. Miso is the result of an ancient food-processing technology. Other traditional foods are simply unprocessed source-foods such as vegetables, fruits, and animal foods. My nutritional philosophy places greater emphasis on foods that have stood the test of time, while also withstanding modern scientific inquiry.

Self-Sufficiency

The healthiest people I know regularly cook for themselves and their families. Perhaps not every meal is home cooked, but certainly most are prepared at home. Cooking for yourself allows you to customize your meals according to your needs. Additionally, you can choose higher-quality foods and make sure they are prepared properly. Although some restaurants offer high-quality, health-conscious food, most do not. The restaurant industry is indeed trending towards healthier concepts, but most restaurant menus are not yet designed by nutrition experts.

In the future, I predict that doctors will work closely with chefs. Restaurants will merge food with medicine. The doctor-chef relationship will replace the doctor-pharmacist relationship. Doctors will write prescriptions not for pharmaceutical drugs, but for medicinal food. People will take these prescriptions not to pharmacies, but to supermarkets, farmers' markets, and special restaurants where knowledgeable chefs prepare dietary medicine.

Being healthy in this proposed future will not involve dependency. In other words, knowledge about medicinal food and its preparation will be widely available. Being healthy will not mean being dependent on doctors, health institutions, or pharmaceutical drug companies, as the contemporary healthcare system would have us believe. The opportunity to prepare effective, homemade medicine—food—will be available to everyone. Doctors will provide guidance, advice, and troubleshooting, but the responsibility for primary healthcare, through diet and lifestyle choices, will fall upon each individual.

Eating healthy requires learning which foods are healthy and which are not. Next, you must learn how to prepare the healthy foods. You don't have to become a master chef, nor must you block many hours per day for cooking. This book teaches simple recipes, basic techniques, and smart concepts for making sublime culinary creations, even with limited available time. By cooking regularly, you connect with your food. You actively participate in your own health. You become self-sufficient.

Freedom

Nutrition must be empowering. Nutrition must promote mental and physical harmony, thus enabling spiritual development. Learning about nutrition, through theory and direct experience—cooking and eating—raises awareness while fostering connectivity to nature and our higher Selves. Making educated and informed food choices furthers this connectivity. This is what the grail quest is all about—learning and then implementing what you learn. This process helps you serve others, serve the planet, and serve your own spiritual development. For better or for worse, your food choices can profoundly affect your life, your community, and your world.

The realities of today's geopolitical landscape have pushed nutrition far beyond its conventional boundaries. Special corporate-governmental relationships, for example, have resulted in topsy-turvy dietary recommendations. Dangerous, unhealthy foods are promoted while traditional, healthy foods are discouraged. The modern health advocate must understand not only what makes us healthy, but also what makes us sick. Regarding the latter, we can certainly implicate processed, synthetic foods. But how and why did such foods end up on our plates? A truly holistic perspective should acknowledge not only the problem, but also the problem's roots.

What does it mean when the world's largest biotechnology firm, through cozy government relationships and pure economic might, can block consumer-demanded labeling of GMO foods? What does it mean when the world's largest food and drug safety agency consistently puts corporate interests ahead of public health? Our food choices have enormous implications. Our food choices today can even affect our civil liberties tomorrow. As discussed throughout this book, we must be aware of these larger issues. We must see health and disease not only from medical and nutritional perspectives, but also from historical, cultural, and geopolitical perspectives. During times of ubiquitous disease, eating healthy becomes a revolutionary act.

Notes

[1] John Featherstone, "The Science and Practice of Caries Prevention," *The Journal of the American Dental Association*, July 2000, vol. 131, no. 7, pg. 887–899; Centers for Disease Control, "Achievements in Public Health, 1900–1999: Fluoridation of Drinking Water to Prevent Dental Caries," *MMWR Weekly*, October 22, 1999, vol. 48, no. 41, pg. 933–940; Centers for Disease Control, "Recommendations for Using Fluoride to Prevent and Control Dental Caries in the United States," *MMWR Recommendations and Reports*, August 17, 2001, vol. 50, no. RR14, pg. 1–42

[2] Centers for Disease Control, "Ten Great Public Health Achievements—United States, 1900–1999," *MMWR Weekly*, April 2, 1999, vol. 48, no. 2, pg. 241–243

[3] Press release, "Academy of Nutrition and Dietetics and Proposition 37: The Facts," The Academy of Nutrition and Dietetics, October 8, 2012

[4] "American Dietetic Association/Commission on Dietetic Registration Code of Ethics for the Profession of Dietetics and Process for Consideration of Ethics Issues," *Journal of the American Dietetic Association*, August 2009, vol. 109, no. 8, pg. 1461–1467

[5] The Academy of Nutrition and Dietetics, "Who Are the Academy's Corporate Sponsors?" Eatright.org; The Academy of Nutrition and Dietetics, *Foundation Matters*, May 2013

[6] Stephanie Strom, "Report Faults Food Group's Sponsor Ties," *New York Times*, January 23, 2013

[7] Christopher Cook, "Nutrition, Inc.," *The Progressive*, July 2013; Dayle Hayes et al., "Summary: Presentations from the Kellogg-Sponsored Symposium at the Academy of Nutrition and Dietetics Kids Eat Right Summit," Kelloggsnutrition.com

[8] Commission on Dietetic Registration, Continuing Professional Education Accredited Providers; Cdrnet.org/about/accredited-providers

[9] Commission on Dietetics Registration, Benefits of Becoming a CPE Accredited Provider; Cdrnet.org/accredited-provider-benefits

[10] Jeffrey Koplan and Kelly Brownel, "Response of the Food and Beverage Industry to the Obesity Threat," *Journal of the American Medical Association*, October 6, 2010, vol. 304, no. 13, pg. 1487–1488

[11] Fitch C et al., "Position of the Academy of Nutrition and Dietetics: Use of Nutritive and Nonnutritive Sweeteners," *Journal of the Academy of Nutrition and Dietetics*, May 2012, vol. 112, no. 5, pg. 750

[12] The Coca-Cola Company Beverage Institute for Health & Wellness, CPE Programs, Webinars & Podcasts; Beverageinstitute.org

[13] Fitch C et al., "Position of the Academy of Nutrition and Dietetics: Use of Nutritive and Nonnutritive sweeteners," *Journal of the Academy of Nutrition and Dietetics*, May 2012, vol. 112, no. 5, pg. 739–758

[14] Institute of Medicine of the National Academies, Dietary Reference Intakes for Energy, Carbohydrate, Fiber, Fat, Fatty Acids, Cholesterol, Protein, and Amino Acids, published by National Academies Press, 2002, pg. 323

[15] US Department of Agriculture and US Department of Health and Human Services, *Dietary Guidelines for Americans*, 2010, 7th Edition, US Government Printing Office, December 2010, pg. 28

[16] The Coca-Cola Company Beverage Institute for Health & Wellness, Biotechnology and Genetically-Modified Foods: A Look at Safety and the Peer-Reviewed Science

[17] Press release, "Academy of Nutrition and Dietetics and Proposition 37: The Facts," The Academy of Nutrition and Dietetics, October 8, 2012

[18] Bruhn C et al., "Position of the American Dietetic Association: Agricultural and food biotechnology," *Journal of the American Dietetic Association*, February 2006, vol. 106, no. 2, pg. 285–293

[19] Stephanie Strom, "Food Politics Creates Rift in Panel on Labeling," *New York Times*, April 10, 2013

[20] Michael Asten, "Climate claims fail science test," *The Australian*, December 9, 2009

[21] David Baker, "Animal Models in Nutrition Research," *Journal of Nutrition*, February 2008, vol. 138, no. 2, pg. 391–396

[22] Todd Datz and Harvard School of Public Health Communications, "Red meat raises red flags," *Harvard Gazette*, March 12, 2012

[23] Nicholas Bakalar, "Risks: More Red Meat, More Mortality," *New York Times*, March 12, 2012

[24] Doll R and Hill AB, "Smoking and carcinoma of the lung; preliminary report," *British Journal of Medicine*, September 30, 1950, vol. 2, no. 4682, pg. 739–748

[25] Gary Taubes and Charles Mann, "Epidemiology faces its limits," *Science*, July 14, 1995, vol. 269, no. 5221, pg. 164

[26] Ibid.

[27] Gary Taubes, "Chocolate & Red Meat Can Be Bad for Your Science: Why Many Nutrition Studies Are All Wrong," *Discover*, April 5, 2012

CHAPTER TWO

My Approach

The following is a brief encapsulation of my approach to nutrition. It has no slogans, no logos, no maxims, no mantras, and certainly no gurus. Simply put, my approach embraces basic, authentic, natural foods. Synthetic foods are out. Nontraditional foods are generally out. I focus on macronutrients—protein, fat, and carbohydrates—consuming them intelligently, from the best sources, in proper proportions, and properly prepared. I focus on micronutrients—vitamins, minerals, phytonutrients—primarily obtained through food but occasionally through supplements. Beyond this, I emphasize detoxification, preventing inflammation, increasing antioxidants, and strengthening the digestion. Food must be inspiring and satisfying, but also simple and practical.

Back To Basics

Once upon a time, food was food. Some was derived from plants, some was from animals, but all was from nature. The synthetic-food revolution of the past century changed everything. The widespread embrace of both artificial and nontraditional foods exacerbated existing diseases while making once-obscure diseases common. The pivotal first steps towards improved health and wellness are eliminating, without exception, all of the following:

- Processed foods
- Genetically modified foods
- Chemically refined fats (trans fats, hydrogenated fats, and industrial seed oils, including canola, corn, and soybean oils)

- Artificial sweeteners (aspartame, neotame, saccharin, and sucralose)

- Artificial flavor enhancers (MSG, E621, etc.)

- Artificial colorings

- Artificial preservatives (BHA, BHT, E320, sulfur dioxide, sodium sulfite, E220, E221)

- All other artificial ingredients

Note: Nitrites and nitrates were intentionally excluded from this list (see Chapter 5).

Learning and applying the simple *Nutritional Grail* cooking techniques makes eliminating the aforementioned synthetic ingredients easy. Eliminating vegetables, fruits, and animal foods grown with synthetic pesticides, herbicides, insecticides, growth hormones, and antibiotics, however, can be more challenging. By definition, these latter foods are "artificial" because they contain harmful residues of synthetic chemicals. If you cannot buy solely organically grown foods, prioritize which foods you buy organic based on the Environmental Working Group's (EWG) analysis of pesticide residues in fruits and vegetables. The EWG is a consumer advocacy group that regularly publishes their "Dirty Dozen" and "Clean Fifteen" lists, showing which fruits and vegetables contain the most and least amounts of pesticide residues.[1] For foods on the Dirty Dozen list, always buy them organic. Foods on the Clean Fifteen list can be bought nonorganic, if necessary.

EWG 2013 Guide to Pesticides in Produce – Figure 2.1

Dirty Dozen Plus		Clean Fifteen	
Apples	Nectarines	Asparagus	Mushrooms
Celery	Peaches	Avocados	Onions
Cherry Tomatoes	Potatoes	Cabbage	Papayas
Collard Greens	Spinach	Cantaloupe	Pineapples
Cucumbers	Strawberries	Eggplant	Sweet Corn*
Grapes	Sweet Bell Peppers	Grapefruits	Sweet Peas
Hot Peppers	Summer Squash	Kiwi	Sweet Potatoes
Kale	Zucchini	Mangos	

* Non-GMO only (most corn is genetically modified)

After addressing synthetic foods, the next step is nontraditional foods. Nontraditional foods are natural insofar as they require no chemical processing, but they are nontraditional based on historical precedence. These are foods people have indeed consumed traditionally, but in significantly different ways than do modern humans. Nontraditional foods pose serious nutritional challenges. Some provide adequate, though not ideal, nourishment when properly prepared and moderately consumed. But when improperly prepared and excessively consumed, they promote numerous degenerative diseases. Sugar and wheat are the most relevant examples.

Nontraditional Wheat

Wheat largely enabled the rise of civilization. Population growth, organized cities, large building projects, regional trading, and technological progress were all made possible by agriculture. The cultivation of cereal grains, particularly wheat, allowed for secure food supplies and surpluses, which enabled social differentiation as well as economic specialization. Relieved of the burdens of food production, nonfarmers could focus on other commodities, including clothes, pottery, and leather goods. Wheat made much of this possible, yet from a nutritional perspective wheat is far from ideal.

All seeds, but especially cereal grains and legumes, contain problematic chemical compounds, including phytates, lectins, and enzyme inhibitors. Collectively known as anti-nutrients, these compounds serve as evolutionary defense mechanisms for seeds. For humans, however, they can inhibit mineral absorption and interfere with the digestion. Wheat is particularly troublesome because it also contains gluten and an especially inflammatory lectin called wheat germ agglutinin (WGA). Consequently, frequent wheat consumption can cause digestive interference, gut permeability, and allergies (see Chapter 5).[2]

Traditional cultures learned to minimize anti-nutrients through food-processing techniques, especially through sourdough fermentation. During fermentation, cereal grains undergo biochemical changes, which make their proteins more digestible and their nutrients more bioavailable. Traditional sourdough bread ferments as long as twenty-four hours prior to baking. Fermentation improves the nutritional profile of wheat, but not enough to make it a top-tier, staple food. Nevertheless, fermented wheat is a traditional food and is nutritionally superior to unfermented wheat, a nontraditional food. Wheat has become a nutritional scourge mostly because we have abandoned traditional sourdough fermentation.

Modern bread is typically leavened using fast-rising commercial yeast, not through traditional sourdough fermentation. Other popular wheat products (cakes, cookies, crackers) are unfermented. Furthermore, most modern wheat products are made from refined, stale flour, as opposed to freshly milled flour. Another serious problem with modern wheat began during the Green Revolution of the 1950s and 1960s when traditional wheat species were phased out in favor of semi-dwarf, high-yield cultivars. These newer varieties have significantly lower amounts of minerals and significantly more protein.[3] Additionally, they are much higher in alpha-gliadin, an especially reactive gluten peptide.[4] Modern wheat is therefore very different from traditional wheat, both biochemically and based on its preparation.

A final problem with modern wheat, and with cereal grains in general, is excessive consumption. Today, people in Western nations consume upwards of 24 percent of total calories as cereal grains, mostly refined wheat.[5] Grains are becoming more and more prominent in modern diets, replacing nutritionally superior foods, including fish, meat, eggs, vegetables, and fruits. By the year 2000, Americans were eating 45 percent more grains than they were during the 1970s.[6] The problems with wheat are therefore threefold—improper preparation, detrimental hybridization, and excessive consumption. In short, you should remove modern, nontraditional wheat from your diet altogether. Other cereal grains are discussed in Chapter 4.

Sweet Poison

Sugar is another natural though completely nontraditional food. Humans have been collecting honey since the Stone Age, but during the nineteenth century, sugar became man's sweetener of choice. For most of history and prehistory, honey was only sporadically available and was thus very moderately consumed. Sugar changed everything. By 1822, the average American was eating 6.3 pounds of sugar per person per year.[7] By the turn of the century, this figure increased sevenfold (roughly 43 pounds). By 2012, according to the USDA, the average American was consuming an astonishing 97 pounds of sugar per year, representing a 39 percent increase since the 1950s and a 23 percent increase since the 1970s.[8]

At these consumption levels, sugar is highly inflammatory, promoting metabolic syndrome, nonalcoholic fatty liver disease, and diabetes.[9] Some people characterize sugar as "empty calories," meaning it contains no beneficial nutrients and therefore displaces nutrient-dense foods. While this is indeed true, the problem is much more severe. Sugar, quite simply, is toxic, especially at typical Western consumption levels.

A critical steppingstone towards improving your health and boosting your vitality is dramatically reducing, then eliminating, all synthetic and nontraditional foods. This book helps you identify these foods while developing transitional strategies. You will learn which foods are healthy and which are not. You will learn simple, effective preparation techniques. You will learn how to identify toxic and synthetic ingredients in perhaps nonobvious places. Essentially, you will learn a powerful, straightforward, back-to-basics approach towards eating smarter and living better.

Smart Macronutrients

Protein, fat, and carbohydrates (and water) are the basic, essential macronutrients. Micronutrients include vitamins, minerals, and phytonutrients. If you master the macronutrients, the micronutrients pretty much fall into place. In other words, if you choose high-quality sources of protein, fat, and carbohydrates, and consume them in optimal proportions for your unique physiology, you will probably automatically be consuming sufficient quantities of micronutrients. This is a soft rule, to which there are of course some exceptions.

Some nutritionists advocate heavy supplementation of various minerals, vitamins, and plant extracts. I contend that whole foods provide superior-quality nutrients and can provide these nutrients in sufficient quantities. Nature's complex arrangement of macronutrients and micronutrients within whole foods creates nutritional synergies, which supplements are typically incapable of replicating. In special cases, specific mineral deficiencies for example, supplements may be appropriate. But in general, food is primary and consuming smart macronutrients is essential.

This book is largely about macronutrients because the common perception of them is entirely warped. Consequently, most people are eating the wrong fats, the wrong carbohydrates, and the wrong protein. The importance of pure, unadulterated water also cannot be overemphasized. Even many health-conscious people make the mistake of drinking and cooking with impure tap water. Vegetarianism and veganism are also hot issues, with many people choosing these lifestyles for a variety of reasons, including nutrition. A very critical look at the evidence, however, strongly supports the consumption of animal foods for optimal health.

In this book you will learn the critical differences between saturated, monounsaturated, and polyunsaturated fat. You will learn to evaluate meat, fish, eggs, milk, cereals, and legumes with respect to protein quality. You will learn why sugar and some simple carbohydrates are so destructive, and why cereal grain consumption should be minimized (with a few exceptions). You will learn why meat, fish, eggs, vegetables, fruits, coconut, avocado, fermented dairy, and many more superfoods are the best sources of macronutrients and, by extension, micronutrients.

Ongoing Detoxification

Persistent, low-dose exposure to environmental toxins such as pesticides, dioxins, polychlorinated biphenyls (PCBs), food-processing residues, prescription drugs, heavy metals, and industrial waste is an unfortunate, yet wholly unavoidable, reality of modern living. Whether ingested, inhaled, or absorbed through the skin, toxins are continually entering our bodies and accumulating therein. Some toxins disrupt the endocrine system while others damage the reproductive system, gradually leading to infertility. Some toxins are carcinogenic; others weaken the liver and kidneys. As one's cumulative toxic load increases, the body absorbs and assimilates nutrients less efficiently. Detoxification is therefore part and parcel of healthy living.

Many people think of detoxing as short-term, temporary fasting or cleansing. While such regimes are indeed beneficial, detoxification is an ongoing process, which involves every cell in the body. Your detox regime should be gentle, effective, and sustainable. The primary objective is establishing dietary habits that strengthen and support the critical detoxification organs, primarily the liver, kidneys, and intestines, but also the blood, lymph, and lungs. Foods and herbs that support these organs should be consumed regularly, not periodically. When the primary detoxification organs are strong and unburdened, they function much more efficiently.

Ongoing detoxification involves minimizing toxic inputs, increasing antioxidants, supporting glutathione production, consuming foods and herbs that chelate heavy metals, and consuming foods that support the primary detoxification organs. Chapter 6 describes in detail how to make detoxification part of your regular dietary regime.

Preventing Inflammation

Inflammation is a physiological response to physical, chemical, and biological stimuli. Acute inflammation is a completely normal, and indeed essential, reaction to injuries, infections, and pathogens. Chronic inflammation, conversely, disrupts the immune system and certain metabolic processes. Whereas acute inflammation is temporary and localized, chronic inflammation is prolonged and systemic. Eventually the blood vessel linings become inflamed, which ultimately leads to impaired organ function. Cancer, heart disease, diabetes, leukemia, lymphoma, kidney diseases, liver diseases, and metabolic syndrome are all related to chronic, systemic inflammation.[10] Metabolic syndrome is a combination of concurrent conditions—insulin resistance, glucose intolerance, obesity, and hypertension—that collectively increases one's risk for heart disease, diabetes, and stroke. In a landmark 2003 scientific statement, the AHA and CDC concluded,

> *"Basic science and epidemiological studies have developed an impressive case that atherogenesis is essentially an inflammatory response to a variety of risk factors and the consequences of this response lead to the development of acute coronary and cerebrovascular syndromes."*[11]

Chronic inflammation primarily results from oxidative damage, which is a classic consequence of unhealthy diets and lifestyles.[12] The top five factors promoting chronic inflammation are:

1. Poor nutrition (gluten, industrial seed oils, trans fats, sugar)
2. Environmental toxins (xenoestrogens, heavy metals, pesticides, phthalates)
3. Recurrent stress (emotional, psychological, environmental)
4. Smoking
5. Sedentary lifestyle (high energy intake with low physical activity)

Regarding nutrition, most people eat far too much omega-6 fat and not enough omega-3 (see Chapter 3). We require only very small amounts of each. The ratio of omega-6 to omega-3 should also be very small. One to one is ideal, but Western diets typically range from ten to one to thirty to one (omega-6 to omega-3).[13] High omega ratios and high absolute intakes of omega-6 promote many diseases, including heart disease, cancer, and various inflammatory and autoimmune diseases.[14]

Those who suffer from chronic inflammatory conditions including rheumatoid arthritis should be particularly diligent regarding the omega ratio. A study published in *Biomedicine & Pharmacotherapy* in 2002 observed that rheumatoid arthritis patients maintaining omega ratios equal to or lower than three to one experience significantly decreased levels of inflammation.[15] Hydrogenated fats, trans fats, sugar, and gluten all factor heavily into diet-induced inflammation.

Increasing Antioxidants

Oxygen free radicals are a primary cause of inflammation. Normal aerobic cellular metabolism causes oxidative stress through free radical chain reactions (see Chapter 6). Many external influences, including environmental pollution, emotional stress, physical stress, pharmaceutical drugs, cigarette smoke, electromagnetic pollution, denatured foods, artificial preservatives, herbicides, pesticides, and common household chemicals, also promote oxidative stress and damage. According to a 2013 article published in *Critical Reviews in Food Science and Nutrition*, "Oxidative stress is rapidly gaining recognition as a key phenomenon in chronic diseases."[16]

Free radicals are unstable molecules that can accelerate aging, denature DNA strands, degrade fat cells by attacking cell membranes, and damage protein cells by inactivating certain enzymes.[17] Cancer, atherosclerosis, myocardial infarction, senile cataracts, acute respiratory distress syndrome, and rheumatoid arthritis are just some of the conditions caused by free radicals.[18] Free radicals also promote neurological disorders, including Alzheimer's disease and Parkinson's disease.[19] Furthermore, the free radical theory of aging, supported by some studies but refuted by others, points to free radical reactions as the fundamental cause and accelerant of aging.

Antioxidants are the body's primary defense against free radicals. As the name suggests, antioxidants inhibit free radical oxidation reactions. When stable molecules interact with free radicals, they themselves become free radicals. Chain reactions are then set in motion capable of damaging many more cells. Because antioxidants are extremely stable, they can donate electrons to free radicals without actually becoming free radicals. When this happens, the antioxidant becomes inactive, necessitating even more antioxidants to ward off other free radicals. We can curb free radicals by:

1. Implementing healthy diet and lifestyle changes
2. Increasing antioxidant consumption

Although the body has certain endogenous free radical defense mechanisms, they cannot completely prevent and protect against oxidative damage. Consuming plenty of dietary antioxidants is therefore essential.[20] Foods high in vitamin E, vitamin C, and carotenoids are important dietary sources of antioxidants.

Certain phytochemicals contained in many fruits and vegetables also behave like antioxidants. Phytochemicals are bioactive plant compounds that promote an array of extraordinary therapeutic effects. The most important classes of phytochemicals are polyphenols and flavonoids (a subcategory of polyphenols). Polyphenols are abundant in many fruits, including apples, berries, grapes, pears, and pomegranates, and many vegetables, including broccoli, cabbage, celery, and parsley. Regarding flavonoids, green tea, olive oil, red wine, cacao, and various superfoods like bee pollen are potent sources. Polyphenols are the richest source of dietary antioxidants.[21] A balanced diet typically provides ten times more polyphenols than it does vitamin C and roughly one hundred times more polyphenols than it does vitamin E and carotenoids.[22] Since dietary antioxidants are so essential, we should regularly consume antioxidant-rich foods including fruits, vegetables, and olive oil.

Strengthening Digestion

Digestive strength and efficiency are key indicators of overall health and wellness. During digestion, food is chemically (enzymes) and physically (chewing) broken down, assimilated into the blood, and subsequently transported throughout the body, providing nourishment for the cells. Impaired, weakened, and otherwise inefficient digestion can compromise the immune system, as the two are closely interrelated. Indeed, many immune cells reside within the gastrointestinal tract, specifically within the gut-associated lymphoid tissue (GALT), which represents about 70 percent of the entire immune system.[23] A weakened immune system sets the stage for many serious degenerative diseases.

The primary causes of impaired digestion are improper diet and poor nutrition. Food preparation methods are also vitally important regarding digestion. Soaking seeds, nuts, cereals, and legumes for 8 to 24 hours, for example, dramatically increases their digestibility. Fermentation, low-temperature cooking, raw preparations, and many other food preparation methods discussed throughout this book also make food more digestible. Other causes of impaired digestion include, chronic stress, excessive alcohol consumption, antibiotics, and imbalanced intestinal flora.

One consequence of prolonged digestive neglect is gut permeability, meaning the intestinal lining becomes damaged, which allows undigested food particles, bacteria, and toxins to enter the bloodstream. Since these substances are not normally present within the blood, the immune system recognizes them as antigens. This triggers the immune system to release antibodies and signaling molecules, called cytokines, which alert the white blood cells to fight the antigens. This process causes both local and systemic inflammation and is associated with the following conditions:

- Allergies

- Autoimmune diseases

- Celiac disease and Crohn's disease

- Inflammatory joint diseases, including arthritis

- Chronic fatigue syndrome

- Acne, eczema, and psoriasis

- Food allergies and sensitivities

- Liver dysfunction

- Rheumatoid arthritis

- Irritable bowel syndrome

Simply put, you cannot be healthy without a healthy gut. Bowel movements are a good indicator of gut health. If they aren't regular, well formed, and buoyant, then your gut probably needs some attention. The intestines house a vibrant, dynamic ecosystem consisting of some 500 different bacterial species. Known as gut flora (or intestinal flora), these microorganisms coexist with humans (and other animals) in symbiotic relationships. The gut flora performs many important functions, including assisting digestion, warding off pathogenic bacteria, training the immune system to respond only to pathogens, regulating gut development, and synthesizing essential vitamins. Bacterial cells are so prolific that within every human, they outnumber human cells ten to one.[24] Not all these bacteria, however, are necessarily good.

Dysbiosis is an imbalance of bad bacteria caused by antibiotic abuse, pesticides, and improper diet. Excessive sugar, for example, feeds bad bacteria (fungi, yeast, and anaerobic bacteria) to the detriment of the good. Pesticides, herbicides, insecticides, and fungicides also damage good bacteria. Fermented foods, including yogurt, kefir, lacto-fermented vegetables (sauerkraut and kimchi), and miso, are rich sources of probiotics, which promote healthy gut flora. The foods and preparation techniques discussed throughout this book promote strong, efficient digestion.

Notes

[1] Press Release, "Apples Top EWG's Dirty Dozen," Environmental Working Group, April 22, 2013

[2] Karen Lammers et al., "Gliadin Induces an Increase in Intestinal Permeability and Zonulin Release by Binding to the Chemokine Receptor CXCR3," *Gastroenterology*, July 2008, vol. 135, no. 1, pg. 194–204

[3] Fan MS et al., "Evidence of decreasing mineral density in wheat grain over the last 160 years," *Journal of Trace Elements in Medicine and Biology*, 2008, vol. 22, no. 4, pg. 315–324

[4] HC van den Broeck et al., "Presence of celiac disease epitopes in modern and old hexaploid wheat varieties: wheat breeding may have contributed to increased prevalence of celiac disease," *Theoretical and Applied Genetics*, November 2010, vol. 121, no. 8, pg. 1527–1539

[5] Loren Cordain et al., "Origins and evolution of the Western diet: health implications for the 21st century," *American Journal of Clinical Nutrition*, February 2005, vol. 81, no. 2, pg. 341–354

[6] United States Department of Agriculture, Agriculture Fact Book 2001–2002, March 2003, Office of Communications

[7] Henry Blodget, "CHART OF THE DAY: American Per-Capita Sugar Consumption Hits 100 Pounds Per Year," *Business Insider*, February 19, 2012

[8] United States Department of Agriculture, Agriculture Fact Book 2001–2002, March 2003, Office of Communications, pg. 20; Stephanie Strom, "U.S. Cuts Estimate of Sugar Intake," *New York Times*, October 26, 2012

[9] Carlos Roncal-Jimenez et al., "Sucrose induces fatty liver and pancreatic inflammation in male breeder rats independent of excess energy intake," *Metabolism*, September 2011, vol. 60, no. 9, pg. 1259–1270

[10] Rosário Monteiro and Isabel Azevedo, "Chronic Inflammation in Obesity and the Metabolic Syndrome," *Mediators of Inflammation*, July 14, 2010, vol. 2010, no. 289645

[11] Thomas Pearson et al., "AHA/CDC Scientific Statement: Markers of Inflammation and Cardiovascular Disease," *Circulation*, 2003, vol. 107, pg. 499–511

[12] Daniel Closa and Emma Folch-Puy, "Oxygen Free Radicals and the Systemic Inflammatory Response," *IUBMB Life*, April 2004, vol. 56, no. 4, pg. 185–191

[13] Artemis Simopoulos, "The importance of the ratio of omega-6/omega-3 essential fatty acids," *Biomedicine & Pharmacotherapy*, October 2002, vol. 56, no. 8, pg. 365–379

[14] William Lands, "Dietary fat and health: the evidence and the politics of prevention: careful use of dietary fats can improve life and prevent disease," *Annals of the New York Academy of Sciences*, December 2005, vol. 1055, pg. 179–192; Hirohmi Okuyama et al., "ω3 fatty acids effectively prevent coronary heart disease and other late-onset diseases: the excessive linoleic acid syndrome," *World Review of Nutrition and Dietetics*, 2007, vol. 96, pg. 83–103; Joseph Hibbeln, "Healthy intakes of n–3 and n–6 fatty acids: estimations considering worldwide diversity," *American Journal of Clinical Nutrition*, June 2006, vol. 83, pg. 1483S–1493S

[15] Artemis Simopoulos, "The importance of the ratio of omega-6/omega-3 essential fatty acids," *Biomedicine & Pharmacotherapy*, October 2002, vol. 56, no. 8, pg. 365–379

[16] Landete JM, "Dietary intake of natural antioxidants: vitamins and polyphenols," *Critical Reviews in Food Science and Nutrition*, 2013, vol. 53, no. 7, pg. 706–721

[17] Robert Floyd and John Carney, "Free radical damage to protein and DNA: Mechanisms involved and relevant observations on brain undergoing oxidative stress," *Annals of Neurology*, 1992, vol. 32, pg. S22–S27

[18] Bagachi and Puri, "Free radicals and antioxidants in health and disease," *Eastern Mediterranean Health Journal*, 1998, vol. 4, no. 2, pg. 350–360

[19] Uttara B et al., "Oxidative stress and neurodegenerative diseases: a review of upstream and downstream antioxidant therapeutic options," *Current Neuropharmacology*, March 2009, vol. 7, no. 1, pg. 65–74

[20] Landete JM, "Dietary intake of natural antioxidants: vitamins and polyphenols," *Critical Reviews in Food Science and Nutrition*, 2013, vol. 53, no. 7, pg. 706–721

[21] Augustin Scalbert et al., "Polyphenols: antioxidants and beyond," *American Journal of Clinical Nutrition*, January 2005, vol. 81, no. 1, pg. 215S–217S

[22] Ibid.

[23] Vighi G et al., "Allergy and the gastrointestinal system," *Clinical and Experimental Immunology*, Sep 2000, vol. 153, Supplement 1, pg. 3–6

[24] Melinda Wenner, "Humans Carry More Bacterial Cells than Human Ones," *Scientific American*, November 30, 2007

CHAPTER THREE

Fat

During the last century, a radical nutritional theory regarding dietary fat emerged, gained traction, and became dogma. During the 1930s and 1940s, degenerative disease rates, especially cardiovascular disease, were rapidly increasing. The theory that fat, particularly saturated fat, elevates cholesterol and subsequently promotes cardiovascular disease was proposed and popularized. Other dietary factors such as trans fats and reckless sugar consumption were all but ignored.

To make matters worse, industrial seed oils were portrayed and promoted as healthy alternatives to supposedly unhealthy traditional fats like butter and coconut oil. Most industrial seed oils contain excessive amounts of omega-6 polyunsaturated fat. Omega-6 is an essential fatty acid (EFA), meaning we are unable synthesize this nutrient and must therefore obtain it through food. But we need only very small amounts, and overconsumption causes many problems. When consumed in excess, omega-6 promotes inflammation and prevents the absorption of omega-3, a critical nutrient for cognitive development and function. Diets rich in omega-6 promote chronic, systemic inflammation, the underlying cause of many degenerative diseases, including heart disease. To the detriment of untold millions, prominent institutions, including the American Medical Association (AMA), the American Heart Association (AHA), and others, have unintentionally exacerbated the scourge of cancer, diabetes, and heart disease by discouraging traditional, healthy foods while simultaneously promoting dangerous, industrial pseudo-foods.

Despite the past century's disastrous nutritional misdirection, there are currently many encouraging trends and developments. First and foremost, nutritional science has exhaustively disproven the theory that saturated fat and dietary cholesterol cause heart disease. Fat metabolism and basic fat chemistry are much better understood now. We understand the differences, for example, between short-chain, medium-chain, and long-chain fatty acids. We understand the differences between saturated, monounsaturated, and polyunsaturated fats. We know about omega-6 fat versus omega-3. We know about heated fat versus raw fat. We know about trans fats. We have a much better understanding of cholesterol, including the differences between HDL, small-particle LDL, and large-particle LDL. In short, modern science strongly supports the consumption of traditional fat sources, which are dominant in saturated and monounsaturated fat. Conversely, science does not support consuming foods rich in polyunsaturated omega-6. The old nutritional paradigm is crumbling while a new one, rooted in tradition and validated by modern scientific research, is emerging. So how did these changes come about? How were entire nations convinced to swap sound dietary traditions for radically ill-conceived diets?

A Brief History Of Fat

By the 1920s, dieting was firmly entrenched in US culture, mostly among middle class and upper class women, and generally motivated by vanity rather than wellness. Women's magazines regularly featured dieting columns, which typically advocated low-calorie diets. Since each gram of fat has 9 calories, as opposed to 4 calories for each gram of protein or carbohydrate, diet gurus concluded that losing weight was best accomplished by consuming less fat. By the 1950s, against this cultural backdrop, some scientists and physicians began promoting low-fat diets for cardiovascular health. Coronary heart disease was already the leading cause of death in the US and had been since the beginning of the century.[1] Americans were consuming copious amounts of sweetened beverages and sugar-heavy desserts, and lower amounts of fruits and vegetables. A dietary link was implicit, but for many reasons, saturated fat became the scapegoat, whereas sugar was all but ignored.

By 1961, the AHA was actively encouraging Americans to replace saturated fat with unsaturated fat.[2] Instead of butter, they recommended margarine, and instead of animal fats, they recommended vegetable oils. Many people blame the prominent American scientist Ancel Keys for this monumental dietary error. Since the 1950s, Keys had been promoting low-fat diets. His enthusiasm and outspokenness finally landed him on the cover of *Time* magazine's January 1961 issue. In the corresponding article, Keys expressed his conviction that saturated fat increases blood cholesterol levels, damages the arteries, and eventually leads to coronary heart disease.[3]

Keys later published his famous Seven Countries Study, a highly influential yet heavily criticized analysis of diet and lifestyle trends around the world. Keys' critics accused him of intentionally skewing his results because he possessed data from twenty-two countries, yet excluded fifteen. Regardless, a critical trend emerged from both the full dataset as well as the seven-country dataset: the consumption of sugar was almost equally predictive of heart disease as was the consumption of saturated fat.[4] According to Keys,

"The fact that the incidence rate of coronary heart disease was significantly correlated with the average percentage of calories from sucrose in the diets is explained by the inter-correlation of sucrose with saturated fat."[5]

In other words, people who were eating higher amounts of saturated fat also were eating higher amounts of sugar. And these people had higher rates of heart disease. But what was driving the disease, fat or sugar? According to Keys, sugar was simply along for the ride. Saturated fat was the bad guy. But perhaps the reverse was true.

During the 1960s and early 70s, neither the public nor the medical establishment was firmly convinced that saturated fat promotes heart disease. Even the AHA in their 1961 report included the following caveat:

"It must be emphasized that there is as yet no final proof that heart attacks or strokes will be prevented by such [dietary] measures."[6]

Also during these years, distinguished scientists, including Margaret Albrink, John Gofman (who worked on the Manhattan Project), and Peter Kuo, were criticizing, to varying degrees, the low-fat theory. Instead, these scientists were focusing on high-carb diets, which they believed increase triglycerides, thereby increasing the risk of heart disease.

The most formidable adversary of Keys turned out to be John Yudkin, a leading nutritionist and physiologist from the UK. Yudkin was the first prominent scientist to implicate sugar as the primary driver of heart disease. Through his experiments, Yudkin demonstrated that sugar raises blood triglyceride levels and insulin levels, eventually causing type 2 diabetes and heart disease. He became world-famous by publishing his 1972 book, *Pure, White, and Deadly*. Yudkin was far ahead of his time and was constantly butting heads with Keys and other mainstream personas. His 1995 obituary in the *Independent* observed,

> *"His idea that too much sugar is harmful brought him into conflict with powerful lobbies but he was never afraid to question established dogma."*[7]

Yudkin also argued that saturated fat, far from promoting heart disease, is actually a necessary, health-supportive nutrient. Today, Yudkin seems like a visionary. During the 1970s, however, he was ridiculed and ostracized, at least within the US; his views were more widely accepted in Europe.[8]

During the 1970s, US public opinion gradually shifted towards the low-fat theory popularized by Keys. In 1977, the US government issued its first ever comprehensive, unambiguous dietary recommendations. The Senate Select Committee on Nutrition and Human Needs published a report, "Dietary Goals for the United States," which fully embraced the low-fat diet. This report led to US Dietary Guidelines, which are revised every five years. During the 1980s and 1990s, the low-fat theory became the prevailing dogma of the medical establishment. Doctors, health pundits, teachers, and media personalities subsequently echoed this dogma ad nauseam.

Political and economic policies have also influenced dietary recommendations. During the early 1970s, the US government began heavily subsidizing corn. Several years later, the US implemented a series of sugar tariffs and quotas. Domestic sugar prices subsequently soared, as did corn production. From 1973 until 1979, US corn production rose 40 percent, resulting in huge surpluses and effectively catalyzing a massive shift towards high fructose corn syrup (HFCS).[9] The food industry embraced the government's low-fat guidelines. Simply by emphasizing sugar (especially cheap HFCS) over fat, manufacturers could reap huge profits. With corn and soy becoming progressively cheaper, manufacturers started replacing costly animal fats with corn- and soy-based hydrogenated vegetable oils, which greatly promote heart disease. The 1980s began the low-saturated fat, high-sugar era. The "low in saturated fat" label adorned endless boxes of crackers, cookies, and other processed foods.

To this day, heart disease remains the leading cause of death in the United States. So were the government and the leading medical and nutritional institutions correct? Is saturated fat unhealthy? Does it promote heart disease? A definitive 2010 meta-analysis published in the *American Journal of Clinical Nutrition* examined twenty-one epidemiological studies following nearly 350,000 subjects for intervals ranging from five to twenty-three years. Absolutely no association between saturated fat intake and coronary heart disease could be established. The authors concluded,

"There is no significant evidence for concluding that dietary saturated fat is associated with an increased risk of coronary heart disease or coronary vascular disease." [10]

The US government spends roughly $1.2 billion per year studying heart disease.[11] During the past five years, the EU has chipped in an additional €163 million.[12] With so much money being thrown at research, why are governments still drawing the wrong conclusions? A 2012 study published in *Nutrition* examined inconsistencies between US/EU dietary recommendations and published nutritional research. The study's author, Robert Hoenselaar, analyzed three important government reports concerning dietary fat, one from the USDA, one from the Institute of Medicine, and one from the European Food Safety Authority. Hoenselaar concluded,

"All three reports included the effect of saturated fat on low-density lipoprotein cholesterol in the evidence linking saturated fat to cardiovascular disease, but the effect on high-density lipoprotein cholesterol was systematically ignored. Both US reports failed to correctly describe the results from the prospective studies. Results and conclusions about saturated fat intake in relation to cardiovascular disease, from leading advisory committees, do not reflect the available scientific literature." [13]

The relationship between cholesterol, dietary fat, and cardiovascular disease is much better understood today than it was fifty years ago. The concept of good and bad cholesterol has been refined and revised. Breakthrough research proves that LDL, the so-called "bad cholesterol," is not necessarily bad. Saturated fat increases large, buoyant LDL particles, but not small, dense LDL particles.[14] Saturated fat also increases HDL levels, colloquially known as "good cholesterol." Strong predictors of cardiovascular disease include low HDL levels and high small, dense LDL levels. Large, buoyant LDL is not associated with cardiovascular disease.[15] For a variety of reasons, governments and certain health institutions have not yet assimilated this modern understanding of cholesterol. They continue encouraging people to replace healthy traditional foods rich in saturated fat with omega-6-rich industrial seed oils. This amounts to replacing heart-supportive foods with inflammatory foods that promote cardiovascular disease.

The notion that saturated fat promotes cardiovascular disease is a flawed theory that became conventional wisdom. The time has come for a new understanding of dietary fat and cholesterol, an understanding that values sound scientific research and timeless dietary wisdom over dogma and the fiscal wellness of select corporations and industries.

The Basic Chemistry

Fats are poorly understood. Our food supply consists of many types of fats from many different sources. Some fats are health supportive and indeed essential, while others wreak havoc and promote disease. A basic understanding of fats and how the body processes them will enable you to choose the best sources while eliminating the worst. Fats are classified in two basic ways:

1. According to hydrogen saturation levels
2. According to chain length

From a biochemical perspective, fats are chemical compounds consisting of fatty acids. Fatty acids are chains of carbon atoms with hydrogen atoms attached. The three primary varieties of fatty acids are:

1. Saturated
2. Monounsaturated
3. Polyunsaturated

Saturated fatty acids have the maximum number of hydrogen atoms attached to each carbon atom. The carbon atoms attach to each other via single bonds, thereby creating straight fatty acid chains. This is why saturated fats remain solid at room temperature. Unsaturated fatty acids have at least one hydrogen pair missing from their carbon chains. This creates gaps whereby two carbon atoms must connect by double rather than single bonds. Subsequently, these fatty acid chains become kinked, or bent. The more bent the molecules are, the more space they occupy. This is why unsaturated fats are liquid at room temperature. Monounsaturated fatty acids are missing only one pair of hydrogen atoms, whereas polyunsaturated fatty acids are missing two or more pairs. As stated above, fatty acids are also classified according to carbon chain length:

- Short-chain fatty acids (SCFA) have 6 or fewer carbon atoms.
- Medium-chain fatty acids (MCFA) have 8 to 12 carbon atoms.
- Long-chain fatty acids (LCFA) have more than 12 carbons.

SCFAs and MCFAs are rapidly absorbed and efficiently converted into energy, unlike LCFAs, which require bile salts for digestion. SCFAs and MCFAs are absorbed into the bloodstream by the intestinal capillaries and the portal vein. Once there, SCFAs and MCFAs proceed directly to the liver where they rapidly and efficiently convert into energy. In many ways, the digestion of SCFAs and MCFAs resembles carbohydrate digestion, without the associated blood sugar swings.

The digestion of LCFAs is less efficient and more time consuming. LCFAs are not directly absorbed by the small intestines, as are SCFAs and MCFAs. To pass through the intestinal walls, LCFAs require the action of pancreatic lipase enzymes and bile salts from the liver. Next, LCFAs are incorporated into chylomicrons (lipoproteins), which travel through the lymphatic system en route to the liver.[16] Whereas SCFAs and MCFAs are always healthy, LCFAs are sometimes healthy but sometimes not. SCFAs and MCFAs have antimicrobial, antiviral, and antifungal properties, which LCFAs do not. Whereas SCFAs and MCFAs are always saturated, LCFAs can either be saturated, monounsaturated, or polyunsaturated. Most sources of dietary fat, whether saturated or unsaturated, and whether derived from animal or vegetal sources, consist primarily of LCFAs. To determine whether or not a particular source of dietary fat is healthy, the entire fatty acid profile must be assessed.

Every food has its own unique fatty acid profile, including a unique saturation profile (the ratio of saturated to monounsaturated to polyunsaturated fatty acids) and a unique chain-length profile (the distribution of particular fatty acids within each saturation category). The entire profile must be considered when determining which fat sources are healthy and which are not. Figure 3.2 (pg. 74) details the composition of common dietary sources of fat. The analysis is based solely on the fat portion of each food. In other words, water, carbohydrate, and protein data have been discarded so the fat data can be analyzed independently.

The PUFA Problem

Misconceptions about saturated fat have resulted in radical dietary shifts towards unsaturated fatty acids, and specifically polyunsaturated fatty acids (PUFAs), during the past fifty-plus years. Most significantly, traditional, health-supportive animal fats have been replaced by cheap, unhealthy vegetable oils, the worst of which include canola, corn, safflower, sunflower, and soybean oil. All these vegetable oils are rich in PUFAs, especially the inflammation-inducing omega-6 variety.

Diets rich in omega-6 PUFAs promote heart disease, cancer, various autoimmune diseases, digestive disorders, and other serious health issues.[17] The widespread switch from saturated fat to supposedly heart-healthy omega-6 PUFAs was perhaps the most misguided dietary adjustment of the past century. The notion that saturated fat clogs arteries, thus promoting heart disease, simply does not withstand rigorous scientific inquiry. In fact, a 1994 study published in *The Lancet* found that aortic plaque levels are primarily associated with PUFAs, not with saturated fat:

> *"These findings imply a direct influence of dietary polyunsaturated fatty acids on aortic plaque formation and suggest that current trends favouring increased intake of polyunsaturated fatty acids should be reconsidered."* [18]

PUFAs are problematic for many reasons, especially because they are inherently unstable from a molecular perspective. When exposed to heat, light, and air, PUFAs oxidize and become rancid, thus creating free radicals. Because most polyunsaturated vegetable oils are extracted using intense heat, as well as chemical solvents, they are already denatured and chemically reactive before even reaching your supermarket shelves. Once purchased and brought home, they are typically subjected to more heat through cooking. By the time they are consumed, PUFAs are rife with inflammatory free radicals.

Differentiating Between 6 and 3

There are two basic types of PUFAs—omega-6 and omega-3. Whereas small amounts of omega-6 are necessary, Western diets commonly provide far too much. Omega-3 PUFAs, also necessary in small amounts, are integral to brain development, cognitive function, skin health, bone health, proper metabolism, and reproductive capacity. The differences between omega-6 and omega-3 are critically important, but commonly misunderstood. Opportunistic marketers exploit this misunderstanding by using the word "omega" whenever possible. Typical product labels include phrases like "rich in omega-3" or "great source of omega essential fatty acids." Such product labels are worthless, however, unless they convey two essential pieces of information: 1) the absolute amount of omega-6, and 2) the omega-6 to omega-3 ratio. Product labels featuring the word "omega," but failing to provide this information should arouse suspicion. For those who understand the relationship between omega-6 and omega-3, the most informative phrases would be something to the effect of "very low in omega-6" and "very low omega-6 to omega-3 ratio."

The most important concept regarding PUFAs is that both omega-6 and omega-3 fatty acids compete for the same rate-limiting enzymes. Simply upping your daily omega-3 intake does not necessarily mean you assimilate these fatty acids. When you consume too much omega-6, as most people do, you assimilate proportionally more omega-6 and less omega-3. In other words, increasing dietary omega-3 or taking omega-3 supplements is futile unless you concurrently restrict your daily omega-6 intake. Thus the problem is twofold:

1. Western diets are entirely deficient in omega-3.

2. Western diets are disproportionally high in omega-6 compared to omega-3.

According to numerous studies, the ideal omega-6 to omega-3 ratio is 1:1, which means equal amounts of both.[19] Humans maintained this ratio for the vast majority of history and prehistory. Around 150 years ago, however, at the onset of the Industrial Revolution, fat consumption patterns started shifting dramatically. By 1939, the omega ratio for the average American was 8.4:1, which increased to 10.3:1 by 1985.[20] Whereas any ratio less than 3:1 (three times as much omega-6 as omega-3) generally promotes good health, today's Western diets typically yield omega ratios ranging from 10:1 to 30:1.[21]

Excessive consumption of omega-6 fatty acids (and high 6 to 3 ratios) leads to chronic inflammation, while also promoting many diseases, including heart disease, cancer, and various inflammatory and autoimmune diseases.[22] Relatively higher amounts of omega-3, and thus lower 6 to 3 ratios, help prevent these diseases.[23] Those who suffer from chronic inflammatory diseases and conditions including rheumatoid arthritis should be particularly diligent regarding the omega ratio.

Figure 3.2 provides detailed fat profiles for most commonly consumed sources of dietary fat. Foods with high absolute levels of PUFAs and poor omega ratios should be strictly avoided. Foods with higher absolute levels of PUFAs but beneficial omega ratios, fish oil for example, can be consumed regularly but only in small quantities. We need only very small amounts of daily PUFAs. The problem is not only the ratio, but also the absolute amount. Regarding omega-3 fatty acids, 1 gram of combined DHA and EPA per day is optimal, plus another gram or two of ALA. DHA, EPA, and ALA are subcategories of omega-3 PUFAs, described below. With the optimal 1:1 omega ratio, you're looking at 6 total grams per day of PUFAs (3 grams omega-6 and 3 grams omega-3). The 3:1 ratio would bring you up to 12 total grams per day (9 grams omega-6 and 3 grams omega-3).

Eating fatty fish such as salmon, mackerel, or sardines three times per week should satisfy your omega-3 requirements. Supplementation with small amounts of chia seeds, flax seeds, or fish oil can also be beneficial. Chia and flax seeds, however, contain ALA, not DHA and EPA. This necessitates endogenous conversion, which can be complicated (see below). Therefore, whole fish and high-quality fish oils are superior. Raw fish preparations are best, such as ceviche or sashimi.

Don't worry about getting enough omega-6. Olive oil alone gives you plenty. Adding eggs and avocados to your diet, as I highly recommend, also ensures you are getting adequate amounts of omega-6. By eating nuts and seeds regularly, you can easily consume too much omega-6, thereby skewing your omega ratio and decreasing your omega-3 uptake. You need not worry about getting enough omega-6. The three basic challenges regarding PUFAs are:

1. Limiting omega-6 consumption

2. Getting sufficient omega-3

3. Limiting total polyunsaturated fat

Subcategories of 3 and 6

Besides understanding the crucial omega 6 to 3 ratio, you should also understand the differences between the various subcategories of omega fatty acids. In other words, there are different types of omega-6 and different types of omega-3. Both omega-6 and omega-3 are commonly classified as essential fatty acids (EFAs) because the body cannot produce them endogenously. The most important long-chain omega fatty acids are:

Omega-6 fatty acids

- Linoleic acid (LA)
- Gamma-Linolenic acid (GLA)
- Arachidonic acid (AA)

Omega-3 fatty acids

- Alpha-Linolenic acid (ALA)
- Docosahexaenoic acid (DHA)
- Eicosapentaenoic acid (EPA)

Technically, only LA and ALA are essential because the body can convert these parent EFAs into the other omega fatty acids. This conversion, however, is unreliable and inefficient, especially concerning the critical omega-3 fatty acids DHA and EPA, which are essential for brain, eye, and nerve health. Under optimal conditions, only about 6 percent of ALA converts into EPA and only 3.8 percent of ALA converts into DHA.[24] Eating a typical Western diet lowers these conversion rates approximately 40 to 50 percent. In other words, don't bank on these conversions. Go directly to the DHA and EPA source foods instead.

The best sources of DHA and EPA are cold-water, oily fish, including salmon, mackerel, herring, anchovies, and sardines. The oils from these fish typically have ratios around 1:7 (seven times *more* omega-3 than 6). Also, eggs from hens fed special diets consisting of greens, insects, flax seeds, and fish oils have significantly higher percentages of omega-3 fatty acids (ALA and DHA, but not EPA) compared to eggs from hens fed conventional corn- and soy-based diets.[25] Whereas the omega ratio for conventional eggs ranges from 11:1 to 16:1, a 2009 study published in *Food Chemistry* observed a much healthier 2.27:1 ratio for omega-3-enriched eggs.[26]

Vegetarian sources of DHA and EPA are rare, but some varieties of microalgae do provide these nutrients and are becoming increasingly available in supplement form. In 2012, a team of researchers published a meta-analysis concerning algal DHA oil and its impact on heart health. They discovered that algal DHA, like fish oil, reduces triglycerides, raises HDL cholesterol (good), and raises large-particle LDL (which is benign).[27] Most plant sources of omega-3 contain ALA, not DHA or EPA. Besides the conversion inefficiency problem, most plant sources of ALA also contain far too much omega-6. Flax and chia seeds are best because both are high in ALA and low in omega-6. Although these foods don't promote inflammation, they might not provide enough ALA to satisfy DHA and EPA requirements.

Rethinking Saturated Fat

There are two kinds of dietary SCFAs—butyric acid and caproic acid—and three kinds of dietary MCFAs—caprylic acid, capric acid, and lauric acid. As discussed above, SCFAs and MCFAs are highly digestible, highly nourishing, and health-protective. Butyric acid, for example, is particularly important for colon health and has been shown to kill colon cancer cells.[28] Butyric acid is abundant in dairy products. MCFAs aid weight loss (due to their ease of digestion), promote healthy HDL to LDL cholesterol ratios, and have potent antiviral and antimicrobial properties.[29]

A study published in the *American Journal of Clinical Nutrition* in 2000 found that lauric acid oxidizes extremely efficiently. Monounsaturated, polyunsaturated, and longer-chain saturated fatty acids, according to this study, oxidize considerably less efficiently.[30] This means the body efficiently burns lauric acid for energy, as opposed to storing it as fat. Lauric acid also has significant antibacterial properties, particularly against helicobacter pylori bacteria, which is associated with gastritis, ulcers, stomach cancer, and heart disease.[31] Furthermore, lauric acid elevates HDL cholesterol levels, thus decreasing the risk of coronary heart disease.[32]

Common Dietary Fatty Acids – Figure 3.1

Saturated Fatty Acids		*Unsaturated Fatty Acids*	
Name	C:D	Name	C:D
Butyric acid	4:0	Palmitoleic acid	16:1
Caproic acid	6:0	Oleic acid	18:1
Caprylic acid	8:0	Gadoleic acid	20:1
Capric acid	10:0	*Polyunsaturated Fatty Acids*	
Lauric acid	12:0	Linoleic acid (LA)	18:2 (ω-6)
Myristic acid	14:0	Alpha-Linolenic acid (ALA)	18:3 (ω-3)
Palmitic acid	16:0	Gamma-Linolenic acid (GLA)	18:3 (ω-6)
Stearic acid	18:0	Arachidonic acid (AA)	20:4 (ω-6)
Arachidic acid	20:0	Eicosapentaenoic acid (EPA)	20:5 (ω-3)
Lignoceric acid	24:0	Docosahexaenoic acid (DHA)	22:6 (ω-3)

C = number of carbon atoms, D = number of double bonds, ω-6 = omega-6, ω-3 = omega-3

SCFAs and MCFAs, both of which are always saturated, are healthy and totally undeserving of anti-saturated-fat hysteria. But what about saturated LCFAs? The three most common saturated LCFAs are myristic acid, palmitic acid, and stearic acid. Even more so than oleic acid (the primary component of olive oil), stearic acid has been shown to lower LDL cholesterol.[33] Even the AHA acknowledges that stearic acid has no negative effect on cholesterol levels.[34] According to the AHA, WHO, and other advocates of low-saturated-fat (high-PUFA) diets, myristic and palmitic acids are the worst types of saturated fat. But are they really so bad?

Some studies have indeed linked myristic and palmitic acids to increased LDL cholesterol levels and decreased HDL to LDL ratios.[35] These and other saturated fatty acids, however, only increase large-particle, benign LDL (discussed below), not the dangerous small-particle LDL.[36] Also, palmitic acid generally elevates bad cholesterol only when combined with trans fats.[37] The saturated fatty acid most abundant in plants and animals is palmitic acid. Of the total fat contained in human breast milk, for example, 20.5 percent is palmitic acid—a good indication it plays an important role in human nutrition.[38] Saturated fat is indeed necessary and completely beneficial. Ironically, after being implicated for causing cardiovascular disease, it was replaced by fats that actually do, namely omega-6 fatty acids (in excess) and trans fats.

Trans Fats: The Worst Of The Worst

Trans fats are created through hydrogenation, a process whereby unsaturated fat molecules gain extra hydrogen atoms, thus losing their characteristic double bonds and subsequently becoming partially or completely saturated. Since their commercial debut in 1911 as Proctor & Gamble's Crisco product, hydrogenated fats have been causing immense health problems. For the food industry, however, hydrogenation has been extremely lucrative. Hydrogenation increases product shelf life, decreases the need for refrigeration, and enables huge cost savings by making cheap vegetable oils behave like butter and other expensive animal fats.

To convert liquid oils into solid or semisolid fats, food manufacturers combine vegetable oils with nickel oxide, a strong catalyst for chemical reactions. These oils, typically from corn, soybeans, and cottonseed (the top three GMO crops), are already rancid due to high-heat and hexane-solvent extraction methods. Next, manufacturers subject these oils to hydrogen gas inside high-temperature, high-pressure reactors. Then they add chemical emulsifiers to create desirable textures and consistencies. The final stages include bleaching, deodorizing, and flavoring. High temperatures and high pressure cause atomic repositioning along the fatty acid chain, which results in exotic toxins not recognized by the digestive system. Trans fats, consequently, are only partially absorbed; they interfere with cell metabolism and eventually lead to numerous diseases and disorders.

Coronary heart disease is the primary and most acknowledged risk of trans fats. The AHA explains that trans fat consumption "increases your risk of developing heart disease and stroke. It's also associated with a higher risk of developing type 2 diabetes."[39] A 2006 study published in *Nutrition in Clinical Practice* attributed as many as 100,000 deaths per year in the US to trans fats from hydrogenated oils.[40] Also in 2006, a study published in the prestigious *New England Journal of Medicine* drew the following emphatic conclusion:

> *"On a per-calorie basis, trans fats appear to increase the risk of CHD [coronary heart disease] more than any other macronutrient, conferring a substantially increased risk at low levels of consumption (1 to 3% of total energy intake)."* [41]

Studies published in other journals have linked trans fats to Alzheimer's disease,[42] liver dysfunction,[43] female infertility,[44] and depression.[45]

People are gradually becoming more and more aware of the dangers posed by trans fats. Consequently, many cities, states, and entire nations are implementing partial or total bans. Food manufacturers are responding by introducing trans-fat-free products. On this initiative, they have been greatly assisted by characteristically lax US Food and Drug Administration (FDA) regulations. Beginning in 2008, the FDA imposed mandatory trans fat labeling regulations, ostensibly to protect public health. In reality, however, these laws protect corporate profits while potentially harming consumers. Under the new laws, foods with 0.5 grams trans fat per serving can legally be labeled "zero grams trans fats."[46] The AHA recommends no more than 2 grams trans fats per day. Thus, consuming "zero grams trans fats" several times per day can quickly amount to dangerous, disease-promoting levels.

While trans fat consumption is declining, as of 2005 the average American was still eating 5.8 grams daily.[47] The most obvious trans fat sources are processed foods, including chips, crackers, and cookies; deep fried foods, including French fries and doughnuts; margarines and shortenings; pastries and baked goods; etc. You should eliminate trans fats from your diet, without exception.

Cholesterol Clarity

What we've been told about cholesterol is inaccurate and completely misleading. Take eggs, for example, one of the foods highest in dietary cholesterol with roughly 185 mg per egg. The AHA recommends no more than 300 mg of cholesterol per day, effectively limiting egg consumption to one per day. But does consuming cholesterol increase blood cholesterol levels? Does eating fat make you fat? Does eating spinach make you green? While the idea that dietary cholesterol (cholesterol contained in food) translates into serum cholesterol (cholesterol contained in your blood) may seem plausible, it lacks scientific support. Even Ancel Keys, the famous progenitor of the lipid hypothesis of coronary heart disease, discussed this noncausal relationship as early as 1953:

"Repeated careful dietary surveys on large numbers of persons in whom blood cholesterol was measured consistently fail to disclose a relationship between the cholesterol in the diet and in the serum." [48]

In short, you can eat eggs and other cholesterol-rich foods. Eggs do contain dietary cholesterol, but they don't affect blood cholesterol levels negatively. Understanding why dietary cholesterol doesn't negatively affect serum cholesterol requires a basic understanding of the various types of cholesterol.

Cholesterol is a liver-generated lipid (fat), which exists in every cell. A necessary precursor for numerous hormones, including testosterone, estrogen, and cortisol, cholesterol is essential for optimal health.[49] Cholesterol is lipid based, whereas blood is water based. Since cholesterol is not water soluble, it requires transport proteins to move it through the blood. Thus when we speak about cholesterol, we're actually speaking about transport proteins, which move cholesterol around. Most people have heard about good and bad cholesterol. High-density lipoprotein (HDL) is called good cholesterol and low-density lipoprotein (LDL) is called bad cholesterol. This view, however, is oversimplified because both HDL and LDL are necessary and beneficial.

LDL varies by particle size, only becoming problematic when small, dense LDL particles, known as type-b, accumulate under the blood vessel linings. Large, buoyant LDL particles, known as type-a, are non-inflammatory and essentially benign.[50] Type-a LDL floats easily through the bloodstream; type-b sinks, accumulates, and subsequently contributes to atherosclerotic plaque. Damage to arterial walls triggers inflammation, which leads to plaque development.[51] This damage has many causes including smoking, psychological stress, nitric oxide depletion, microbial infections, trans fats, excessive carbohydrates, and excessive omega-6.[52] A 1994 study published in the *Lancet* found aortic plaque formation is directly influenced by dietary omega-6 fatty acids. No associations were found with saturated fatty acids.[53]

Saturated fat raises type-a LDL, the benign variety, but doesn't significantly affect type-b. Dietary carbohydrates, especially sugars, are the primary drivers of type-b LDL.[54] Refined carbohydrates have been shown to increase triglycerides, increase type-b LDL, and decrease beneficial HDL.[55] While LDL cholesterol has long been linked to heart disease and type 2 diabetes, numerous modern studies suggest that type-b, not type-a LDL, promotes these diseases.[56] In other words, eat saturated fat, but be more discerning with carbohydrates. As John Yudkin explained four decades ago, sugar, not fat, is the primary driver of heart disease.

So what about eggs and other high-cholesterol foods? Eggs increase healthy HDL levels while changing type-b cholesterol into type-a, a decidedly win-win scenario.[57] A recent meta-analysis published in the *British Medical Journal* concluded that high egg consumption is associated neither with increased risk of heart disease, nor with stroke.[58] Besides being loaded with vitamins, minerals, and antioxidants, eggs contain high-quality fat and protein. Quite simply, they are among the planet's best foods.

Now back to dietary cholesterol. The only firmly established cholesterol-related risk factor for coronary heart disease is elevated circulating levels of small, dense type-b LDL. As Keys discussed more than sixty years ago, dietary cholesterol does not increase serum cholesterol levels. Dietary cholesterol actually improves the serum cholesterol profile. Modern research shows that dietary cholesterol decreases the harmful type-b LDL.[59] The conventional view of cholesterol, having misunderstood the relationship between dietary and serum cholesterols, as well as the differences between type-a and type-b LDL, clearly must be reconsidered.

Mad Statins

Traditional cholesterol tests, not surprisingly, do not differentiate between type-a and type-b LDL. Only modern, sophisticated tests (cholesterol fractionation tests and subfractionated lipid panels) measure both varieties. Many progressive doctors are now replacing traditional cholesterol tests with modern tests, thus providing their patients with more informative advice. Other doctors are deriving incomplete and misleading information from traditional tests and subsequently prescribing statin drugs, generally for nonexistent cholesterol problems.

Statins are drugs that lower cholesterol by blocking an enzyme responsible for LDL cholesterol production within the liver. The main problem with statins is they indiscriminately reduce all LDL, not just the inflammatory type-b variety. Research published by the *Texas Heart Institute Journal* in 2010 shows that while statins reduce absolute levels of both type-a and type-b LDL, statin therapy proportionally increases type-b.[60] In 2004, the US National Cholesterol Education Program (NCEP) reduced target LDL levels for high-risk patients from an already too-low 100 to a potentially dangerous 70. This was a boon for statin manufacturers because achieving this new target essentially requires statin drugs. What could be driving such a dramatic and seemingly irrational recommendation? Even the NCEP acknowledged that only 5 percent of US women and 2 percent of US men have LDL levels at or below 70.[61] Does more than 95 percent of the population really require statins?

A 2006 review in the *Annals of Internal Medicine* deemed the new government LDL recommendation neither beneficial nor safe.[62] The NCEP recommendation serves as yet another example of the fine line between corporate interests and public health policies. Following an investigation, the *Associated Press* revealed that eight of the nine doctors on the panel tasked with devising the new cholesterol guidelines were financially entwined with various manufacturers of statin drugs.[63] As a direct result of their recommendations, 33 percent of the US population and 24 percent of the UK population are currently taking statin drugs.[64]

Statins are unnecessary and potentially dangerous, except perhaps for people with a rare genetic condition called familial hypercholesterolemia. The documented risks of statins are overwhelming. Side effects include muscle problems and cognition problems. Statins can also amplify metabolic syndrome, thyroid disease, and certain genetic mutations linked to mitochondrial dysfunction.[65] According to a review of the medical literature recently published in the *American Journal of Cardiovascular Drugs*, more than 900 studies have identified adverse reactions to statins.[66] Some of the greatest dangers include:

- Statins increase the risk of diabetes, especially in postmenopausal women (71 percent increase) and women in general (48 percent increase).[67] Even the FDA acknowledges, "People being treated with statins may have an increased risk of raised blood sugar levels and the development of type 2 diabetes."[68]

- The FDA also warns, "Cognitive (brain-related) impairment, such as memory loss, forgetfulness and confusion, has been reported by some statin users."[69]

- Frequent statin use is associated with accelerated coronary artery and aortic artery calcification, a highly predictive factor of cardiovascular disease.[70]

- Statins block the production of coenzyme Q_{10}, an endogenous antioxidant critical to cellular functions and particularly beneficial for heart health.[71]

- Statins decrease testosterone levels, can lower libido, and can induce erectile dysfunction.[72]

Again, allopathic medicine has responded to cardiovascular disease with advice that actually amplifies the problem. Cholesterol is in fact good for you. Your body uses cholesterol, for example, as a precursor to vitamin D obtained through natural sunlight. When your cholesterol levels are too low, you cannot adequately synthesize vitamin D from sunlight.[73] While elevated levels of small-particle LDL are indeed problematic, saturated fat is not the cause, nor are statins the solution. For decades, doctors and dieticians have imprecisely understood the crucial relationship between saturated fat consumption and cholesterol levels. Saturated fat does indeed raise beneficial HDL levels while changing type-b LDL into benign type-a.[74] Saturated fat, therefore, has a net-positive, health-supportive effect on cholesterol.

To conclude, HDL cholesterol has definite health benefits, whereas large-particle type-a LDL is benign. Saturated fat, monounsaturated fat, and small amounts of poly-unsaturated fat do not promote unhealthy serum cholesterol levels. The commonly perceived negative effects of cholesterol are actually the combined effects of small-particle type-b LDL and inflammation. Type-b LDL can readily enter arterial walls, thereby triggering an inflammatory response. Inflammation speeds up cholesterol accumulation, which eventually hardens into plaque.[75] The best strategy for avoiding cholesterol problems is avoiding inflammatory foods, especially sugar, processed foods, and excessive omega-6 PUFAs.

During the twentieth century, the now-disproved theory that saturated fat raises bad cholesterol, thus promoting heart disease, resulted in disastrous dietary advice. People began avoiding heart-healthy saturated fats, while embracing polyunsaturated seed oils. Returning to traditional fats is an essential step towards preventing and treating heart disease, and improving overall health.

Give It To Me Raw

As discussed above, PUFAs are extremely heat sensitive. Logically, they should only be cold-extracted, though most are not. Monounsaturated and saturated fats, while more stable than polyunsaturated, should also ideally be cold-extracted. When fats are heated, their protective enzymes and antioxidants are damaged. Thus you must always pay careful attention to product labels and choose only truly cold-extracted oils. This is not necessarily an easy task, as product descriptions are often confusing, sometimes intentionally so. The onus is on you to learn the jargon and recognize the deceptive marketing tactics.

Many terms are used to describe the extraction processes of oil. Sometimes these terms are unregulated, making them imprecise and confusing. The most commonly used terms are expeller pressed, cold pressed, virgin, and extra-virgin. Expeller-pressed oil is the contrary of refined oil. Expeller-pressed oils are extracted solely through mechanical means. Refined oils use chemical solvents and typically involve bleaching and deodorizing. But unrefined, expeller-pressed oil is not necessarily healthy. Expeller-pressed oils can reach high temperatures during extraction, which creates free radicals and denatures their sensitive PUFAs. Extraction temperatures depend mostly on the hardness of the seed or fruit. The harder the seed, the more pressure is required, which creates more friction and more heat, sometimes as much as 243°C (470°F). Because an almond, for example, is harder than the fleshy part of an avocado, expeller-pressed almond oil reaches much higher temperatures during processing than does expeller-pressed avocado oil.

Unrefined expeller-pressed oil is clearly better than refined, chemically extracted oil. The term expeller pressed, however, is sometimes a false-positive marketing trick, especially absent an accompanying, qualifying term such as virgin. In other words, there is a massive difference between expeller-pressed olive oil and expeller-pressed, extra-virgin olive oil. Some consumers wrongly assume that expeller pressed means no-heat extraction. That's why the term can be a false positive. It tells you that no chemicals were used during extraction, which is great, but more information is needed. Only the terms cold pressed and virgin provide truly relevant information. All cold-pressed oils and virgin oils are necessarily expeller pressed. Therefore, there is no difference between virgin olive oil and expeller pressed virgin olive oil.

So all cold pressed and virgin oils are expeller pressed, but all expeller-pressed oils are not necessarily cold pressed or virgin. To add another layer of complexity, the term cold pressed is strictly regulated in Europe, but not in the US. In Europe, cold pressed means fully unrefined, mechanical extraction (no chemicals involved) with temperatures never exceeding 50°C (122°F).[76] In the US, the term is unregulated and can therefore be used by unprincipled companies to deceive consumers. In the US, there is technically no difference between cold pressed and expeller pressed. Thus, consumers can buy "cold pressed" oils, believing they are no-heat extractions when in fact they are.

In the US, the only relevant terms are virgin and extra-virgin. Although these terms are both strictly regulated, they do not actually specify maximum extraction temperatures. In a roundabout manner, however, they do. These terms are measures of quality and taste based on acidity. Virgin olive oil contains no more than 2 percent free oleic acid, and extra-virgin olive oil contains no more than 0.8 percent free oleic acid. Practically speaking, these acidity levels can only be achieved through no-heat extraction. Cold-pressed olive oil sold in Europe is therefore not precisely the same as virgin or extra-virgin olive oil sold in the US, but from a health perspective, they are comparable. Also from a health perspective, extra-virgin is not significantly better than virgin olive oil as both are cold extractions.

There is yet another layer of complexity regarding labeling and quality. By the late 1990s, olive oil was the most adulterated agricultural product in the entire European Union.[77] Despite the establishment of an olive oil task force by the EU's antifraud office, olive oil fraud remains a major problem today, especially within the EU, and also in the US. In his acclaimed book, *Extra Virginity: The Sublime and Scandalous World of Olive Oil*, Tom Mueller describes the diametrically opposing trends of the olive oil industry. On the one hand, modern technology is now making possible the production of the most exquisite, most complex olive oils in history. On the other hand, the lucrative, improperly regulated industry is attracting dishonest producers and distributors.

Olive oil is commonly cut with cheap oils, including soybean oil and sunflower oil. Other illegal practices include chemical deodorization to remove sensory defects from inferior oils, then selling those oils as extra virgin. The FDA claims their resources are too limited and their responsibilities too great to police the olive oil industry.[78] To avoid being cheated, try buying olive oil from specialty shops. Look for olive oil produced by a single estate, single producer, or single place of production. Also look on the package for a harvest date, as opposed to a "best by" date, which is arbitrary and essentially meaningless. Also, you should expect to pay more for good-quality olive oil. Truly organic, truly cold-pressed olive oil is costly to produce. Fraud and deception have made the situation appear otherwise.

Coconut oil, my other highly recommended oil for regular use, also has labeling peculiarities. Like olive oil, coconut oil can be refined through chemical extraction methods, or unrefined and extracted solely mechanically. Refined coconut oil is very heavily processed, bleached, and deodorized. Also, refined coconut oil is sometimes hydrogenated or partially hydrogenated, resulting in trans fats. Unrefined coconut oil, like olive oil, can be expeller pressed with temperatures reaching 100°C (212°F), or truly cold pressed. The terms cold pressed and virgin are used to describe no-heat expeller-pressed coconut oil. Neither term is strictly regulated, yet coconut oil is much less susceptible to cheating than is olive oil.

Truly cold-pressed (virgin) coconut oil has a sweet, tropical fragrance. In warm temperatures, coconut oil should be liquid and translucent. When cold, it should be solid with a soft white color. There is no such thing as extra-virgin coconut oil. Put another way, virgin coconut oil and extra-virgin coconut oil are exactly the same. I prefer to buy virgin because extra-virgin suggests disingenuousness. Manufacturers know the term is meaningless, but still they manipulate consumers who justifiably presume extra-virgin is somehow superior and worth its premium pricing.

Winners and Losers

As indicated in Figure 3.2, sunflower oil, safflower oil, corn oil, and soy oil all have excessive omega-6 PUFAs. To make matters worse, these oils are extracted with high heat and chemical solvents. This denatures the oil and creates free radicals. Without exception, you should completely eliminate these oils from your diet. If you have them in your pantry, throw them away. Get into the habit of reading product labels at the supermarket. Don't buy products with these oils as ingredients. Eating in restaurants can be more difficult. Always avoid fried foods because the frying oil will almost certainly be one of these dangerous vegetable oils.

The best fats for everyday consumption are olive oil, coconut oil, and butter. You could also add avocados to this list. Coconut oil is extremely heat-stable (due to its saturated fat content) and is therefore best for cooking. Olive oil, which is primarily monounsaturated fat, is best raw but acceptable for occasional low-heat preparations. Butter is also an excellent heat-stable fat. Many people are fond of cooking in duck fat, goose fat, or pig fat. I'm not entirely against the concept. Certainly these fats are much better than seed oils. But as demonstrated in Figure 3.2, these fats have proportionately more monounsaturated and less saturated fat than coconut oil and butter. Monounsaturated fatty acids are less heat-stable than their saturated counterparts. Therefore coconut oil and butter are far better choices.

As discussed above, raw fat is always preferable. For example, I would rather toss steamed vegetables with unpasteurized raw butter than cook those same vegetables with butter. Technically, you could also slather duck, goose, or pig fats on cooked vegetables, except for one important detail. Coconut oil and unpasteurized raw butter are truly raw fats. The extraction of coconut oil and the churning of raw cream into butter do not involve heat. But the rendering of duck, goose, and pig fats requires prolonged boiling of various animal parts in water, thus damaging the unsaturated fatty acids. Making ghee from butter also requires prolonged heating. Butter oil, on the other hand, involves an advanced no-heat, molecular extraction of raw cream. Butter oil is therefore truly raw, like coconut oil and unpasteurized butter.

If you cannot find unpasteurized butter, pasteurized butter is perfectly acceptable. Pasteurization involves rapidly heating milk to 72°C (162°F) for twenty seconds, then rapidly cooling it below 7°C (45°F). This likely does not significantly damage butter's monounsaturated fat and certainly does not damage its saturated fat. Butter is relatively higher in saturated fat than are rendered animal fats. With proportionally higher saturated fat and less heat exposure, pasteurized butter is top tier, whereas rendered animal fats are tier three (see Figure 3.2). In short, ghee, duck fat, goose fat, and pig fat are decent, but olive oil, coconut oil, and butter are superior. Raw butter is best, but when unavailable, pasteurized butter is the next best thing.

The best sources of omega-3 fatty acids are fish and fish oils. Flax and chia are best for ALA, but fish and fish oils are best for the critical DHA and EPA. Wild salmon and small, cold-water fish, including sardines and mackerel, are excellent sources. Raw fish preparations (sashimi and ceviche) are better than cooked preparations. This is because all PUFAs are heat-sensitive. It's okay to lightly cook sardines, tuna, salmon, and other fatty fish, but the PUFAs will be affected. Nevertheless, you can avoid raising internal temperatures too high via quick-cooking methods like searing. For some people, obtaining sufficient omega-3 only through food might be difficult. Therefore, fish oil supplements can be beneficial. Look for blends high in DHA and EPA, tested for purity, and refrigerated to avoid oxidative damage. But because all PUFAs are inherently unstable, whole fish is preferable to fish oils.

Just Say No To Canola

Understanding extraction methods is even more important regarding PUFA-rich oils. Canola oil is 28 percent PUFAs, two-thirds of which are omega-6. Canola almost always undergoes high-heat extraction, thus damaging the PUFAs and creating free radicals. Virgin canola does exist but is rare and expensive. Many people wrongly assume canola is healthy. High-heat extraction notwithstanding, canola is indeed high in omega-3 (ALA), and does have a favorable 2:1 omega ratio. Nevertheless, canola simply has far too much total polyunsaturated fat.

The body does not need large amounts of PUFAs, and overconsumption promotes inflammation, even when proper omega ratios are maintained. Virgin canola is better than heat-extracted canola, but still contains unhealthy absolute PUFA levels. Olive oil, conversely, is only 11 percent polyunsaturated fat. Indeed, canola has a better omega ratio, but olive oil is superior overall, both for its absolute PUFA quantity and many other reasons, including its antioxidant and phytonutrient profile.

Vegetable Oil

It sounds so nonthreatening. Vegetable oil must be healthy, right? Unfortunately, vegetable oil is a highly misrepresentative marketing term. First of all, as a matter of accuracy, vegetable oil is extracted from seeds, not vegetables. Second, sometimes the seeds are not even seeds of vegetable plants, and occasionally not even food plants. Vegetable oil is typically a blend of various oils, including corn oil, soybean oil, and sometimes cottonseed oil. Is cotton food? Is it a vegetable? Manufacturers use the term vegetable oil because cottonseed oil naturally arouses suspicion. Nonfood crops such as cotton are not regulated as food crops and can thus be grown with higher amounts of chemicals. Cottonseeds therefore contain chemical pesticide residues. To make matters worse, cottonseeds also contain an endogenous toxin called gossypol.

The European Union Food Safety Authority recognizes gossypol as a moderate acute toxin and a reproductive toxin.[79] Prolonged feeding to various animals induces anorexia, decreased growth rate, and death. Reducing gossypol content requires chemical refinement using hexane solvents, bleaching, deodorizing, and decolorizing using ferric chloride (a highly toxic, highly corrosive industrial chemical). According to FDA regulations, refined cottonseed oil sold as food can legally contain 450 ppm of gossypol.[80] Cotton is also the third-biggest genetically modified crop, whereas soy and corn are numbers one and two. The health effects of genetically modified foods are beyond the scope of this book, but in general, you should avoid them. And you should avoid so-called "vegetable oil" absolutely.

Recommended Fats: Butter

Unpasteurized butter is an excellent source of healthy, highly digestible, raw fat. Butter has an excellent fatty acid profile with 68 percent saturated and only 3 percent polyunsaturated fat. This makes butter stable for cooking, though not quite as ideal as coconut oil. Butter is also very rich in the retinol form of vitamin A, which is critical for vision and eye health. The vitamin A contained in vegetables is beta-carotene and other carotenoids, which must be converted into retinol. The conversion of beta-carotene into absorbable, retinol-type vitamin A is inefficient, ranging from 3.8 to 28 units of beta-carotene for an equivalent unit of retinol-type vitamin A, according to a recent study published in the *American Journal of Clinical Nutrition*.[81]

Recommended Fats: Coconut Oil

Coconut oil is a truly remarkable, wholly unique food. Its nutritional profile and culinary versatility make it the preferred cooking oil. Unsaturated fats, and especially polyunsaturated fats, are unsuitable for cooking because heat quickly degrades and denatures them. Coconut oil consists of 87 percent (or more) saturated fat, which makes it ideal for sautéing and baking.

Fatty Acid Composition of Common Dietary Fats – Figure 3.2

Food	Total Fat	Saturated	Mono	Poly	ω-6	ω-3	6:3 Ratio
Top-Tier Fats							
Coconut oil	100	92	6	2	1.9	-	-
Palm kernel oil	100	86	12	2	1.7	-	-
Butter oil	100	66	30	4	2.4	1.5	1.6
Cacao butter	100	63	34	3	3.0	-	-
Cod liver oil	100	22	33	45	2.0	43.1	0.1
Sardine oil	100	31	35	33	2.6	30.8	0.1
Olive oil	100	14	75	11	10.0	0.8	12.8
Avocado oil	100	12	74	14	13.1	1.0	13.1
Hazelnut oil	100	8	81	11	10.7	-	-
Butter	81	68	28	4	3.6	0.4	8.7
Macadamia nuts	76	17	81	2	1.8	0.3	6.3
Hazelnuts	61	8	81	11	10.7	-	-
Goat cheese, semisoft	30	74	24	2	2.4	-	-
Parmesan cheese	27	64	31	4	3.5	0.7	5.0
Lamb	22	46	46	8	6.2	1.6	3.8
Feta	21	74	23	3	1.6	1.3	1.2
Sour cream	20	66	29	5	3.6	0.5	7.2
Beef	20	46	50	4	3.0	1.2	2.6
Pork	15	40	49	11	10.5	0.7	14.6
Avocado	15	12	74	14	13.1	1.0	13.1
Mackerel	14	27	46	27	2.1	25.2	0.1
Eggs	10	37	46	17	15.8	1.0	15.5
Salmon	6	18	37	45	3.5	41.1	0.1
Anchovy	5	32	29	39	2.4	36.6	0.1
Tuna, bluefin	4	30	37	33	1.2	30.2	0.1
Chicken, without skin	1	33	33	33	27.0	6.3	4.6
Second-Tier Fats							
Ghee	100	66	30	4	2.4	1.5	1.6
Palm oil	100	51	39	10	9.5	0.2	45.5
Flaxseed oil	100	10	21	69	13.3	55.8	0.2
Almonds	50	9	73	18	18.2	-	-
Cashews	44	20	60	20	19.6	0.2	125.5
Flax seeds	42	9	19	72	14.8	57.1	0.3
Chia seeds	31	11	8	81	20.2	61.3	0.3

Fatty Acid Composition of Common Dietary Fats – Figure 3.2 (continued)

Food	Total Fat	Saturated	Mono	Poly	ω-6	ω-3	6:3 Ratio
Third-Tier Fats							
Lard	100	41	47	12	10.7	1.0	10.2
Duck fat	100	35	52	13	13.4	-	-
Goose fat	100	29	59	12	11.0	0.6	19.6
Argan oil	100	18	46	36	36	-	-
Sesame oil	100	15	41	44	43.4	0.3	137.7
Mustard oil	100	13	64	23	16.6	6.4	2.6
Walnut oil	100	10	24	66	55.6	10.9	5.1
Sunflower oil, high oleic	100	10	86	4	3.7	0.2	18.8
Almond oil	100	9	73	18	18.2	-	-
Hemp oil	100	9	11	80	59.3	20.7	2.9
Canola oil, virgin	100	8	64	28	19.1	9.4	2.0
Safflower oil, oleic	100	7	78	15	15.0	-	-
Pecan nuts	72	9	59	32	30.1	1.4	20.9
Pine nuts	68	8	33	59	58.8	0.2	300.1
Brazil nuts	66	25	41	34	34.1	-	-
Walnuts	65	10	14	76	61.3	14.6	4.2
Sunflower seeds	52	10	40	50	49.9	-	-
Pumpkin seeds	46	20	32	48	47.2	0.4	114.4
Pistachio nuts	44	13	55	32	31.4	0.6	52.0
Chicken, with skin	9	32	44	24	22.0	1.5	14.5
Fourth-Tier Fats							
Cottonseed oil	100	27	19	54	53.9	0.2	257.5
Rice bran oil	100	21	42	37	35.5	1.7	20.9
Wheat germ oil	100	20	15	65	57.3	7.2	7.9
Peanut oil	100	18	48	34	33.6	-	-
Soybean oil	100	16	24	60	52.9	7.1	7.4
Corn oil	100	14	29	57	56.2	1.2	46.1
Sunflower oil, linoleic	100	11	20	69	68.8	-	-
Grapeseed oil	100	10	17	73	73	-	-
Canola oil, standard	100	7	64	29	19.1	9.4	2.0
Safflower oil, linoleic	100	7	15	78	78.4	-	-

Total fat gives the percentage of each food's total calories that are derived from fat.[82] *The other numbers show the percentages of each variety of fat contained in each food. The 6:3 ratio is omega-6 divided by omega-3.*

In contrast, butter (the second-best cooking fat) is 68 percent saturated fat and 28 percent oleic acid (the monounsaturated fatty acid predominant in olive oil). Butter is an excellent food, but coconut oil has a better fatty acid profile. Whereas butter has 14 percent combined SCFAs and MCFAs (the fat portion of butter, disregarding its water content), coconut oil contains an unparalleled 59 percent. This makes coconut oil highly digestible. The MCFAs in coconut oil also provide beneficial antimicrobial, antibacterial, and antifungal properties. Furthermore, due to its unique chemical composition, coconut oil also benefits the treatment and prevention of many types of cancer,[83] cardiovascular disease,[84] diabetes,[85] liver diseases,[86] and other conditions.

Coconut oil resists rancidity and should remain nutritionally potent for two years or more with proper maintenance. Simply store the oil in a cool, dark place and also take precautions regarding germ transfer. In other words, especially when purchasing bulk quantities and transferring to smaller jars for near-term use, always make sure you use clean utensils. It is important to buy cold-pressed virgin coconut oil. Low-quality coconut is made from copra, which is dried coconut meat from which oil is extracted using hexane. Oil extracted from copra is refined, bleached, deodorized, and sometimes hydrogenated (creating trans fats).

Alongside coconut oil, we should also recognize virgin palm kernel oil as another top tier fat, similarly rich in SCFAs and MCFAs. There seems to be confusion in the health food community regarding the differences between palm oil and palm kernel oil. Both come from palm trees but the former comes from palm fruit, whereas the latter comes from palm seeds. Palm oil has no SCFAs nor MCFAs and is roughly 43 percent palmitic acid (and 36 percent oleic acid). Palm kernel oil, on the other hand, contains an impressive 54 percent combined SCFAs and MCFAs, and only 8 percent palmitic acid. The health advantages of SCFAs and MCFAs compared to palmitic acid are what makes palm kernel oil a top tier fat and palm oil only second tier.

Recommended Fats: Olive Oil

Olive oil is the cornerstone of the renowned Mediterranean diet. Besides its heart-healthy monounsaturated fat, olive oil's impressive polyphenol profile (at least two dozen compounds) greatly benefits the cardiovascular system. Polyphenols are phyto-chemicals with powerful antioxidant and anti-inflammatory properties. Two primary underlying causes of heart disease are oxidative stress and chronic inflammation. Avoiding oxidative stress necessitates eating foods rich in antioxidants and low in free radicals. The phenolic content of olive oil increases HDL cholesterol levels, while reducing inflammation and oxidative damage.[87] Research has also demonstrated both the anticancer and antimicrobial effects of polyphenols contained in virgin olive oil.[88] Extra-virgin and virgin olive oil has a higher polyphenol content than heat-processed olive oil, which is yet another reason to use olive oil only for salads and other raw preparations, not for cooking. Olive oil should be stored only in cool, dark places, preferably in dark glass bottles or metal containers. Because oxygen, time, heat, and light all degrade polyphenols while promoting peroxide free radicals, olive oil should not be stored more than two months.

Fats To Avoid

Many misinformed nutritionists and dieticians recommend cooking oils based on smoke point, which is the temperature at which fats and oils begin breaking down into glycerol, acrolein, and free fatty acids, thereby creating visible smoke. Different fats and oils have different smoke points. Those with high smoke points are often promoted for cooking, especially high-heat cooking. This designation, however, gives a false impression of safety and stability. It ignores the fact that detrimental changes happen at temperatures far below the smoke point. Most oils with high smoke points are also rich in extremely heat-sensitive PUFAs. Therefore, regardless of smoke point, heat denatures these oils and creates free radicals. Regrettably, many people promote grapeseed oil as a superior cooking oil. Indeed, grapeseed oil has a high smoke point. But grapeseed oil is nearly 70 percent omega-6 polyunsaturated fat, making it one of the worst possible oils for human consumption and certainly an oil that should never be heated. Forget about smoke point. Unless you are in the business of selling unhealthy oils, smoke point is irrelevant.

Everyone Loves Chocolate

Let's be honest. Chocolate is perhaps the most revered food on the planet and life without it would be considerably different. People are always happy when science indicates that chocolate is healthy. But is this really so? What are the bottom-line facts? Chocolate is typically comprised of two ingredients, cacao and sugar. The cacao portion can include cacao butter, cacao mass, cacao solids, or some combination thereof. Cacao butter is pure cacao fat. Cacao mass is the leftover portion when cacao butter is extracted from cacao seeds. Cacao mass can include some portion of cacao butter. Cacao solids are the non-fatty portions of the cacao seed. Cacao solids are rich in flavonols and other antioxidants, which confer an array of health benefits.

Cacao is primarily saturated and monounsaturated fat. Its two biggest components are heart-healthy stearic acid and heart-healthy oleic acid. It is these fatty acids that make cacao an overall healthy food, when consumed in moderation. Raw cacao is even better than traditionally roasted cacao based on its higher antioxidant potential and greater fatty acid integrity. The main problem with cacao is its fellow travelers, which typically include sugar and milk. For reasons discussed in upcoming chapters, I recommend avoiding both these problematic foods. If you eliminate the milk and minimize the sugar, chocolate becomes a reasonably healthy food.

Another fellow traveler to watch out for is soy lecithin, a stabilizing ingredient commonly used in inferior-quality chocolate. Soy lecithin is a byproduct of hexane-extracted soybean oil (usually GMO). If you pay close attention to chocolate labels, you will notice that many high-end, artisanal chocolatiers spend more money on marketing and packaging than on chocolate. Almost invariably, luxury, high-end chocolates contain soy or sunflower lecithin. The reason is simple. Cacao butter is expensive. Lecithin is cheap. Adding lecithin enables chocolatiers to reduce cacao butter by 8 percent.[89] Do you suppose they adjust their prices accordingly, passing on these savings to their customers?

You should also be aware that cacao naturally contains caffeine and theobromine (a central nervous system stimulant about one-fourth as powerful as caffeine). Cacao is an overall reasonably health-conscious indulgence when consumed in moderation, and with as little sugar as possible. It's best to consume raw cacao and avoid lecithin, also known as "soy sludge." Most organic food shops carry high-quality, lecithin-free chocolate. Try 85 percent cacao (which means 15 percent sugar), or better yet, make your own raw chocolate sweetened with stevia or erythritol (see Chapter 4).

Fat Conclusions

The ill-conceived, low-fat diets popularized during the previous century for the treatment and prevention of heart disease have actually made things much worse. I distinctly remember the low-fat marketing campaigns of the 1980s. Like many people in the US, I foolishly believed I was protecting my heart and improving my general health by eating low-fat cookies and snack foods. Thanks to the past twenty years of nutritional research, we now have a much more sophisticated view of dietary fat. No longer must we endure feelings of guilt and wrongdoing when eating fatty foods, provided they are high-quality, traditional fats and not modern, industrial seed oils. The primary problems with low-fat diets are:

- Increased consumption of simple sugars
- Excessive levels of polyunsaturated fat
- Limited omega-3 assimilation
- Insufficient levels of beneficial saturated fat

As medicine and nutritional science have become more advanced, awareness about PUFAs has increased significantly. But many prominent health institutions are still promoting outdated dietary advice. The Academy of Nutrition and Dietetics (AND), for example, which calls itself "the world's largest organization of food and nutrition professionals," offered the following recommendation in its most recent dietary guidelines, published in 2010:

"Most fats should be polyunsaturated or monounsaturated such as liquid vegetable oils like canola, olive, corn, peanut and soybean." [90]

This advice is bewildering. While they are correct to recommend monounsaturated fats such as olive oil, their remaining recommendations are completely contrary to modern nutritional knowledge. Canola, corn, peanut, and soybean oils contain far too much polyunsaturated fat, especially the inflammatory omega-6 variety. Usually these oils involve high-heat extraction, which creates free radicals, thus promoting even more inflammation. Almost never are these oils virgin/cold pressed.

Polyunsaturated fat is particularly prone to oxidative damage from heat, light, and air. High-heat extraction, along with prolonged shelf lives, creates free radicals, which damage and denature cells, causing inflammation and accelerated aging while promoting various degenerative diseases. The AND has also completely overlooked the crucial omega 6:3 ratio. When we consume too much omega-6, we assimilate far less omega-3, which is an essential nutrient for brain development and function, skin and hair health, and reproductive capacity.

Besides encouraging excessive quantities of omega-6 PUFAs, many prominent health organizations also discourage heart-healthy saturated fat. The US Department of Agriculture, for example, refers to saturated fat as "empty calories." Incredibly, they claim that solid fats like butter and coconut oil "add calories to the food but few or no nutrients."[91] Saturated fat, especially SCFAs and MCFAs, is extremely beneficial and health supportive. Butter and coconut oil provide easily digestible energy and potent antimicrobial, antiviral, and antifungal protection. Additionally, butter and various other animal fats provide fat-soluble vitamins, including A, D, E, and K.

Decades of dogma based on ill-conceived studies and the lobbying efforts of many corporations convinced the world that saturated fat promotes heart disease and should be replaced with unsaturated fat. We now know, based on extensive research, including a definitive 2010 meta-analysis published in the *American Journal of Clinical Nutrition*, that saturated fat is not associated with coronary heart disease. We also know that saturated fat positively affects serum cholesterol, unlike omega-6 PUFAs, which cause dangerous inflammation and promote atherosclerotic plaque.

In terms of quantity consumed, saturated and monounsaturated fats are the most important types of fat. Polyunsaturated fat is also important, but we require only very small amounts, generally less than 12 grams daily. As a macronutrient, our diets should consist of 35 to 65 percent total calories from fat. Whenever possible, fat should be raw and unheated. Fat used for cooking should be predominantly saturated. Avoid heating monounsaturated fats, and especially polyunsaturated fats.

My primary cooking fats are coconut oil and butter. For salads and other raw preparations, olive oil is the undisputed king. We should consume fat from a wide variety of sources, but olive oil generally surpasses all others, both for its versatility and health properties. In moderation, you can enjoy seeds and nuts and their oils, but give preference to those rich in monounsaturated fats and lower in polyunsaturated fats. The best include macadamias, hazelnuts, cashews, and almonds. Also, avocados are rich in monounsaturated fat and perfect for regular consumption. Other excellent sources of high-quality fat include various types of cheese, full-fat yogurt (especially unpasteurized), fish, beef, lamb, pork, and eggs. Flaxseeds and chia seeds are excellent sources of ALA, whereas fish and fish oils are the best sources of DHA and EPA. Most importantly, enjoy some cacao from time to time.

Notes

[1] Ann LaBerge, "How the Ideology of Low Fat Conquered America," *Journal of the History of Medicine*, April 2008, vol. 63, no. 2, pg. 139–177; Centers for Disease Control, "Leading Causes of Death, 1900–1998," Cdc.gov/nchs/data/dvs/lead1900_98.pdf

[2] Irvine Page et al., "Dietary Fat and Its Relation to Heart Attacks and Strokes," *Journal of the American Heart Association*, January 1961, vol. 23, pg. 133–136

[3] "Medicine: The Fat of the Land," *Time*, January 13, 1961

[4] Gary Taubes, "Is Sugar Toxic?" *New York Times*, April 13, 2011

[5] Ancel Keys, *Seven Countries: A Multivariate Analysis of Death and Coronary Heart Disease*, published by Harvard University Press, 1980, pg. 262

[6] Irvine Page et al., "Dietary Fat and Its Relation to Heart Attacks and Strokes," *Journal of the American Heart Association*, January 1961, vol. 23, pg. 133–136

[7] Louise Davies, "Obituary: John Yudkin," *Independent*, July 25, 1995

[8] Gary Taubes, "Is Sugar Toxic?" *New York Times*, April 13, 2011

[9] Index Mundi, Indexmundi.com

[10] Patty Siri-Tarino et al., "Meta-analysis of prospective cohort studies evaluating the association of saturated fat with cardiovascular disease," *American Journal of Clinical Nutrition*, March 2010, vol. 91, no. 3, pg. 535–546

[11] National Institutes of Health, "Estimates of Funding for Various Research, Condition, and Disease Categories (RCDC)," April 10, 2013; Shelly Wood, "Part 2: Money—Is cancer beating cardiovascular disease?" *Heart Wire*, August 6, 2011

[12] European Commission, Research and Innovation, Medical Research, Cardiovascular Diseases, Ec.europa.eu

[13] Robert Hoenselaar, "Saturated fat and cardiovascular disease: The discrepancy between the scientific literature and dietary advice," *Nutrition*, February 2012, vol. 28, no. 2, pg. 118–123

[14] DM Dreon et al., "Change in dietary saturated fat intake is correlated with change in mass of large low-density-lipoprotein particles in men," *American Journal of Clinical Nutrition*, May 1998, vol. 67, no. 5, pg. 828–836

[15] Chris Packard et al., "The role of small, dense low density lipoprotein (LDL): a new look," *International Journal of Cardiology*, June 30, 2000, vol. 74, supplement 1, pg. S17–S22

[16] AA Papamandjaris et al., "Medium chain fatty acid metabolism and energy expenditure: obesity treatment implications," *Life Sciences*, 1998, vol. 62, no. 14, pg. 1203–1215

[17] William Lands, "Dietary fat and health: the evidence and the politics of prevention: careful use of dietary fats can improve life and prevent disease," *Annals of the New York Academy of Sciences*, December 2005, vol. 1055, pg. 179–192; Hirohmi Okuyama et al., "ω3 fatty acids effectively prevent coronary heart disease and other late-onset diseases: the excessive linoleic acid syndrome," *World Review of Nutrition and Dietetics*, 2007, vol. 96, pg. 83–103; Joseph Hibbeln, "Healthy intakes of n–3 and n–6 fatty acids: estimations considering worldwide diversity," *American Journal of Clinical Nutrition*, June 2006, vol. 83, pg. 1483S–1493S

[18] CV Felton et al., "Dietary polyunsaturated fatty acids and composition of human aortic plaques," *The Lancet*, October 1994, vol. 344, no. 8931, pg. 1195–1196

[19] Artemis Simopoulos, "The importance of the ratio of omega-6/omega-3 essential fatty acids," *Biomedicine & Pharmacotherapy*, October 2002, vol. 56, no. 8, pg. 365–379; PM Kris-Etherton et al., "Polyunsaturated fatty acids in the food chain in the United States," *American Journal of Clinical Nutrition*, January 2000, vol. 71, no. 1, 179S–188S

[20] PM Kris-Etherton et al., "Polyunsaturated fatty acids in the food chain in the United States," *American Journal of Clinical Nutrition*, January 2000, vol. 71, no. 1, 179S–188S

[21] Artemis Simopoulos, "The importance of the ratio of omega-6/omega-3 essential fatty acids," *Biomedicine & Pharmacotherapy*, October 2002, vol. 56, no. 8, pg. 365–379

[22] William Lands, "Dietary fat and health: the evidence and the politics of prevention: careful use of dietary fats can improve life and prevent disease," *Annals of the New York Academy of Sciences*, December 2005, vol. 1055, pg. 179–192; Hirohmi Okuyama et al., "ω3 fatty acids effectively prevent coronary heart disease and other late-onset diseases: the excessive linoleic acid syndrome," *World Review of Nutrition and Dietetics*, 2007, vol. 96, pg. 83–103; Joseph Hibbeln, "Healthy intakes of n–3 and n–6 fatty acids: estimations considering worldwide diversity," *American Journal of Clinical Nutrition*, June 2006, vol. 83, pg. 1483S–1493S

[23] Artemis Simopoulos, "The importance of the ratio of omega-6/omega-3 essential fatty acids," *Biomedicine & Pharmacotherapy*, October 2002, vol. 56, no. 8, pg. 365-379

[24] H. Gerster, "Can adults adequately convert alpha-linolenic acid (18:3n-3) to eicosapentaenoic acid (20:5n-3) and docosahexaenoic acid (22:6n-3)?" *International Journal for Vitamin and Nutrition Research*, 1998, vol. 68, no. 3, pg. 159–173

[25] Samir Sammana et al., "Fatty acid composition of certified organic, conventional and omega-3 eggs," *Food Chemistry*, October 15, 2009, vol. 116, no. 4, pg. 911–914

[26] Ibid.

[27] Janet Smith et al., "A Meta-Analysis Shows That Docosahexaenoic Acid from Algal Oil Reduces Serum Triglycerides and Increases HDL-Cholesterol and LDL-Cholesterol in Persons without Coronary Heart Disease," *Journal of Nutrition*, vol. 142, no. 1, pg. 99–104

[28] Wallace Yokoyama et al., "Butyric Acid from the Diet: Actions at the Level of Gene Expression," *Critical Reviews in Food Science and Nutrition*, 1988, vol. 38, no. 4, pg. 259–297

[29] St-Onge MP et al., "Weight-loss diet that includes consumption of medium-chain triacylglycerol oil leads to a greater rate of weight and fat mass loss than does olive oil," *American Journal of Clinical Nutrition*, March 2008, vol. 87, no. 3, pg. 621–625

[30] James DeLany et al., "Differential oxidation of individual dietary fatty acids in humans," *American Journal of Clinical Nutrition*, October 2000, vol. 72, no. 4, pg. 905–911

[31] BW Petschow et al., "Susceptibility of Helicobacter pylori to bactericidal properties of medium-chain monoglycerides and free fatty acids," *Antimicrobial Agents and Biochemistry*, February 1996, vol. 40, no. 2, pg. 302–306

[32] Ronald Mensink et al., "Effects of dietary fatty acids and carbohydrates on the ratio of serum total to HDL cholesterol and on serum lipids and apolipoproteins: a meta-analysis of 60 controlled trials," *American Journal of Clinical Nutrition*, May 2003, vol. 77, no. 5, pg. 1146–1155

[33] Andrea Bonanome et al., "Effect of Dietary Stearic Acid on Plasma Cholesterol and Lipoprotein Levels," *New England Journal of Medicine*, May 12, 1988, vol. 318, pg. 1244–1248

[34] American Heart Association, Heart.org/HEARTORG/General/Frequently-Asked-Questions-About-Bad-Fats_UCM_306349_Article.jsp

[35] PL Zock et al., "Impact of myristic acid versus palmitic acid on serum lipid and lipoprotein levels in healthy women and men," *Arteriosclerosis, Thrombosis, and Vascular Biology*, 1994, vol. 14, pg. 567–575

[36] Dreon DN et al., "Change in dietary saturated fat intake is correlated with change in mass of large low-density-lipoprotein particles in men," *American Journal of Clinical Nutrition*, May 1998, vol. 67, no. 5, pg. 828–836

[37] MA French et al., "Cholesterolaemic effect of palmitic acid in relation to other dietary fatty acids," *Asia Pacific Journal of Clinical Nutrition*, 2002, vol. 11, pg. S401–407

[38] CJ Lammi-Keefe et al., "Lipids in human milk: a review. 2: Composition and fat-soluble vitamins," *Journal of Pediatric Gastroenterology and Nutrition*, March 1984, vol.3, no. 2, pg. 172–198

[39] Heart.org/HEARTORG/GettingHealthy/FatsAndOils/Fats101/Trans-Fats_UCM_301120_Article.jsp

[40] Zaloga et al., "Trans fatty acids and coronary heart disease," *Nutrition in Clinical Practice*, October 2006, vol. 21, no. 5, pg. 505–512

[41] Dariush Mozaffarian et al., "Trans Fatty Acids and Cardiovascular Disease," *New England Journal of Medicine*, April 13, 2006, vol. 354, pg. 1601–1613

[42] Martha Clare Morris et al., "Dietary Fats and the Risk of Incident Alzheimer Disease," *Archives of Neurology*, February 2003, vol. 60, no. 2, pg. 194–200

[43] M. Mahfouz, "Effect of dietary trans fatty acids on the delta 5, delta 6 and delta 9 desaturases of rat liver microsomes in vivo," *Acta Biologica et Medica Germanica*, 1981, vol. 40, no. 12, pg. 1699–1705

[44] Jorge Chavarro et al., "Dietary fatty acid intakes and the risk of ovulatory infertility," *American Journal of Clinical Nutrition*, January 2007, vol. 85, no. 1, pg. 231–237

[45] Almudena Sánchez-Villegas et al., "Dietary Fat Intake and the Risk of Depression: The SUN Project," *PLoS One*, January 26, 2011, vol.6, no. 1

[46] Associated Press, "Zero trans fat doesn't always mean none," August 19, 2007

[47] Revealing Trans Fats, US Food and Drug Administration, Publications.usa.gov/epublications/reveal-fats/reveal-fats.htm

[48] Ancel Keys, "Prediction and Possible Prevention," *American Journal of Public Health and the Nation's Health*, November 1953, vol. 43, no. 11, pg. 1399–1407

[49] Hume R et al., "Cholesterol metabolism and steroid-hormone production," *Biochemical Society Transactions*, 1978, vol. 6, no.5, pg. 893–898

[50] Rafael Carmena et al., "Atherosclerosis: Evolving Vascular Biology and Clinical Implications," *Circulation*, June 15, 2004, vol. 109, pg. III-2–III-7; Jonny Bowden and Stephen Sinatra, The Great Cholesterol Myth: Why Lowering Your Cholesterol Won't Prevent Heart Disease—and the Statin-Free Plan That Will, published by Fair Winds Press, November 2012

[51] Luigi Spagnoli et al., "Role of Inflammation in Atherosclerosis," *Journal of Nuclear Medicine*, November 2007, vol. 48, no. 11, pg. 1800–1815

[52] Ambrose JA et al., "The pathophysiology of cigarette smoking and cardiovascular disease: an update," *Journal of the American College of Cardiology*, May 19, 2004, vol. 43, no. 10, pg. 1731–1737; Alan Rozanski et al. "Impact of Psychological Factors on the Pathogenesis of Cardiovascular Disease and Implications for Therapy," *Circulation*, 1999, vol. 99, no. 2192–2217; Ignarro LJ et al., "Novel features of nitric oxide, endothelial nitric oxide synthase, and atherosclerosis," *Current Diabetes Reports*, February 2005, vol. 5, no. 1, pg. 17–23

Fred Kummerow et al., "Effect of trans fatty acids on calcium influx into human arterial endothelial cells," *American Journal of Clinical Nutrition*, November 1999, vol. 70, no. 5, pg. 832–838; Turpeinen AM et al., "A high linoleic acid diet increases oxidative stress in vivo and affects nitric oxide metabolism in humans," *Prostaglandins, Leukotrienes and Essential Fatty Acids*, September 1998, vol. 59, no. 3, pg. 229–233

[53] Felton CV et al., "Dietary polyunsaturated fatty acids and composition of human aortic plaques," *Lancet*, October 29, 1994, vol. 344, no. 8931, pg. 1195–1196

[54] Krauss RM, "Atherogenic lipoprotein phenotype and diet-gene interactions," *Journal of Nutrition*, February 2001, vol. 131, no. 2, pg. 340S–343S

[55] Siri-Tarino PW, "Saturated fat, carbohydrate, and cardiovascular disease," *American Journal of Clinical Nutrition*, March 2010, vol. 91, no. 3, pg. 502–509

[56] Toft-Petersen AP et al., "Small dense LDL particles—a predictor of coronary artery disease evaluated by invasive and CT-based techniques: a case-control study," *Lipids in Health and Disease,* January 25, 2011, vol. 10, no. 21; Koba S et al., "Small LDL-cholesterol is superior to LDL-cholesterol for determining severe coronary atherosclerosis," *Journal of Atherosclerosis and Thrombosis*, October 2008, vol. 15, no. 5, pg. 250–260; Suh S et al., "Smaller Mean LDL Particle Size and Higher Proportion of Small Dense LDL in Korean Type 2 Diabetic Patients," *Diabetes & Metabolism Journal*, October 2011, vol. 35, no. 5, pg. 536–542

[57] Maria Luz Fernandez, "Dietary cholesterol provided by eggs and plasma lipoproteins in healthy populations," *Current Opinion in Clinical Nutrition & Metabolic Care*, January 2006, vol. 9, no. 1, pg. 8–12; Mutungi G et al., "Eggs distinctly modulate plasma carotenoid and lipoprotein subclasses in adult men following a carbohydrate-restricted diet," *Journal of Nutritional Biochemistry*, April 2010, vol. 21, no. 4, pg. 261–267

[58] Ying Rong et al., "Egg consumption and risk of coronary heart disease and stroke: dose-response meta-analysis of prospective cohort studies," *British Medical Journal*, January 2013, vol. 346:e8539

[59] Fernandez ML et al., "Revisiting dietary cholesterol recommendations: does the evidence support a limit of 300 mg/d?" *Current Atherosclerosis Reports*, November 2010, vol. 12, no. 6, pg. 377–383

[60] Choi CU et al., "Statins do not decrease small, dense low-density lipoprotein," *Texas Heart Institute Journal*, 2010, vol. 37, no. 4, pg. 421–428

[61] Rita Rubin, "Cholesterol guidelines get stricter," *USA Today*, July 12, 2004

[62] Rodney Hayward et al., "Narrative Review: Lack of Evidence for Recommended Low-Density Lipoprotein Treatment Targets: A Solvable Problem," *Annals of Internal Medicine*, October 3, 2006, vol. 145, no. 7, pg. 520–530

[63] "Cholesterol guidelines become a morality play," *USA Today* via *Associated Press*, October 16, 2004

[64] Press release, "Study Finds Statin Costs 400 Percent Higher in US Compared to UK," Boston University, January 12, 2012

[65] Beatrice Golomb and Marcella Evans, "Statin adverse effects: a review of the literature and evidence for a mitochondrial mechanism," *American Journal of Cardiovascular Drugs*, November 2008, vol. 8, no. 6, pg. 373–418

[66] Ibid.

[67] Culver AL et al., "Statin use and risk of diabetes mellitus in postmenopausal women in the Women's Health Initiative," *Archives of Internal Medicine*, January 23, 2012, vol. 172, no. 2, pg. 144–152

[68] FDA, "FDA Expands Advice on Statin Risks," February 2012; Fda.gov/ForConsumers/ConsumerUpdates/ucm293330.htm

[69] Ibid.

[70] Saremi A et al., "Progression of vascular calcification is increased with statin use in the Veterans Affairs Diabetes Trial (VADT)," *Diabetes Care*, November 2012, vol. 35, no. 11, pg. 2390–2392

[71] Leo Marcoff and Paul Thompson, "The Role of Coenzyme Q10 in Statin-Associated Myopathy," *Journal of the American College of Cardiology*, June 2007, vol. 49, no. 23

[72] L De Graaf et al., "Is decreased libido associated with the use of HMG-CoA-reductase inhibitors?" *British Journal of Clinical Pharmacology*, September 2004, vol. 58, no. 3, pg. 326–328; Catherine Do et al., "Statins and Erectile Dysfunction: Results of a Case/Non-Case Study using the French Pharmacovigilance System Database," *Drug Safety*, July 2009, vol. 32, no. 7, pg. 591–597

[73] Bouillon R et al., "Structure-function relationships in the vitamin D endocrine system," *Endocrine Review*, April 1995, vol. 16, no. 2, pg. 200–257

[74] DM Dreon et al., "Change in dietary saturated fat intake is correlated with change in mass of large low-density-lipoprotein particles in men," *American Journal of Clinical Nutrition*, May 1998, vol. 67, no. 5, pg. 828–836; H Campos et al., "Low density lipoprotein particle size and coronary artery disease," *Arteriosclerosis, Thrombosis, and Vascular Biology*, February 1992, vol. 12, no. 2, pg. 187–195

[75] Ray Hainer, "The cholesterol-inflammation connection," *CNN*, October 16, 2008

[76] Spectrum Organics, "Expeller Pressed versus Cold Pressed," Spectrumorganics.com/?id=32

[77] Sally Errico, "Olive Oil's Dark Side," *The New Yorker*, February 8, 2012

[78] Ibid.

[79] "Scientific Opinion of the Panel on Contaminants in the Food Chain on a request from the European Commission on gossypol as undesirable substance in animal feed," *The EFSA Journal*, 2008, vol. 908

[80] United States Food and Drug Administration, Code of Federal Regulations, Title 21, Volume 3, 21CFR172.894

[81] Haskell MJ, "The challenge to reach nutritional adequacy for vitamin A: β-carotene bioavailability and conversion—evidence in humans," *American Journal of Clinical Nutrition*, November 2012, vol. 96, no. 5, pg. 1193S–1203S

[82] Based on analysis of the USDA's National Nutrient Database for Standard Reference via Nutritiondata.com

[83] B Mendez et al., "Effects of different lipid sources in total parenteral nutrition on whole body protein kinetics and tumor growth," *Journal of Parenteral and Enteral Nutrition*, November/December 1992, vol. 16, no. 6, pg. 545–551; BW Petschow et al., "Susceptibility of Helicobacter pylori to bactericidal properties of medium-chain monoglycerides and free fatty acids," *Antimicrobial Agents and Biochemistry*, February 1996, vol. 40, no. 2, pg. 302–306

[84] H Lemieux et al., "Dietary fatty acids and oxidative stress in the heart mitochondria," *Mitochondrion*, January 2011, vol. 11, no. 1, pg. 97–103; F Labarthe et al., "Medium-chain fatty acids as metabolic therapy in cardiac disease," *Cardiovascular Drugs and Therapy*, April 2008, vol. 22, no. 2, pg. 97–106

[85] S Wein et al., "Medium-chain fatty acids ameliorate insulin resistance caused by high-fat diets in rats," *Diabetes/Metabolism Research and Reviews*, February 2009, vol. 25, no. 2, pg. 185–194; JR Han et al., "Effects of dietary medium-chain triglyceride on weight loss and insulin sensitivity in a group of moderately overweight free-living type 2 diabetic Chinese subjects," *Metabolism: Clinical and Experimental*, July 2007, vol. 56, no. 7, pg. 985–991

[86] H Kono et al., "Protective effects of medium-chain triglycerides on the liver and gut in rats administered endotoxin," *Annals of Surgery*, February 2003, vol. 237, no. 2, pg. 246–255; Willem Linscheer et al., "Medium and Long Chain Fat Absorption in Patients with Cirrhosis," *Journal of Clinical Investigation*, 1966, vol. 45, no. 8, pg. 1317–1325

[87] María-Isabel Covas, et al., "The Effect of Polyphenols in Olive Oil on Heart Disease Risk Factors," *Annals of Internal Medicine*, September 5, 2006, vol. 145, no. 5, pg. 333–341

[88] Elisa Tripoli et al., "The phenolic compounds of olive oil: structure, biological activity and beneficial effects on human health," *Nutrition Research Reviews*, 2005, vol. 18, pg. 98–112

[89] Sternchemie Lipid Technology, "Successful trials with dark and milk chocolate: Standardised sunflower lecithin – virtually no flavour differences in chocolate," *Sternchemie News*, November 2011

[90] Academy of Nutrition and Dietetics, Everyday Eating for a Healthier You, 2010 Dietary Guidelines

[91] US Department of Agriculture, "What are Empty Calories?" Choosemyplate.gov/weight-management-calories/calories/empty-calories.html

CHAPTER FOUR

Carbohydrates

With the publication of his 1972 book, *Dr. Atkins' Diet Revolution*, Robert Atkins gradually emerged as the world's most prominent advocate of low-carbohydrate diets (relatively lower amounts of carbohydrates and higher amounts of protein and fat). As the field of nutrition steadily advances, the science increasingly favors this dietary strategy. Initially, however, Atkins endured heavy criticism. The *Journal of the American Medical Association*, for example, said his diet was "without scientific merit," and "grossly unbalanced."[1] Furthermore, they urged physicians to "counsel their patients as to the potentially harmful results that might occur." This was the era of low-fat, high-carb diets. Atkins challenged deeply entrenched conventions and nutritional dogma. For this, he was demonized. His diet was controversial, to be sure, but his assessment of carbohydrates was sound.

Before publishing his book, Atkins was already well known. His popularity surged in 1970 when *Vogue* magazine published his weight loss plan.[2] His book subsequently became an instant bestseller. Nevertheless, despite his progressive educational efforts, carbohydrate consumption skyrocketed during the ensuing decades. Consumption of cereal grains, especially refined grains, increased about 45 percent from 1970 to 2000.[3] Consumption of added sugars increased 23 percent from 1970 to 2000.[4] By 2010, US adults were consuming 13 percent of total calories as added sugars, while children and adolescents were consuming 16 percent as such.[5]

During these years, prominent medical institutions and opportunistic companies repeatedly blamed obesity, cardiovascular disease, and various other conditions on fat consumption, particularly saturated fat. Consequently, society fully embraced low-fat, "heart-healthy" foods. From a palatability perspective, however, reduced fat generally means reduced tastiness. To compensate, manufacturers began adding copious amounts of sugar to their products, especially a cheap, new sugar called high fructose corn syrup (HFCS). Pasta consumption went up. Grain consumption went up. Sugar consumption skyrocketed. Cardiovascular disease rates were supposed to fall, but the opposite happened. By the end of the 1990s, people were growing weary of low-fat diets, which generally don't work. They neither promote weight loss, nor do they prevent cardiovascular disease. It seemed that finally a significant proportion of the population was ready for Atkins' sensible low-carb approach.

The Atkins diet gained considerable traction during the early years of the new century. In 2002, Atkins was among *Time* magazine's ten most influential people of the year. In 2003, the highly regarded *New England Journal of Medicine* published two studies supporting low-carb diets.[6] By 2004, 9 percent of the US population had switched to low-carb diets.[7] Pasta sales subsequently dropped 10 percent.[8] It seemed the low-fat era was over and the low-carb era was beginning. By 2005, however, the story had changed dramatically.

In 2003, Atkins died tragically after slipping on ice and sustaining severe head trauma. By August 2005, Atkins Nutritionals was filing for bankruptcy, citing heavy debt, the death of its founder, and waning consumer interest. By that time, only 2.2 percent of the US population was still on low-carb diets. Industry experts said Atkins products, including low-carb shakes, breads, and bars, failed the taste test. Much more significantly, however, Atkins Nutritionals failed the nutrition test.

Despite the good intentions of its founder, Atkins Nutritionals came to promote quantitative, rather than qualitative, nutrition. They advocated decreased carbs with respect to protein and fat, but failed to differentiate between high-quality and low-quality macronutrients (carbs, protein, fat). Atkins Nutritionals still operates today, selling meal replacement bars, snack bars, and frozen meals. Their highly processed foods contain vegetable oils, soy protein isolate, and other synthetic ingredients.[9] From a nutritional perspective, they cannot be taken seriously.

Atkins Nutritionals completely misses the qualitative aspect of macronutrients while focusing squarely on macronutrient ratios. Successful results cannot reasonably be expected by eating poor-quality ingredients. The company's demise has surely damaged the reputation of low-carb diets in general. The low-carb theory has merit, but results depend both on macronutrient quality as well as macronutrient ratios, not just the latter. Perhaps we should drop the concept of low-carbs altogether and start thinking more in terms of smart-carbs.

Smart-Carbs

When we think carbs, we generally think sugar, pasta, potatoes, cereals, and fruit. We don't typically group vegetables in with carbs. But vegetables are essentially carbs (including fiber), protein, micronutrients, and water. Broccoli, for example, is about 90 percent water. Ignoring its water content, broccoli's remaining nutrients are 70 percent carbs and 30 percent protein. Carrots are 90 percent carbs and 10 percent protein. By comparison, brown rice checks in at 88 percent carbs, 9 percent protein, and 3 percent fat. Quinoa is 76 percent carbs, 17 percent protein, and 7 percent fat. Vegetables and cereals are very different for many reasons. And there are many good reasons for reducing or eliminating cereals and all sugar from your diet. Doing so, however, means replacing these foods with healthier foods. By focusing on higher amounts of protein and fat, vegetables sometimes get overlooked. This is a mistake.

Don't confuse low-carb diets with no-carb or very-low-carb diets. We can and should eat carbs, but we should choose them wisely. In other words, replace high-carb cereals and sugars with smart-carb foods. Vegetables are smart-carbs. Vegetables contain an abundance of vitamins, minerals, antioxidants, and phytonutrients. High-quality fat, high-quality protein, and vegetables are the three core components of healthy, sensible cuisine.

Although vegetables should be the primary carbohydrate source, we need not eliminate all other carbs. Gluten-free cereals, especially quinoa and buckwheat, can be healthy, assuming you prepare them properly. Fruits, in moderation, are also great for daily consumption. Carbs can be categorized as follows:

Superior-carbs for everyday consumption:

- Leafy green vegetables
- Cruciferous vegetables
- Other vegetables

Good-carbs for moderate consumption:

- Berries
- Other fruits
- Potatoes, sweet potatoes, and other starchy tubers

Decent-carbs for less-frequent consumption (assuming proper preparation):

- Non-gluten grains (quinoa, amaranth, buckwheat)
- Beans and lentils (if you digest them easily)

Bad-carbs for avoidance or complete elimination:

- Refined sugars
- Gluten-containing grains (except sourdough fermentations)

Carbohydrates provide glucose, which nearly all cells require for energy. The body, however, can efficiently make glucose from protein and fat. Cereals are not necessary for energy. Carbs also provide fiber, which promotes digestive regularity and metabolic harmony. Dietary carbs without fiber—sugar, for example—can trigger adverse insulin reactions because the carbs metabolize too quickly. Simple carbs have single or double bonds, called monosaccharides and disaccharides, whereas complex carbs have triple or higher bonds, called oligosaccharides and polysaccharides.

Single-bond sugars include:

- Fructose (found in fruits)
- Glucose (primary source of energy, metabolized by all cells)
- Galactose (found in dairy)

Double bond sugars include:

- Lactose (found in dairy)
- Maltose (found in certain vegetables and beer)
- Sucrose (common table sugar)

Long chain complex sugars include:

- Starches (cereals, legumes, root vegetables)
- Cellulose (main component of dietary fiber)

Starchy foods include cereal grains, potatoes, and root vegetables. Vegetables such as leafy greens and cruciferous vegetables contain some starch, but much more fiber. Comparing simple and complex carbs can be somewhat confusing since the digestion and assimilation of different saccharides varies considerably. For example, simple carbs generally digest faster, raising blood sugar levels more rapidly than complex carbs. Some complex carbs (such as starches), however, also raise blood sugar rapidly, and some simple carbs digest more slowly. Fructose digestion can be problematic, especially without dietary fiber. Differentiating between simple and complex carbs is therefore not entirely useful. Total daily carb consumption can include both simple and complex carbs, with the following general stipulations:

- Eat whole foods, not refined foods (white rice is acceptable).
- Eat plenty of vegetables from each of the primary categories (root vegetables, leafy greens, cruciferous vegetables).
- Be somewhat restrictive with high-starch vegetables like sweet potatoes.
- Eat whole fruit, as opposed to fruit juice, giving preference to berries.
- If you are inclined to eat cereals, choose gluten-free varieties such as quinoa, buckwheat, rice, and amaranth.
- Minimize anti-nutrients as much as possible through proper preparation methods (discussed below).
- Eliminate all gluten-containing cereals (unless properly fermented).
- Avoid sugar, or better yet, eliminate sugar completely (discussed below).

Glycemic Index and Load

The glycemic index (GI) ranks various foods according to blood-glucose-raising potential. The GI compares blood-sugar-level increases relative to pure glucose, which has a GI of 100. Low-GI foods digest slowly, increasing blood sugar levels slightly, thus provoking mild insulin responses. High-GI foods digest rapidly, spiking blood sugar levels, thereby provoking more extreme insulin responses. Chronically elevated insulin leads to insulin resistance, which is one of the primary risk factors for diabetes, heart disease, cancer, and metabolic syndrome. Numerous studies have linked high-GI diets to diabetes and heart disease.[10] GI scores are classified as follows:

- Low GI = less than 55
- Medium GI = 56 to 70
- High GI = more than 70

Glycemic index is informative, but can be misleading. Some high GI foods are healthy, while some low GI foods promote disease. Fructose, for example, despite having a low GI, burdens the liver, increases blood triglyceride levels, and indirectly promotes insulin resistance. A more relevant, though also imperfect, indicator of metabolic impact is glycemic load (GL), which accounts for serving size as well as fiber content. GL can be calculated as follows:

GL = GI/ 100 x Net Carbs

To calculate Net Carbs, subtract Dietary Fiber from Total Carbs. As demonstrated in Figure 4.1, when GI goes up, GL doesn't necessarily follow.[11] Many fruits and some vegetables, for example, have higher GI values, but lower GL scores. Carrots have a GI of 47, but a very low GL of just 2. This is due to serving size and fiber content. Sugar is another story altogether. Why does sugar have such a low GL?

GI and GL of Common Foods – Figure 4.1

Food	GI	Serving Size	Net Carbs	GL
Grapefruit	25	½ large (166g)	11	3
Fructose	23	50 grams	50	12
Low-fat yogurt	33	1 cup (245g)	47	16
Apples	38	1 medium (138g)	16	6
Carrots	47	1 large (72g)	5	2
Oranges	48	1 medium (131g)	12	6
Bananas	52	1 large (136g)	27	14
Brown rice	55	1 cup (195g)	42	23
Honey	55	1 tablespoon (21g)	17	9
Oatmeal	58	1 cup (234g)	21	12
Raisins	64	1 small box (43g)	32	20
White rice	64	1 cup (186g)	52	33
Sugar (sucrose)	68	1 tablespoon (12g)	12	8
White bread	70	1 slice (30g)	14	10
Watermelon	72	1 cup (154g)	11	8
Baked potato	85	1 medium (173g)	33	28
Glucose	100	50 grams	50	50

Sugar is 50 percent glucose and 50 percent fructose. Sugar has a low GL because of its fructose content. A 12-gram serving of fructose has a GL just shy of 3. A 12-gram serving of glucose has a GL of 12. Pure fructose, therefore, has much lower GI and GL scores than does pure glucose. Does this mean fructose is healthy and safe? The answer, discussed below, is decidedly no. GI and GL both have serious limitations, especially concerning foods high in fructose yet low in fiber. This includes fruit juice. Most people presume fruit juice is healthy. Though it does provide some beneficial vitamins, its fiber-less fructose is particularly disruptive.

The Fructose Story

In 2002, the US National Research Council established "a comprehensive set of reference values for nutrient intakes for healthy US and Canadian individuals."[12] Their highly influential report established "a maximal intake level of 25 percent or less of energy from added sugars."[13] This excludes naturally occurring sugars from fruits, vegetables, and cereals. Can "healthy individuals" really thrive on 25 percent sugar? In 2013, researchers fed mice 25 percent sugar diets for a study published in *Nature Communications*. The male mice became less territorial and significantly less fertile, while the female mice had fewer offspring and significantly higher mortality rates.[14] Most people are not eating such extreme quantities of sugar—the average for US adults is 13 percent—but sugar consumption has skyrocketed to dangerous levels in just the past two centuries. How and why did this happen?

For most of human history, the only available sweetener was honey. Although man has collected honey at least since the Stone Age, consumption rates are difficult to estimate.[15] Historians say the amber nectar was relatively scarce throughout most of human history, but a 1996 study published in the *British Journal of Nutrition*, argues that honey was widely available and profusely consumed. The authors explain,

"A reappraisal of the evidence from the Stone Age, Antiquity, the Middle Ages and early Modern times suggests that ordinary people ate much larger quantities of honey than has previously been acknowledged. Intakes at various times during history may well have rivaled our current consumption of refined sugar."[16]

Sugar came on the scene much later than honey. Although production began around 500 BC in India, sugar was unknown in Europe until the eleventh century when crusaders brought it back from the Middle East. During the sixteenth century, sugar became the cash crop of most New World colonies and, regrettably, the engine of the slave trade. By the eighteenth century, "white gold" was highly coveted. In Britain, consumption increased fivefold from 1710 to 1770.[17] Nevertheless, sugar was still too expensive for most people during this era. Historian Sidney Mintz explains,

> *"During the period 1750–1850 every English person, no matter how isolated or how poor, and without regard to age or sex, learned about sugar. Most learned to like it enough to want more than they could afford."* [18]

During the nineteenth and twentieth centuries, sugar became cheap, which made consumption swell. The average Briton was eating 15 to 18 pounds annually from 1800 to 1815, and upwards of 35 pounds by 1850.[19] In the US, consumption rose from 6 to 43 pounds from 1822 to 1900 and has more than doubled since, reaching an astonishing 97 pounds per person, annually, today.[20]

The primary factors driving sugar's rise to prominence were price, availability, and perception. The 1970s was a pivotal decade. John Yudkin and Ancel Keys were famously debating the causes of cardiovascular disease (see Chapter 3). Yudkin put the blame on sugar, whereas Keys inculpated cholesterol and saturated fat. Keys eventually won, not because he was right, but because the powerful sugar industry, and by extension the US government, were behind him.

The fight was no knockout. Both fighters—sugar and fat—were severely weakened before sugar prevailed. Eventually, the great sugar versus fat debate made people weary and suspicious of both. Consequently, during the 1970s, the sugar industry faced massive public perception problems. To convince people that eating sugar is safe, the Sugar Association, an industry front-group, launched an exceptional public relations campaign.

In 1976, the Sugar Association received the Public Relations Society of America's (PRSA) coveted Silver Anvil award. According to the PRSA, the annual Silver Anvil award celebrates "the forging of public opinion" while recognizing "organizations that have successfully addressed contemporary issues with exemplary professional skill, creativity and resourcefulness."[21] Regarding the Sugar Association's mid-1970s public relations campaign, the PRSA recalls, "The objectives of the program were to reach target audiences with the scientific facts concerning sugar, enlist their aid in educating the consuming public, and to establish with the broadest possible audience the safety of sugar as a food."[22] Having secured this victory, the Sugar Association began encouraging US health agencies and various health institutions to officially recognize sugar as safe for regular consumption.

In 1976 the FDA gave sugar GRAS status—generally recognized as safe. In making their determination, they relied heavily on "Sugar in the Diet of Man," a white paper produced by the Sugar Association, with major contributions by Edwin Bierman and Fred Stare.[23] Bierman was the sugar industry's top diabetes expert; Stare founded the department of nutrition at the Harvard School of Public Health. Between 1952 and 1956, the sugar industry funded thirty research papers within Stare's department.[24] Throughout the 1970s, Stare testified many times before Congress on sugar safety while promoting sugar through various Sugar Association campaigns.

Despite the Association's triumphant public relations campaign, sugar's perceived link to diabetes wasn't going away. Stare and Bierman were instrumental in rectifying this situation for the industry. The USDA published its first opinion on sugar in 1980, concluding that tooth decay is sugar's primary risk and "contrary to widespread opinion, too much sugar in your diet does not seem to cause diabetes."[25] The USDA based their conclusions on "Carbohydrates, sucrose, and human disease," an article written by Bierman and published by the *American Journal of Clinical Nutrition.*[26] Five years later, the USDA was due to update their opinion. By this time, Stare was on the USDA's dietary guidelines advisory committee. Their updated opinion largely echoed their 1980 opinion, but became much more resolute: "too much sugar in your diet does not cause diabetes."[27] By the 1990s, government-backed research into the effects of sugar effectively ceased. Favorable public perception was secure, at least for several more decades.

The USDA's cozy relationship with the sugar industry continues to this day. In 2012, when Americans were consuming an astounding 97 pounds of sugar per year, top sugar executives started worrying. They weren't worrying, however, about the health and wellbeing of their customers. They were worrying, again, about public perception. By 2012, more than three decades after the industry's successful coup over science and commonsense, most people finally realized that sugar is unhealthy, especially in large quantities. But recognizing a substance as harmful and overcoming dependencies are quite different things. If only the industry could again manipulate public perception to their advantage. It was too late to argue that sugar is harmless, but perhaps they could lobby for reduced per capita consumption estimates. Suppose you wanted to convince some alcoholics that they were drinking much less than they actually were. Suppose you showed them charts and graphs and complex calculations. To keep their addictions going, they would be inclined to believe you. They wouldn't need to understand your calculations, provided they seemed authoritative.

This, essentially, was the sugar industry's strategy—to persuade the USDA to use a new calculation methodology, one that would drastically reduce sugar consumption estimates. If Americans could be told they were eating less than they actually were, their sugar addictions could be prolonged. According to emails acquired through a Freedom of Information Act request, Jack Roney, director of economics and policy analysis at the American Sugar Alliance, candidly wrote in March 2011,

> *"We perceive it to be in our interest to see as low a per-capita sweetener consumption estimate as possible."* [28]

Roney's wish was granted. In October 2012, unannounced and without fanfare, the USDA shaved 20 pounds off its official consumption estimate. From one day to the next, Americans went from eating 97 to 77 pounds of sugar per person annually. Speaking to *The New York Times*, Roney said he was pleased to have "more accurate" information available. "If folks are assuming there is much greater consumption than there really is," Roney asserted, "then we are misleading the public unnecessarily."[29] Misleading the public—indeed.

While the sugar industry's spin machine clearly facilitated sugar's meteoric rise, economic factors were also essential. If sugar had never become so cheap, it would never have become so prevalent. Economic policies enacted during the Nixon and Carter administrations paved the way for a new form of sugar, HFCS, to flood the market. The sugar and corn industries were technically competitors, but the success of both depended on favorable assessments of glucose and fructose. Sugar and HFCS, from molecular and nutritional perspectives, are essentially the same. Therefore, the sugar industry's public relations campaigns greatly benefitted HFCS, and vice versa.

In the early 1970s, the Nixon administration dismantled New Deal farm subsidy programs, which had been in effect since World War II. Whereas New Deal policies favored farmers and rural economies, Nixon administration policies favored corn and big agribusiness. Previously, when corn prices fell too low, the government bought up the surpluses and removed them from the market, effectively preventing prices from falling even lower. But since Nixon, the government has been giving farmers direct payments, thus ensuring artificially low prices and abundant supplies. Current payments are granted under the *Food, Conservation, and Energy Act of 2008*, also known as the farm bill. Large-scale commodity producers of genetically modified corn and soy receive $4.9 billion per year in free handouts, effectively driving down the price of all corn- and soy-based products.[30]

A steady supply of cheap corn meant cheap HFCS. Whereas Nixon policies made corn cheaper, Carter policies made sugar more expensive. When Carter first took office in 1977, cheap sugar imports were driving down domestic sugar prices. But by the end of 1977, his administration implemented a series of sugar quotas and tariffs, which effectively increased domestic sugar prices, thereby making HFCS even more attractive to US food manufacturers. By 1980, Coca-Cola was partially sweetening its beverages with HFCS, before fully converting in 1982.[31] The rest of the industry soon followed suit. From 1970 until 2000, HFCS consumption rose tenfold.[32] Cane sugar consumption decreased, but overall sugar consumption increased 23 percent.

It's All Sugar

During the 1980s, HFCS became the sweetener of choice in the US, mostly for economic reasons. Corn was cheap. Sugar was relatively more expensive. The taste was similar. Over the decades, however, consumers grew wary of both HFCS and sugar as both became increasingly associated with degenerative diseases and various health problems. Consequently, demand has steadily increased for healthy, practical sugar substitutes. Without fail, year after year, "healthy" alternative sweeteners come to market. Despite many false and inaccurate claims about these products, sugar is sugar. And more to the point, fructose is fructose.

In the late 1990s, seemingly from nowhere, an "all-natural" sweetener called agave syrup emerged as the new darling of sugar alternatives. The health-food community eagerly embraced this low GI "healthy" sweetener. For many years, agave was the sweetener of choice for health-conscious consumers. As demand steadily increased, manufacturers began sweetening teas, energy drinks, energy bars, desserts, and many other products with agave. From 2003 to 2007, the number of agave-sweetened products more than tripled.[33] Nevertheless, the truth about agave was bound to come out sooner or later.

Agave is simply another fructose-rich sweetener, not much different from HFCS. Agave ranges from 55 to 97 percent fructose.[34] Marketing descriptions such as "pure agave nectar" lead people to believe agave is naturally extracted, like pressing oil from olives. In reality, however, the situation is radically different. Agave extraction is a chemically intensive process involving caustic acids, clarifiers, filtration chemicals, and genetically modified enzymes.[35] Because it's so heavily refined, agave has few, if any, minerals. Organic, raw agave syrup is naturally processed and does have slightly more minerals than mass-produced versions, but in the end it's still fructose.

The most ironic thing about agave is its reputation as an alternative to both sugar and HFCS. Sucrose, the organic compound commonly known as table sugar, contains 50 percent glucose and 50 percent fructose. The two most common varieties of HFCS, HFCS-55 and HFCS-42, contain 55 and 42 percent fructose, respectively (the remaining sugars are glucose). Yet agave, supposedly the alternative, actually has more fructose than both sugar and HFCS. But why is fructose unhealthy? Doesn't fruit contain fructose? Isn't fruit healthy?

Yes, fruit is healthy. And yes, fruit contains fructose. Nevertheless, refined, "free fructose" is altogether different from unrefined fructose consumed as whole fruit. Whole fruit contains a harmonious balance of enzymes, vitamins, minerals, pectin, and fiber. The fiber aspect is particularly important. Whereas every cell in the body metabolizes glucose, the liver bears most of the fructose metabolism burden. Free fructose, devoid of fiber, hits the liver faster and stronger than fiber-bound fructose in whole fruit. Beyond certain person-specific thresholds, the liver converts fructose into fat. Fat droplets form and accumulate within the liver cells, eventually leading to nonalcoholic fatty liver disease.

According to Harvard Medical School, nonalcoholic fatty liver disease was very rare before 1980. Today it affects 30 percent of adults in developed countries, and 70 to 90 percent of diabetics and obese people.[36] If addressed early enough, the condition can be reversed. But should the liver become inflamed, cirrhosis can result. Excessive fructose consumption also promotes many other diseases. The liver converts fructose into fatty acids, storing some as fat while releasing some as triglycerides into the bloodstream. This leads to insulin resistance and metabolic syndrome (a combination of disorders leading to heart disease and diabetes).[37]

Most people benefit from moderate whole-fruit consumption—one or two small servings per day. Berries are particularly beneficial because they are antioxidant-rich and lower in fructose than other fruits. Additionally, all fruit contains therapeutic phytonutrients and fiber, which slows down the rate of fructose absorption. Fruit juice, on the other hand, is concentrated fructose without accompanying fiber. A glass of fruit juice requires three to four times the amount of whole fruit one would normally eat. Green vegetable juice is much better than fruit juice because vegetables contain far less fructose, sometimes none. All fruit juice and fructose-containing sweeteners (common sugar and most sugar substitutes) should be avoided.

The Hormone-Sugar Connection

Simple table sugar is 50 percent fructose and 50 percent glucose. Nearly every cell in the body can metabolize and use glucose for energy, especially brain cells. Fructose, however, breaks down into many toxins and produces many adverse side effects. Both glucose and fructose act on several key metabolism-regulating hormones, the most significant of which are insulin and leptin.

Insulin, produced by the beta cells of the pancreas, is the energy storage hormone. Insulin allows the body to store energy as fat. From an evolutionary perspective, the abundance of food enjoyed today is completely abnormal. Insulin enabled our distant ancestors to eat when food was plentiful and survive when food was scarce. Insulin also balances blood sugar levels. When blood sugar rises, the pancreas responds by releasing insulin. Whereas chronically elevates blood sugar levels were once rare, today they are common.

Above certain person-specific thresholds, insulin directs the cells to store energy as fat rather than burn energy. Chronically elevated insulin leads to insulin resistance, a condition whereby the cells no longer respond to appropriate levels of insulin. Even higher levels of insulin then become necessary to elicit the proper response. This leads to greater and greater accumulation of body weight. Insulin resistance, through a variety of mechanisms, promotes liver disease, heart disease, diabetes, and cancer. The two primary dietary drivers of insulin are glucose and fructose, but the effects of fructose are much more severe.

The liver bears about 20 percent of the glucose metabolism burden and almost 100 percent of the fructose metabolism burden.[38] Let's suppose you consume 100 calories of pure glucose. Glucose metabolism depends on insulin, thus the pancreas releases an appropriate amount. Roughly 20 percent (20 calories) of the glucose goes to the liver. The remaining 80 percent goes to other organs. The liver turns the majority of its allotted glucose into glycogen, which is like liver starch, a non-harmful energy reserve. For immediate energy, the liver mitochondria burn a small amount of the liver's glucose. The liver converts any remaining glucose into triglycerides. Elevated triglycerides promote cardiovascular disease, so here we have one potential danger of glucose metabolism. Another potential danger is free radical damage, which occurs when the other organs metabolize the other 80 percent of the glucose.

The metabolism of fructose is entirely different. Let's suppose you consume 100 calories of sugar (50 percent glucose and 50 percent fructose). As before, the liver will metabolize about 20 percent of the glucose, or 10 calories. Regarding the fructose, however, the liver must metabolize pretty much everything. So now the liver faces 60 calories, or triple the burden of an equal caloric intake of pure glucose. Furthermore, fructose cannot be converted into glycogen. Consequently, the liver converts fructose into fat. Fructose metabolism also activates a liver enzyme, which indirectly leads to liver insulin resistance. Liver insulin resistance puts extra stress on the pancreas. The detrimental effects of fructose metabolism are dose-dependent. In other words, the more you consume, the bigger your liver's burden.

The liver can effectively handle small amounts of fructose consumed as whole fruit. Since the fiber is still intact, the rate of absorption is much slower compared to processed sugar. The liver can also handle modest amounts of glucose. In general, starchy, glucose-rich foods like potatoes, white rice, and pasta may promote weight gain, but they don't make you sick the way fructose does.[39] If weight gain becomes excessive, of course, insulin resistance and metabolic disease can follow. But fructose metabolism is much more taxing on the liver and is a much quicker route to insulin resistance and a related condition called leptin resistance.

Leptin is a protein hormone made and released by fat cells. Leptin travels through the bloodstream en route to the brain, specifically to the hypothalamus. Once there, leptin tells the brain whether or not the fat cells have enough stored energy.[40] This signal tells the body how much to eat, when to stop eating, and how much energy to store as fat. When leptin functions normally, we feel good, experience an appropriate appetite, and enjoy good energy levels. When leptin functions abnormally (leptin resistance), the hypothalamus interprets starvation, and therefore directs the body to store more energy. This manifests as decreased physical activity, increased appetite, and unabated fat storage, particularly around the stomach.[41]

What causes leptin resistance? Leptin expert Dr. Ron Rosedale believes the same mechanisms that cause insulin resistance are also responsible for leptin resistance:

> *"It has been shown that as sugar gets metabolized in fat cells, fat releases surges of leptin. Those surges result in leptin-resistance, just as insulin over-exposure results in insulin resistance. Insulin resistance leads to high glucose that then contributes to high leptin and leptin resistance, and they both conspire to make you fat and accelerate your rate of aging."[42]*

In other words, excessive carbohydrate consumption, and especially excessive sugar consumption, leads to increased insulin production and increased fat storage, which eventually triggers the overproduction of leptin. Chronically elevated leptin leads to leptin resistance, or impaired brain function whereby the brain cannot decipher the leptin signal. The brain therefore interprets starvation, which triggers a vicious cycle of more appetite, more food, more sugar, more insulin, and more fat. Through its hormonal effects, sugar can literally reprogram your brain. Adopting a healthy low-carb, extremely low-sugar diet with high-quality protein, fat, and vegetables is the best strategy towards establishing healthy, balanced insulin and leptin levels.

Kicking The Habit

Quitting sugar or reducing sugar consumption requires an effective strategy. We must recognize that certain foods trigger sugar cravings. We must identify these foods and replace them with foods that do not trigger cravings. Cereals, especially refined and highly processed cereals, are the primary culprits. Eating a balanced diet with more vegetables, fewer cereals (or none), and more high-quality fat and protein is effective for most people. Sugar cravings gradually diminish. While transitioning to a low-carb diet, alternative sweeteners with better nutritional profiles can replace white sugar and HFCS, both of which should be strictly avoided.

HFCS is not much different from sucrose. The fructose content is roughly the same. The metabolism is the same. HFCS does, however, almost always come from GMO corn. Consuming GMO foods opens a Pandora's box of health risks, an issue beyond the scope of this book, yet vitally important to inform yourself about. Some alternative sweeteners are slightly better than sugar or HFCS, but the differences are generally negligible. Most sweeteners contain various combinations of glucose and fructose. Some grain-based sweeteners, barley malt for example, contain maltose, which is simply a disaccharide consisting of two glucose molecules. Other grain-based sweeteners contain maltotriose, a trisaccharide consisting of three glucose molecules. The problem with these glucose sweeteners is they are much less sweet than fructose-containing sweeteners. Therefore, achieving a desirable sweetness requires higher quantities, which results in excessive free glucose (devoid of fiber).

Basically, don't get too excited about alternative sweeteners. Some are of course slightly better than others. But the differences between a cake made with coconut sugar and the same cake made with cane sugar are trivial. Stevia and erythritol are probably the safest sweeteners, but still I encourage you to focus on food rather than desserts. It's better to address the source of your sugar cravings than to appease those cravings with sugar substitutes, many of which are simply fructose in disguise. By eating healthy, balanced meals with higher quantities of protein and fat and lower quantities of carbs, you can gradually bring your sugar cravings under control.

Fructose-Free Substitutes: Good and Bad

Although most sweeteners contain different proportions of glucose and fructose, some have absolutely nothing to do with these molecules. In theory, they seem to be miraculous. In practice, however, most have serious shortcomings. I'm speaking about stevia and sugar alcohols. We'll also put synthetic sweeteners in this category. For a quick synopsis, stevia is good, at least nutritionally speaking, but the taste can be off-putting. As for sugar alcohols, the body cannot absorb them; some promote digestive distress. Regarding synthetic sweeteners, forget about them—very bad idea.

Synthetic Sweetness

Synthetic sweeteners are zero-calorie, zero-GI, chemically derived molecules with sweetness indices many times that of sucrose. The most popular synthetic sweeteners are aspartame (Equal and NutraSweet), neotame, sucralose (Splenda), and saccharin (Sweet'N Low). While each synthetic sweetener has its own issues, in general they are pernicious and altogether unadvisable. Aspartame, for example, is 10 percent methanol. According to research published by the *European Journal of Clinical Nutrition*, the body converts methanol into formate, "which can either be excreted or can give rise to formaldehyde, diketopiperazine (a carcinogen), and a number of other highly toxic derivatives."[43] In mice studies, aspartame has been shown to impair memory performance and increase brain oxidative stress.[44] Rat studies have shown aspartame to be carcinogenic at low doses, especially when exposure begins during prenatal life.[45] Additionally, people with mood disorders and histories of depression are particularly vulnerable to adverse aspartame reactions.[46]

Sucralose has been shown to alter gut flora while raising fecal pH at commonly ingested levels.[47] Sucralose has never been subjected to independent, long-term safety studies measuring cumulative toxicity. Such studies are important, especially since sucralose has been shown to cause liver and kidney damage at higher doses.[48] In 2013, the Center for Science in the Public Interest (CSPI) finally downgraded sucralose from "safe" to "caution," pending a review of a yet-unpublished Italian study showing that sucralose causes leukemia in mice.[49] Artificial sweeteners have no place within a healthy diet and should therefore be eliminated entirely.

Sugar Alcohols: Let's Party?

Sugar alcohols are carbohydrates that structurally resemble sugar and alcohol, but technically are neither. Bloating and diarrhea are the most common side effects of sugar alcohols. The intestines cannot completely absorb these sugars. Consequently, they ferment, causing gastrointestinal distress. Sorbitol and mannitol are particularly disruptive.[50] Products containing higher amounts of sorbitol are required by US law to carry the disclaimer, "Excess consumption may have a laxative effect."

Derived from birch trees or corn, xylitol is becoming an increasingly popular sweetener. As shown in Figure 4.2, xylitol has 2.4 calories per gram, a low GI score of 13, and a sweetness index comparable to sugar.[51] Some research suggests that xylitol prevents dental caries. The sweetener is therefore commonly added to chewing gums. Most sugars interact with oral bacteria to form acid, which can damage the teeth. Oral bacteria, however, cannot metabolize xylitol. Nevertheless, I recommend you avoid partying with this sugar alcohol. There aren't enough long-term safety studies. Also, xylitol sometimes comes from corn, which suggests GMO. And while not as bad as sorbitol or mannitol, xylitol can cause significant digestive distress.

The best sugar alcohol is erythritol, a substance occurring naturally in some fruits and some fermented foods including soy sauce, wine, and some cheeses. Industrial erythritol production involves a simple fermentation of glucose. Erythritol has only 0.24 calories per gram, a GI of 1, and a sweetness index of 0.65 (65 percent as sweet as sugar). The small intestines readily absorb erythritol. The molecule is excreted through the urine, having no adverse gastrointestinal effects.[52] Many studies show erythritol does not increase serum glucose or insulin levels, even in diabetics.[53] A double-blind study on human volunteers, for example, showed remarkable tolerances with repeated daily doses of 1 gram per kilogram of body weight.[54] Some of the better alternative sugar products available today are combinations of erythritol and stevia.

Stevia: The De Facto Winner

Stevia is a zero-calorie, zero-GI, natural herb. Natural extracts of the stevia plant, called steviol glycosides, are 250 to 300 times sweeter than sucrose. Stevia has been used medicinally and as a sweetener around the world since ancient times. Steviol glycosides have numerous therapeutic benefits. They are anti-hyperglycemic, anti-inflammatory, antihypertensive, antitumor, antidiarrheal, and have various immune-modulatory actions.[55] Despite many years of regulatory chicanery, in 2008 the FDA finally approved steviol glycosides when both Coca-Cola and PepsiCo were seeking approval for stevia-sweetened products. The European Union followed suit in 2011. Stevia has a strong aftertaste, which some people find disagreeable. It can, however, be combined with other sweeteners to improve its taste. This is what Coca-Cola has done with Coca-Cola Life. Launched in Argentina in June 2013, this product is sweetened with sugar and stevia and contains half the calories of the classic version. Stevia is native to this region of the world, which probably influenced the company's decision to launch there.

Whereas erythritol is mostly benign, stevia has some therapeutic benefits, making stevia the winner for best alternative sweetener. Stevia has wonderful properties, but because of its strong taste, I use it more as a sweetness booster rather than a stand-alone sweetener. In other words, stevia is best combined with other sweeteners. As mentioned above, the most health-conscious combination is erythritol plus stevia. You don't have to mix them yourself. Some companies have already developed these products for you. If you are still hooked on fructose, stevia can help.

Start adjusting your recipes such that stevia progressively replaces more and more of your fructose-containing sweeteners. In other words, you can make your favorite chocolate mousse with half its normal sugar or normal maple syrup content, while using an appropriate amount of stevia to fill the sweetness void. This works for many recipes, but less effectively for recipes requiring baking. Use stevia where you can, but remember, your goal should be reducing your sweetness cravings through proper nutrition and wholesome meals, not simply swapping one sweetener for another.

Fructose By Any Other Name

The following popular sweeteners are all variations on a common theme—fructose. Some of these products are slightly better than sugar or HFCS. Honey, for example, does have some redeeming value. But honey, just like all its fellow travelers, is loaded with fructose. And fructose by any other name would taste as sweet—and damage as intensively. Consume the following sweeteners in very small quantities, or better yet, eliminate them completely from your diet.

Coconut Sugar

Coconut sugar, the latest darling sweetener of the health-food community, is 85 percent sucrose, 3 percent fructose, and 2 percent glucose.[56] Case closed. Coconut sugar is sugar. But isn't coconut sugar low GI? As discussed above, low GI does not necessarily signify healthy. After all, fructose is low GI, yet metabolically devastating.

A Comparison of Common Sweeteners – Figure 4.2

Sweetener	Cal. per gram	GI	Sweetness index	Sweetener	Cal. per gram	GI	Sweetness index
Saccharides				Sugar Alcohols			
Maltose	4	105	0.3	Sorbitol	2.6	4	0.55
Glucose	4	100	0.75	Maltitol	2.4	35	0.9
Dextrose	4	100	0.75	Xylitol	2.4	12	1
Sucrose	4	65	1	Lactitol	2	3	0.4
Lactose	4	42	0.15	Mannitol	1.6	2	0.5
Fructose	4	23	1.7	Erythritol	0.24	1	0.65
Galactose	4	23	0.3				
Syrups				Sweet Plants			
Coconut sugar	3.8	35	1	Luo Han Guo	0	0	300
Molasses	3.4	55	0.8	Stevia	0	0	300
Honey	3.4	35–58	1.1	Synthetic Sweeteners			
Sorghum syrup	3.3	50	1	Aspartame	3.5	0	180
Maple syrup	3.2	54	1	Neotame	0	0	8,000
HFCS-42	3.1	68	1.1	Sucralose	0	0	600
HFCS-55	3.1	58	1.2	Saccharin	0	0	300
Agave syrup	3.1	30	1.5	Acesulfame-K	0	0	200
Barley malt	2.9	42	0.5	Cyclamate	0	0	40
Brown rice syrup	2.6	25	0.5				

Notes: Sweetness index quantifies sweetness relative to sucrose. Syrups have less than 4 calories per gram due to water content.

According to the Philippine Coconut Authority, the GI of coconut sugar is 35.[57] Nearly all coconut sugar manufacturers and vendors cite this GI score, all based on the same study. But how can it be? Pure sucrose has a GI of 68 and coconut sugar is 85 to 90 percent sucrose. The numbers don't add up. Coconut sugar does contain a polysaccharide called inulin, which behaves like dietary fiber by slowing down the digestion. This could potentially lower the GI of coconut sugar—but all the way down to 35? While the sweetener does have some trace minerals, including potassium, the bottom line is coconut sugar is luxury sugar—highly priced, but functionally almost identical to cane sugar (sucrose).

Blackstrap Molasses

Sugarcane roots extend deep into the soil, beyond the mineral-depleted topsoil, to depths where minerals are more abundant. When manufacturers process sugarcane into refined sugar (both brown and white), most of these minerals are lost. Blackstrap molasses, however, the byproduct of sugar production, does retain these minerals. Molasses has a GI of 55 and impressive amounts of vitamin B6, magnesium, iron, calcium, and potassium. As a strong-tasting syrup, molasses is perhaps less versatile. Surely it's better than refined sugar, but still molasses contains plenty of fructose.

Honey

Honey is primarily glucose, fructose, and water with some trace minerals. Raw honey has various antibacterial, antiseptic, and other medicinal properties. Manuka and Ulmo are two particularly renowned varieties. The majority of honey consumed in Western nations is refined and processed, having no nutritional value. In 2011, *Food Safety News* conducted an extensive investigation in conjunction with Texas A&M professor Vaughn Bryant, one of the nation's premier investigators of honey pollen. They determined that 75 percent of US honey is not actually honey.[58] In other words, the pollen has been fully removed, leaving only the sugars.

According to FDA regulations, any ultrafiltered "honey" not containing pollen cannot legally be sold as honey. If you use honey therapeutically, purchase genuinely raw honey only, which does have medicinal, healing properties. Trace components of raw honey, for example, have the following nutritional and biological effects: anti-inflammatory, antimicrobial, antioxidant, antiviral, antiparasitic, anti-mutagenic, anticancer and immunosuppressive activities.[59] The bottom line with honey—it's good, but only raw and only in very small amounts.

Barley Malt Syrup

Traditional barley malt syrup is made from germinated and sprouted barley. The traditional germination process generates more than 140 different enzymes, which hydrolyze carbohydrates into simple sugars while breaking down proteins into amino acids. This centuries-old process takes thirty to forty-five days, as opposed to modern methods using artificially produced enzymes, gibberellic acid, and potassium bromate to accelerate the process.[60] Barley malt syrup is approximately 76 percent maltose, 19 percent glucose, and 5 percent fructose.[61] Barley malt syrup has a low GI and some beneficial minerals including magnesium and potassium.

Barley malt is low in fructose and high in glucose. Metabolically, this composition is preferable, but the consequence is reduced sweetness. Barley malt is only half as sweet as sugar. Larger quantities are therefore required to attain adequate sweetness levels. Accordingly, barley malt is a candidate for mixing with stevia. The bottom line: better than sugar or HFCS, but needs a sweetness booster.

Dried Fruits

Dried fruits are concentrated fructose, but with one major redeeming quality—fiber. Fiber slows down digestion, thereby decreasing the liver's fructose burden while minimizing the insulin response. The keys with dried fruits are refraining from eating too many and eating them whole. Blending dried fruits may compromise their fiber. Chopping them into pieces and putting them into cookies or cakes, however, maintains the fiber's integrity.

Dried fruits also have significantly more phenol antioxidants compared to fresh fruits, although this is largely due to the concentration effect. When fresh fruits lose their water content, all the nutrients and sugars become concentrated. Dates have the highest concentration of polyphenols among dried fruits.[62] Dates have a low GI, ranging from 30 to 50 depending on the variety. The bottom line: dried fruits are fine in moderation, as are fresh fruits. Just don't eat too many.

Cereals In Perspective

As with sugar, modern consumption of cereal grains is decidedly incongruous with evolutionary precedents. For about 97 percent of evolutionary history, humans were hunter-gatherers eating low amounts of simple carbohydrates. Whereas early humans ate no cereal grains, modern humans in Western nations consume upwards of 24 percent of total calories as cereals, mostly as refined, unfermented wheat.[63] Americans were eating 45 percent more cereal grains by the year 2000 than they were during the 1970s.[64] Since the human genome has changed very little during the past 40,000 years, eating such large quantities of cereal grains may be misguided.

Low-fat, high-carb diets have been studied extensively with respect to low-carb, high-fat diets, and the latter consistently yields better results. For overweight and obese individuals, numerous studies show low-carb diets to be superior.[65] Those with metabolic syndrome or diabetes also fare considerably better on low-carb diets.[66] Gluten-containing cereals pose additional health challenges. Nevertheless, healthy diets can include some cereal grains, given the following stipulations:

- Reduce or eliminate all gluten-containing grains (see Chapter 5).

- Favor low-GI cereals such as quinoa and buckwheat (neither are actually cereals, although both are typically classified as such).

- Reduce cereal consumption to less than 15 percent of total calories.

- Minimize anti-nutrient content as much as possible (see below).

- Harness the power of fermentation (see page 251).

Kitchen Chemistry

Anti-nutrients are compounds that interfere with the digestion and assimilation of nutrients. They are present, to some degree, in almost all foods. Seeds, nuts, grains, and legumes contain phytic acid, enzyme inhibitors, lectins, and tannins. Unless properly addressed, these anti-nutrients can significantly compromise the nutritional value of otherwise nutrient-dense foods. Health-conscious chefs use many simple techniques, including soaking, sprouting, and fermenting, to minimize these anti-nutrients. Cooking, to some degree, also reduces anti-nutrients.

Phytic Acid

Phytic acid occurs naturally in the bran and hulls of most nuts, seeds, grains, and beans. By attracting and binding to calcium, magnesium, iron, and zinc, phytic acid obstructs mineral absorption, thereby promoting deficiencies.[67] Phytic acid can also inhibit the activity of digestive enzymes such as pepsin (needed for protein digestion in the stomach), amylase (needed for carbohydrate digestion), and trypsin (needed for protein digestion in the small intestines). The World Health Organization says iron deficiency is the world's most widespread nutritional disorder, affecting developing and developed nations.[68] Due to menstruation, women are particularly vulnerable to iron deficiencies and anemia (advanced-staged iron deficiency). Given phytic acid's particularly strong affinity for iron, proactive anti-nutrient reduction is essential.

Enzyme Inhibitors

Enzyme inhibitors are compounds that enable seeds to maintain dormancy until conditions are favorable for germination and growth. Enzyme inhibitors interfere with digestive enzymes produced by the pancreas. Fortunately, enzyme inhibitors are very easy to neutralize through soaking and sprouting (see below). Soaking initiates the germination process, which releases the enzyme inhibitors. Soaking also catalyzes the production of many beneficial enzymes. The action of these enzymes increases certain vitamin levels, especially B vitamins.

Lectins

To protect themselves against fungi, bacteria, and insects, many plants produce carbohydrate-binding "sticky proteins" known as lectins. Being resistant to digestive enzymes and stomach acid, lectins reach the small intestines relatively unscathed. Once there, they bind to specific receptors on the intestinal mucosal cells, thereby triggering mucus production, which can impede nutrient absorption. Lectins also promote gut permeability, a condition whereby various toxins and undigested food particles can enter the bloodstream. This can provoke autoimmune responses and can potentially lead to irritable bowel syndrome (IBS), rheumatoid arthritis, Crohn's disease, chronic fatigue syndrome, and other autoimmune diseases.

Soaking and germinating decrease lectins, but certain lectins are resistant to these processing methods. Wheat germ agglutinin (WGA) is perhaps the most relevant example. WGA is an aggressive, pro-inflammatory lectin capable of bypassing the intestinal lining and provoking immunological and neurological damage. Extensive research, published in prestigious medical journals, indicates that WGA interferes with protein absorption, increases gut permeability, and causes allergic reactions.[69] Wheat, spelt, kamut, barley, and rye all contain WGA. Wheat, however, has the highest levels. For millennia, humans selectively bred wheat for increased protein content. Consequently, we also slowly increased wheat lectin levels. Modern wheat has relatively high lectin levels, but ancient relatives of wheat, such as spelt and kamut, underwent much less selective breeding, and therefore have relatively lower lectin levels.

The effect of sprouting on lectins is not entirely clear. Some research suggests that sprouting neutralizes lectins while other research suggests the opposite, that sprouting actually increases lectin content (so as to protect seedlings against bacteria and mold during this vulnerable period). Fermentation is probably the best way (along with soaking) to reduce lectins. The fermentation of soy while making tempeh, for example, reduces lectins by 95 percent.[70] Soy has high amounts of soybean agglutinin, a lectin that damages the intestines.[71] The best anti-lectin strategy is eliminating all unfermented soy and all WGA-containing grains, especially wheat. If you do eat WGA-containing grains, they should always be soaked, and preferably fermented.

Tannins

Tannins are plant polyphenols (antioxidants) that bind to proteins, amino acids, and other organic compounds. The word tannin comes from tanning, the traditional practice of converting animal skins into leather. This process exploits the intrinsic capacity of tannins to bind with proteins and subsequently convert soft, flimsy animal skins into durable leather, strong enough to make shoes, belts, and coats. Tannins are widely present in the bran of most cereal grains. They also occur in most legumes, seeds, nuts, tea, and red wine. Tannins can deactivate digestive enzymes, interfere with protein absorption, and damage the mucosal lining of the gastrointestinal tract.[72] As antioxidants, however, tannins can protect against oxidative damage when consumed in small quantities.[73] Published in *Trends in Food Science & Technology*, a critical review of the scientific literate concluded, "Ingestion of large quantities of tannins may result in adverse health effects. However, the intake of a small quantity of the right kind of tannins may be beneficial to human health."[74]

Reducing Anti-Nutrients

The most practical and effective techniques for minimizing phytic acid, enzyme inhibitors, lectins, and tannins are soaking, sprouting, fermenting, and cooking. Soaking seeds initiates biotransformational processes whereby anti-nutrients, having served their protective evolutionary purpose, are gradually released. During soaking, lactobacilli and other naturally occurring airborne microorganisms help break down phytic acid. While soaking does not remove anti-nutrients 100 percent, it reduces them significantly, and is therefore essential.

Longer soaking times are best, with twenty-four hour being ideal. Also, the bigger the seed, the longer it should soak. Larger beans like chickpeas and kidney beans should always soak for twenty-four hours. Using an acidic medium is also effective. Simply add a few spoons of lemon juice, apple cider vinegar, yogurt, or kefir to your soaking water. This helps remove even more anti-nutrients. Kefir and yogurt are best because they introduce lactobacilli probiotics, which further neutralize anti-nutrients. Always discard your soaking water and cook with fresh water.

Germinating and Sprouting

Germinating and sprouting are other practical and effective methods for reducing anti-nutrients from seeds, nuts, grains, and beans. Germinating and sprouting also greatly increase beneficial enzymes while improving overall nutrient bioavailability.

Germination involves complex biochemical changes whereby enzymes break down proteins, carbohydrates, and fats into simpler compounds. These changes increase essential fatty acid quantity, improve protein quality, and increase overall vitamin content.[75] Sprouting especially increases B-group vitamins, vitamin E, and beta-carotene, while reducing phytic acid.

Fermentation

Fermentation improves amino acid composition and vitamin content, increases protein and carbohydrate bioavailability, and decreases anti-nutrients.[76] The practice of leavening bread with a sourdough starter extends back to ancient Egypt. Making the starter involves mixing water and flour, then exposing this mixture to natural airborne microorganisms. This process makes a SCOBY (symbiotic colony of bacteria and yeast) consisting of lactobacilli bacteria and various strains of yeasts. Commercial yeast has only one strain, saccharomyces cerevisiae, which acts rapidly and thus does not provide the benefits of traditional, prolonged sourdough fermentation. During traditional fermentation, bacteria and yeast produce enzymes. These enzymes break down proteins into easily digestible and absorbable amino acids.

Fast-rising commercial yeast was invented during the nineteenth century. Before then, almost all bread was made through sourdough fermentation. Sourdough bread always varies regionally based on natural variations of airborne yeasts. Sourdough starters, however, never contains saccharomyces cerevisiae, the ale yeast commonly known as baker's yeast or commercial yeast. Sourdough fermentation improves the nutritional profile of cereal grains significantly. Beneficial microorganisms in the sourdough starter help control against candida albicans, whereas commercial yeast encourages candida growth. Sourdough fermentation also dramatically decreases phytic acid content while increasing mineral bioavailability. A 2003 study of naturally leavened sourdough bread published in the journal *Nutrition* demonstrated 71 percent phytic acid reductions plus significantly greater bioavailability of magnesium, iron, and zinc.[77] Sourdough fermentation also increases soluble protein content while making carbs more digestible (lower glycemic and insulin responses).[78] Furthermore, sourdough fermentation (as well as germination) increases lysine bioavailability, an essential amino acid.[79]

Carb Conclusions

Modern humans consume far too many carbohydrates as sugar (various forms) and improperly prepared cereals. Sugar should be drastically reduced from our diets, if not eliminated entirely. Occasionally, the sugar alternatives discussed above are acceptable, especially when transitioning towards a healthier diet. Cereals should also be drastically reduced, especially gluten-containing cereals.

The best cereal grains for occasional consumption are low-GI cereals including quinoa, buckwheat, amaranth, and teff. White rice is also acceptable, especially for those requiring more starchy carbs. I don't recommend brown rice. Despite being more nutrient dense than white rice, brown rice contains far more anti-nutrients, which adversely affect its nutrient bioavailability. A 1996 Portuguese study showed that nutrient absorption from brown and white rice is comparable.[80] White rice is simply easier to digest and easier to prepare. Cereals require proper preparation. Soaking is an absolute must (except with white rice). Fermentation requires much more time and attention, but results in nutritionally superior foods.

When executed properly, smart-carb diets (also known as low-carb diets) are far superior to low-fat diets. In study after study, they consistently outshine low-fat diets. For example, controlled, randomized studies comparing low-carb diets to low-fat diets have concluded the following:

- Low-carb diets promote significantly more weight loss.[81]

- Low-carb diets improve blood sugar levels and glycemic control, especially for diabetics.[82]

- Low-carb diets change unhealthy small-particle LDL cholesterol into benign large-particle LDL.[83]

- Low-carb diets increase healthy HDL cholesterol levels.[84]

- Low-carb diets drastically lower triglycerides, which is an important gauge of metabolic health.[85] Elevated triglycerides are positively correlated with increased heart disease and stroke, especially when HDL cholesterol levels are low and small-particle LDL levels are high.

Think vegetables, lots of vegetables. Think fat, good-quality fat. Think protein, easily digestible protein. Fill in the gaps with fruit (especially berries), fermented dairy, and occasionally, if you are so inclined, with properly prepared legumes and cereals, preferably gluten-free.

Notes

[1] "A Critique of Low-Carbohydrate Ketogenic Weight Reduction Regimens: A Review of Dr. Atkins' Diet Revolution," *Journal of the American Medical Association*, June 4, 1973, vol. 224, no. 10, pg. 1415–1419

[2] "Beauty: Vogue's Take It Off, Keep It Off Super Diet Devised with the Guidance of Dr. Robert Atkins," *Vogue,* June 1970, vol. 155, no. 10, pg. 84–85

[3] United States Department of Agriculture, Agriculture Fact Book 2001–2002, March 2003, Office of Communications, pg. 19

[4] Ibid., pg. 20

[5] Bethene Ervin et al., "Consumption of Added Sugars Among U.S. Adults, 2005–2010," Centers for Disease Control and Prevention, NCNH Data Brief, May 2013, no. 122

[6] Gary Foster et al., "A randomized trial of a low-carbohydrate diet for obesity," *New England Journal of Medicine*, May 22, 2003, vol. 348, no. 21, pg. 2082–2090; Frederick Samaha et al., "A low-carbohydrate as compared with a low-fat diet in severe obesity," *New England Journal of Medicine*, May 22, 2003, vol. 348, no. 21, pg. 2074–2081

[7] Theresa Howard, "Atkins Nutritionals files for bankruptcy protection," *USA Today*, August 1, 2005

[8] Wendy Kaufman, "Atkins Bankruptcy a Boon for Pasta Makers," *National Public Radio*, August 3, 2005

[9] Atkins.com

[10] Jeroen de Munter et al., "Whole Grain, Bran, and Germ Intake and Risk of Type 2 Diabetes: A Prospective Cohort Study and Systematic Review," *PLoS Medicine*, August 2007, vol. 4, no. 8; Joline Beulens et al., "High Dietary Glycemic Load and Glycemic Index Increase Risk of Cardiovascular Disease Among Middle-Aged Women," *Journal of the American College of Cardiology*, June 2007, vol. 50, pg. 14–21; Thomas Halton et al., "Low-Carbohydrate-Diet Score and the Risk of Coronary Heart Disease in Women," *New England Journal of Medicine*, November 9, 2006, vol. 355

[11] Nutrition Data, Nutritiondata.self.com/topics/glycemic-index

[12] Institute of Medicine of the National Academies, Dietary Reference Intakes For Energy, Carbohydrate, Fiber, Fat, Fatty Acids, Cholesterol, Protein, and Amino Acids, published by National Academies Press, 2002, pg. xv

[13] Ibid., pg. 323

[14] James Ruff et al., "Human-relevant levels of added sugar consumption increase female mortality and lower male fitness in mice," *Nature Communications*, August 13, 2013, vol. 4, no. 2245

[15] Eva Crane, *The Archaeology of Beekeeping*, Cornell University Press, 1983

[16] KA Allsop and JB Miller, "Honey revisited: a reappraisal of honey in pre-industrial diets," *British Journal of Nutrition*, April 1996, vol. 75, no. 4, pg. 513–520

[17] Clive Ponting, *World History: A New Perspective*, published by Pimlico, 2000, pg. 510

[18] Sidney Mintz, *Sweetness and Power: The Place of Sugar in Modern History*, published by Penguin Books, reprint edition, 1986, pg. 148

[19] Loren Cordain et al., "Origins and evolution of the Western diet: health implications for the 21st century," *American Journal of Clinical Nutrition*, February 2005, vol. 81, no. 2, pg. 341–354; Clive Ponting, *World History: A New Perspective*, published by Pimlico, 2000, pg. 698

[20] Henry Blodget, "CHART OF THE DAY: American Per-Capita Sugar Consumption Hits 100 Pounds Per Year," *Business Insider*, February 19, 2012; Stephanie Strom, "U.S. Cuts Estimate of Sugar Intake," *New York Times*, October 26, 2012

[21] Public Relations Society of America, 2013 Silver Anvil Call for Entries, Prsa.org/awards/silveranvil/silveranvilenter/documents/sa%2013.pdf

[22] Ibid.

[23] Gary Taubes, "Big Sugar's Sweet Little Lies," *Mother Jones*, November/December 2012

[24] Ibid.

[25] US Department of Agriculture and US Department of Health, Education and Welfare, *Nutrition and Your Health: Dietary Guidelines for Americans*, 1980

[26] Edwin Bierman, "Carbohydrates, sucrose, and human disease," *American Journal of Clinical Nutrition*, December 1979, vol. 32, no. 12, pg. 2712–2722

[27] US Department of Agriculture and US Department of Health, Education and Welfare, *Nutrition and Your Health: Dietary Guidelines for Americans*, Second Edition, 1985

[28] Stephanie Strom, "U.S. Cuts Estimate of Sugar Intake," *New York Times*, October 26, 2012

[29] Ibid.

[30] Editors, "For a Healthier Country, Overhaul Farm Subsidies," *Scientific American*, April 19, 2012

[31] Allen Amason, *Strategic Management: From Theory to Practice*, published by Taylor & Francis, Dec 9, 2010, pg. 87

[32] United States Department of Agriculture, *Agriculture Fact Book 2001–2002*, March 2003, Office of Communications, Usda.gov

[33] Elena Conis, "Agave syrup's benefits are in debate," *Los Angeles Times*, March 30, 2009

[34] Ibid.

[35] Joseph Mercola, "This Sweetener Is Far Worse Than High Fructose Corn Syrup," *Huffington Post*, April 15, 2010

[36] "Abundance of fructose not good for the liver, heart," *Harvard Heart Letter*, September 2011

[37] Sánchez-Lozada et al., "Comparison of free fructose and glucose to sucrose in the ability to cause fatty liver," *European Journal of Nutrition*, February 2010, vol. 49, no. 1

[38] Robert H. Lustig, *Fat Chance: Beating the Odds Against Sugar, Processed Food, Obesity, and Disease*, published by Hudson Street Press, December 2012, pg. 134

[39] Ibid., pg. 135

[40] Leibel RL, "The role of leptin in the control of body weight," *Nutrition Reviews*, October 2002, vol. 60, pg. S15–S9

[41] Robert H. Lustig, *Fat Chance: Beating the Odds Against Sugar, Processed Food, Obesity, and Disease*, published by Hudson Street Press, December 2012, pg. 56–57

[42] Ron Rosedale, "Insulin, Leptin, Diabetes, and Aging: Not So Strange Bedfellows," *Diabetes Health*, January 13, 2008

[43] Humphries P et al., "Direct and indirect cellular effects of aspartame on the brain," *European Journal of Clinical Nutrition*, April 2008, vol. 62, no. 4, pg. 451–462

[44] Abdel-Salam OM, et al., "Studies on the effects of aspartame on memory and oxidative stress in brain of mice," *European Review for Medical and Pharmacological Sciences*, December 2012, vol. 16, no. 15, pg. 2092–2101

[45] Morando Soffritti et al., "Life-Span Exposure to Low Doses of Aspartame Beginning during Prenatal Life Increases Cancer Effects in Rats," *Environmental Health Perspectives*, September 2007, vol. 115, no. 9, pg. 1293-1297

[46] Robert Walton et al., "Adverse reactions to aspartame: Double-blind challenge in patients from a vulnerable population," *Biological Psychiatry*, July 1993, vol. 34, no. 1, pg. 13–17

[47] Mohamed Abou-Donia, et al., "Splenda Alters Gut Microflora and Increases Intestinal P-Glycoprotein and Cytochrome P-450 in Male Rats," *Journal of Toxicology and Environmental Health*, September 18, 2008, vol. 71, no. 21, pg. 1415–1429

[48] Sharma Ashwani et al., "Studies on the genotoxic effects of sucralose in laboratory mice," *Indian Journal of Animal Research*, 2007, vol. 41, no. 1, pg. 1–8

[49] Press release, "CSPI Downgrades Splenda From 'Safe' to 'Caution,'" *Center for Science in the Public Interest*, June 12, 2013

[50] Walter Glinsmann et al., "Report from the FDA's Sugar Task Force, 1986, Evaluation Of Health Aspects Of Sugars Contained In Carbohydrate Sweeteners," *Journal of Nutrition*, November 1986, vol. 116, no. 11

[51] Geoffrey Livesey, "Health potential of polyols as sugar replacers, with emphasis on low glycaemic properties," *Nutrition Research Reviews*, December 2003, vol. 16, no. 2, pg. 163–91

[52] Eva Arrigoni et al., "Human gut microbiota does not ferment erythritol," *British Journal of Nutrition*, November 2005, vol. 94, no. 5, pg. 643–646

[53] Noda K et al., "Serum glucose and insulin levels and erythritol balance after oral administration of erythritol in healthy subjects," *European Journal of Clinical Nutrition*, April 1994, vol. 48, no. 4, pg. 286–292; Ishikawa M et al., "Effects of oral administration of erythritol on patients with diabetes," *Regulatory Toxicology and Pharmacology*, October 1996, vol. 24, no. 2, pg. S303–308; Bornet FR et al., "Gastrointestinal response and plasma and urine determinations in human subjects given erythritol," *Regulatory Toxicology and Pharmacology*, October 1996, vol. 24, no. 2, pg. S296–302

[54] W. Tetzloff et al., "Tolerance to Subchronic, High-Dose Ingestion of Erythritol in Human Volunteers," *Regulatory Toxicology and Pharmacology*, October 1996, vol. 24, no. 2, pg. S286–295; Tsuneyuki Oku et al., "Laxative threshold of sugar alcohol erythritol in human subjects," *Nutrition Research*, April 1996, vol. 16, no. 4, pg. 577–589

[55] Varanuj Chatsudthipong et al., "Stevioside and related compounds: Therapeutic benefits beyond sweetness," *Pharmacology & Therapeutics*, January 2009, vol. 121, no. 1, pg. 41–54

[56] Naturepacific.com/contents/en-us/d242_Banaban-coconut-sugar.html

[57] Glycemic Index of Coco Sugar, Philippine Coconut Authority, Food and Nutrition Research Institute, Manila, Philippines, Pca.da.gov.ph/pdf/glycemic.pdf

[58] Andrew Schneider, "Tests Show Most Store Honey Isn't Honey," *Food Safety News*, November 7, 2011

[59] Stefan Bogdanov et al., "Honey for Nutrition and Health: A Review," *Journal of the American College of Nutrition*, December 2008, vol. 27, no. 6, pg. 677–689

[60] Eden Foods, http://www.edenfoods.com/store/product_details.php?products_id=104050

[61] Ibid.

[62] Joe Vinson et al., "Dried Fruits: Excellent in Vitro and in Vivo Antioxidants," *Journal of the American College of Nutrition*, February 2005, vol. 24, no. 1, pg. 44–50

[63] Loren Cordain et al., "Origins and evolution of the Western diet: health implications for the 21st century," *American Journal of Clinical Nutrition*, February 2005, vol. 81, no. 2, pg. 341–354

[64] United States Department of Agriculture, Agriculture Fact Book 2001–2002, March 2003, Office of Communications, Usda.gov

[65] Frederick Samaha et al., "A Low-Carbohydrate as Compared with a Low-Fat Diet in Severe Obesity," *New England Journal of Medicine*, May 22, 2003, vol. 348, no. 21, pg. 2074–2081; Iris Shai et al., "Weight Loss with a Low-Carbohydrate, Mediterranean, or Low-Fat Diet," *New England Journal of Medicine*, July 17, 2008, vol. 359, no. 3, pg. 229–241

[66] Jeff Volek et al., "Carbohydrate Restriction has a More Favorable Impact on the Metabolic Syndrome than a Low Fat Diet," *Lipids*, April 2009, vol. 44, no. 4, pg. 297–309; Eric Westman et al., "The effect of a low-carbohydrate, ketogenic diet versus a low-glycemic index diet on glycemic control in type 2 diabetes mellitus," *Nutrition & Metabolism*, December 19, 2008, vol. 5, no. 36

[67] M Torre et al., "Effects of dietary fiber and phytic acid on mineral availability," *Critical Reviews in Food Science and Nutrition*, 1991, vol. 30, no. 1, pg. 1–22

[68] World Health Organization, Who.int/nutrition/topics/ida/en/index.html

[69] Karin Fälth-Magnusson, "Elevated levels of serum antibodies to the lectin wheat germ agglutinin in celiac children lend support to the gluten-lectin theory of celiac disease," *Pediatric Allergy and Immunology*, May 1995, vol. 6, no. 2, pg. 98–102; Daniel Hollander et al., "Increased Intestinal Permeability in Patients with Crohn's Disease and Their Relatives. A Possible Etiologic Factor," *Annals of Internal Medicine*, December 1, 1986, vol. 105, no. 6, pg. 883–885; Bernhard Watzl et al., "Dietary wheat germ agglutinin modulates ovalbumin-induced immune responses in Brown Norway rats," *British Journal of Nutrition*, April 2001, vol. 85, no. 4, pg. 483–490

[70] Reddy and Pierson, "Reduction in antinutritional and toxic components in plant foods by fermentation," *Food Research International*, 1994, vol. 27, no. 3, pg. 281–290

[71] Zang J et al., "Effects of soybean agglutinin on body composition and organ weights in rats," *Archives of Animal Nutrition*, June 2006, vol. 60, no. 3, pg. 245–253

[72] DK Salunkhe et al., *Dietary Tannins: Consequences and Remedies*, published by CRC Press, 1990; NR Reddy et al., *Phytates in Cereals and Legumes*, published by CRC Press, 1989

[73] Giovannelli L et al., "Effect of complex polyphenols and tannins from red wine on DNA oxidative damage of rat colon mucosa in vivo," *European Journal of Nutrition*, October 2000, vol. 39, no. 5, pg. 207–212

[74] Chung KT et al., "Are tannins a double-edged sword in biology and health?" *Trends in Food Science & Technology*, April 1998, vol. 9, no. 4, pg. 168–175

[75] Chavan and Kadam, "Nutritional improvement of cereals by sprouting," *Critical Reviews in Food Science and Nutrition*, 1989, vol. 28, no. 5, pg. 401–437; Stephen Mbithi et al., "Effects of sprouting on nutrient and antinutrient composition of kidney beans (Phaseolus vulgaris var. Rose coco)," *European Food Research and Technology*, January 2001, vol. 212, no. 2, pg. 188–191

[76] Chavan and Kadam, "Nutritional improvement of cereals by fermentation," *Critical Reviews in Food Science and Nutrition*, 1989, vol. 28, no. 5, pg. 349–400

[77] Lopez et al., "Making bread with sourdough improves mineral bioavailability from reconstituted whole wheat flour in rats," *Nutrition*, June 2003, vol. 19, no. 6, pg. 524–30

[78] Jenni Lappia et al., "Sourdough fermentation of wholemeal wheat bread increases solubility of arabinoxylan and protein and decreases postprandial glucose and insulin responses," *Journal of Cereal Science*, January 2010, vol. 51, no. 1, pg. 152–158

[79] Hamad and Fields, "Evaluation of the protein quality and available lysine of germinated and fermented cereals," *Journal of Food Science*, March 1979, vol. 44, no. 2, pg. 456–459

[80] Callegaro Mda D et al., "Comparison of the nutritional value between brown rice and white rice," *Arquivos de Gastroenterologia*, October–December 1996, vol. 33, no. 4, pg. 225–231

[81] Dyson PA et al., "A low-carbohydrate diet is more effective in reducing body weight than healthy eating in both diabetic and non-diabetic subjects," *Diabetic Medicine: Journal of the British Diabetic Association*, December 2007, vol. 24, no. 12, pg. 1430–1435; JS Volek et al., "Comparison of energy-restricted very low-carbohydrate and low-fat diets on weight loss and body composition in overweight men and women," *Nutrition & Metabolism*, November 8, 2004, vol. 1, no. 13

[82] Westman EC et al., "The effect of a low-carbohydrate, ketogenic diet versus a low-glycemic index diet on glycemic control in type 2 diabetes mellitus," *Nutrition & Metabolism*, December 19, 2008, vol. 5, no. 36; William Yancy et al., "A low-carbohydrate, ketogenic diet to treat type 2 diabetes," *Nutrition & Metabolism*, December 1, 2005, vol. 2, no. 34

[83] Krauss RM et al., "Separate effects of reduced carbohydrate intake and weight loss on atherogenic dyslipidemia," *American Journal of Clinical Nutrition*, May 2006, vol. 83, no. 5, pg. 1025–1031

[84] Foster GD et al., "A randomized trial of a low-carbohydrate diet for obesity," *New England Journal of Medicine*, May 22, 2003, vol. 348, no. 21, pg. 2082–2090; Brinkworth GD et al., "Long-term effects of a very-low-carbohydrate weight loss diet compared with an isocaloric low-fat diet after 12 mo.," *American Journal of Clinical Nutrition*, July 2009, vol. 90, no. 1, pg. 23–32

[85] Volek JS et al., "Carbohydrate restriction has a more favorable impact on the metabolic syndrome than a low fat diet," *Lipids*, April 2009, vol. 44, no. 4, pg. 297–309; Jennifer Keogh et al., "Effects of weight loss from a very-low-carbohydrate diet on endothelial function and markers of cardiovascular disease risk in subjects with abdominal obesity," *American Journal of Clinical Nutrition*, March 2008, vol. 87, no. 3, pg. 567–576

CHAPTER FIVE

Protein

Protein always seems to inspire strong opinions. Sometimes these opinions are based on science, sometimes on conjecture, and sometimes on popular opinion. The protein debate typically centers around two basic questions:

1. How much protein do I need?

2. Which source of protein is better, animal or vegetable foods?

Historically, animal protein has been associated with wealth. But today, factory farming has made low-quality meat accessible to most of the world. Some high-quality animal foods, however, still carry significant economic constraints. Grass-fed beef, wild salmon, and free-range organic eggs, for example, all cost significantly more than their chemical-laden, mass-market counterparts. Thankfully, small, oily fish, such as sardines, are still inexpensive and are still among the best sources of high-quality animal protein. This chapter considers scientific data as well as timeless dietary wisdom to critically answer the fundamental questions concerning protein.

Protein Basics

Protein is the basic building material for all body tissue. Protein consists of amino acids linked together by peptide bonds. During digestion, low-pH gastric acid activates three principal protein-digesting enzymes—pepsin, chymotrypsin, and trypsin. These enzymes sever peptide bonds, thus liberating the amino acids. Free amino acids are easily absorbed and assimilated. After water, amino acids are the second largest component of human muscles, cells, and other tissues. There are twenty basic amino acids, which are classified as essential, nonessential, or conditionally essential.

Nonessential amino acids are necessary, but because the body can synthesize them, they need not come from food. Essential amino acids (EAAs), conversely, cannot be synthesized and therefore must come from food. Each EAA is required in sufficient quantities for protein synthesis. Conditionally essential amino acids must come from food under certain special conditions, such as times of illness or high stress. Of the twenty common amino acids, nine are considered absolutely essential, whereas three more are categorized as essential, because for children, they are. The twenty common amino acids are categorized as follows:

Classification of Amino Acids – Figure 5.1

Essential amino acids		Essential for children	Conditionally essential	Nonessential
Histidine	Phenylalanine	Arginine*	Arginine*	Alanine
Isoleucine	Threonine	Cysteine	Glutamine	Aspartic acid
Leucine	Tryptophan	Tyrosine	Glycine	Glutamic acid
Lysine	Valine		Proline	Serine
Methionine			Taurine	

Arginine is both essential for children and conditionally essential for adults.

Most protein sources contain both essential and nonessential amino acids. Unlike fat and carbohydrates, the body cannot store amino acids. Dietary protein is therefore necessary every day. Effective protein metabolism depends on adequate consumption of each EAA. A deficiency in even one EAA causes endogenous protein degradation (such as muscle degeneration) to obtain the deficient amino acid.

Scientists previously believed all EAAs must be consumed during the same meal. Some nutritionists and dieticians still promote this misunderstanding. Mainstream health organizations, including the Academy of Nutrition and Dietetics, Centers for Disease Control, and others, however, acknowledged ten years ago, based on research conducted over two decades ago, that complementary EAAs need only be consumed during the course of the same day.[1]

How Much Is Optimal?

The World Health Organization (WHO) recommends 46 grams of daily protein for average adult females and 56 grams for average males, or 0.8 grams per kilogram of body weight. Regarding calories, they recommend 2,000 per day for moderately active females and 2,600 for moderately active males. Protein provides 4 calories per gram, thus the WHO recommends that just 10 percent of total calories come from protein. The USDA and the US Department of Health and Human Services (HHS) recommend protein consumption ranging from 10 to 35 percent of total calories.[2] Figure 5.2 shows US macronutrient recommendations alongside my *Nutritional Grail* recommendations.

Comparison of Macronutrient Recommendations – Figure 5.2

Macronutrient	USDA/HHS recommendations (%)	NG* recommendations (%)
Carbohydrates	45–65	15–40
Protein	10–35	15–25
Fat	20–25	35–65

* NG = Nutritional Grail

There are different views concerning how much protein is required for optimal health, and surely different people require different amounts. While the 10 percent minimum might suffice for preventing deficiencies, it's probably insufficient for maintaining optimal body composition. On the other hand, the 35 percent maximum is probably too much. On 2,500 calories per day, 35 percent protein equates to 219 grams per day. Lean beef checks in at 27 percent protein, which means you'd need to put down around 800 grams per day, which is rather substantial. You could also achieve this protein intake by eating about thirty eggs. Simply put, for most people, 35 percent protein is excessive. The target zone should be 15 to 25 percent. A meta-analysis published in the *Journal of Nutrition* examined the metabolic effects of high dietary protein and recommended no more than 2 grams per kilogram of body weight.[3] On 2,500 calories per day, this would be 22 percent for someone weighing 70 kilos (154 pounds).

Although protein is an essential macronutrient, protein requirements are highly individualistic. They depend on many factors, including overall muscle mass, lifestyle, and general activity level. Pregnant and nursing mothers, and anyone recovering from an illness, surgery, or trauma, generally require higher amounts. Finding your ideal protein-fat-carb ratio is of paramount importance, but doing so requires some patience, awareness, and experimentation. As a percentage of total calories, shoot for 15 to 25 percent protein. For example, a study published in the *International Journal of Sport Nutrition and Exercise Metabolism* recommends 25 percent maximum.[4]

A safe protein range for peak nutrition is 1 to 1.75 grams per kilogram of body weight per day. This upper limit is completely safe. A 2004 review of the scientific literature published in the *Journal of the International Society of Sports Nutrition* found no adverse effects on liver, renal, or kidney function for protein consumption as high as three times the WHO's 0.8 g/kg level.[5] You can establish your optimal level based on these recommendations and through self-experimentation. Also recognize that some days you may need slightly more protein, and other days slightly less.

Which Sources Are Best?

During the past several decades, many theories have been introduced, promoted, and popularized regarding the supposedly harmful effects of animal foods. Although vegetarianism stretches back to ancient India, only recently has vegetarian dogma veered into the scientific domain. Popular theories and studies, including the blood type diet, the China Study, and acid-alkaline theory, have been offered as scientific proof-positive that animal foods are categorically unhealthy for some or all people. Quite simply, no sound evidence supports this claim. To the contrary, nutritional science strongly supports the consumption of animal foods for optimal health. Some people can certainly enjoy reasonably healthy lives as vegetarians or vegans, but most fare much better with at least some animal protein and animal fat. The contention that animal foods are unhealthy defies ancestral dietary wisdom while contradicting modern nutritional science.

The Blood Type Diet

The blood type diet, created and popularized by Dr. Peter D'Adamo, recommends different dietary regimens—meat consumption, vegetarianism, dairy consumption, or some combination thereof—for each of the four primary blood types. Specific foods are recommended for each blood type and blood type subgroup. According to D'Adamo, blood type O should eat like hunter-gatherers—lean meat, poultry, fish, and vegetables (with some restrictions). Type A, conversely, should be vegetarians, eating plenty of cereals, legumes, and vegetables. Type B thrives on dairy, meat, and vegetables (with restrictions on certain cereals and legumes), while type AB falls somewhere in between types A and B. D'Adamo claims that lectins contained in plant and animal foods affect people differently, based on blood types. Roughly 40 percent of the population is blood type A. If D'Adamo's theory is correct, then these people must become vegetarians or risk increased rates of degenerative disease.

D'Adamo's book, *Eat Right 4 Your Type*, currently has 7 million copies in print, a truly impressive achievement considering the diet has no scientific basis.[6] Regarding lectins, for example, research shows they affect all blood types similarly.[7] No studies support D'Adamo's claim of lectin-blood-type specificity. Since debuting in 1997, the blood type diet has endured heavy criticism. In 2004, for example, a team of Brazilian researchers challenged D'Adamo's contentions that O is the oldest blood type and that A originated fairly recently, when humans became more agrarian.[8] According to research published in *Molecular Biology and Evolution*, type A is actually the oldest and ABO blood types occur not only in humans, but also in apes, chimpanzees, and other primates.[9] This latter point is significant because it suggests blood type differentiation has nothing to do with dietary modifications. Chimpanzees, after all, have never practiced agriculture, nor have they ever domesticated animals.

One reason many people get good results on the blood type diet is because most types and subtypes are encouraged to avoid wheat. As discussed later in this chapter, wheat is an extremely problematic food. Eliminating wheat can dramatically improve your health, but this has nothing to do with your blood type. In 2013, the *American Journal of Clinical Nutrition* published a systematic review of the blood type diet. The study's authors concluded,

> *"No evidence currently exists to validate the purported health benefits of blood type diets. To validate these claims, studies are required that compare the health outcomes between participants adhering to a particular blood type diet (experimental group) and participants continuing a standard diet (control group) within a particular blood type population."*[10]

The China Study

Whereas D'Adamo claims that animal foods are unhealthy only for some people, another researcher, Dr. Colin Campbell, claims that animal foods are harmful and inherently unhealthy for everyone. During the past decade, Campbell has been the most outspoken opponent of animal food consumption. In his book, *The China Study*, he claims that all animal foods promote cancer and other degenerative diseases. His analysis, however, is deeply flawed and his evidence is highly selective. According to Campbell, "Eating foods that contain any cholesterol above 0 mg is unhealthy."[11] As discussed in Chapter 3, some types of cholesterol are unhealthy while others are health supportive and indeed essential. Also, dietary cholesterol does not directly translate into circulating serum cholesterol.

Just as Campbell draws erroneous conclusions about cholesterol, he does the same concerning protein. Having conducted a study on one type of animal protein, casein, Campbell extrapolates his results, ultimately concluding that all animal protein is dangerous. As discussed later in this chapter, however, there are many different types of casein, each of which has very different effects. Campbell does not differentiate between these different types. He draws conclusions based on his pivotal 1989 study, which compared the effects of isolated casein and isolated wheat gluten on rats.[12] Whereas casein encouraged the growth of potentially cancerous liver lesions, wheat did not. But wheat is lysine-deficient, whereas casein is a complete protein. In this study, which Campbell coauthored, the researchers also gave the wheat-eating rats lysine supplementation. When this happened, the lesions grew just as they did with casein. The study concluded that protein quality impacts lesion growth. When all EAAs are consumed, potentially cancerous lesions can grow. When deficiencies exist, they cannot. Are vegans and vegetarians who eat complementary proteins (cereals and legumes) also at risk? How can Campbell reasonably determine that all animal protein, and no vegetable protein, is carcinogenic based on studies of isolated casein?

Acid-Alkaline Theory

Another common argument against animal protein stems from the acid-alkaline theory. The 14-point pH scale measures acidity and alkalinity. The neutral point on this scale is 7 (neither acid nor alkaline). Levels higher than 7 are progressively more alkaline, whereas levels lower than 7 are progressively more acid. The normal pH of the blood is slightly alkaline (around 7.4). According to some studies, including one published in the *American Journal of Clinical Nutrition*, adults eating typical Western diets characteristically develop chronic, low-grade metabolic acidosis.[13] Acidosis promotes numerous diseases, including muscle wasting, bone disease, kidney disease, and growth retardation in children.[14] But which aspects of typical Western diets promote low-grade metabolic acidosis? Can we blame meat? Should we blame cereal grains? Also, alcohol consumption and hypoglycemia have been shown to promote acidosis.[15] Animal protein has not.

Some proponents of acid-alkaline theory claim animal protein damages the bones and kidneys. But again, sound scientific evidence is completely lacking. A 2005 study published in the *Journal of the American College of Nutrition* concluded the opposite, that higher animal protein diets actually promote bone health significantly. The study's author explained,

"In sharp opposition to experimental and clinical evidence, it has been alleged that proteins, particularly those from animal sources, might be deleterious for bone health by inducing chronic metabolic acidosis which in turn would be responsible for increased calciuria and accelerated mineral dissolution. This claim is based on a hypothesis that artificially assembles various notions, including in vitro observations on the physical-chemical property of apatite crystal, short term human studies on the calciuric response to increased protein intakes, as well as retrospective inter-ethnic comparisons on the prevalence of hip fractures." [16]

A 2011 mass-review of the scientific literature, including epidemiological studies, isotopic studies, and meta-analyses, drew the same conclusions. Published in *Current Opinion in Lipidology*, the study concluded that dietary protein works synergistically with calcium to protect the bones. The authors explained,

"The recommendation to intentionally restrict dietary protein to improve bone health is unwarranted, and potentially even dangerous to those individuals who consume inadequate protein." [17]

The acid-alkaline theory is commonly used in support of vegetarianism. But are vegetarian diets any different from low-carb, animal-food diets in terms of net acid load? Figure 5.3 shows potential renal acid loads (PRALs) of selected foods and food groups. [18] Vegetarian diets are typically rich in cereal grains and legumes, both of which, like animal protein, have net positive PRALs. Conversely, vegetables and fruits have net negative PRALs. Acid-alkaline theory is therefore an endorsement of vegetable-rich diets, not of exclusively vegetarian diets. A typical vegetarian diet based on cereals, legumes, and vegetables would have roughly the same PRAL as an animal-food diet complemented by plenty of vegetables.

So does any scientific evidence support the acid-alkaline theory? The *Journal of Environmental and Public Health* published a study in 2012 attempting to answer this question. The study's author, Gerry Schwalfenberg, observed,

"Much has been written in the lay literature as well as many online sites expounding on the benefits of the alkaline diet. This paper is an attempt to balance the evidence that is found in the scientific literature." [19]

There is no evidence, Schwalfenberg concluded, that alkaline foods prevent diseases nor that acidic foods cause them. Eating alkaline foods, however, does have plenty of benefits, including increased intracellular magnesium and improved potassium to sodium ratios (K/Na). Preagricultural humans ate diets featuring net negative PRALs and K/Na ratios around 10:1, much better than typical modern ratios, which average 1:3.[20] Improved K/Na ratios benefit bone health, reduce muscle wasting, and mitigate various chronic diseases. In sum, a healthy diet should include plenty of alkaline foods, especially vegetables, but no healthy diet can exclude protein, and whether protein comes from animal foods or cereals and legumes, its net acid load is always positive. Acid-alkaline theory therefore lacks scientific support and certainly does not prove animal foods are unhealthy.

Potential Renal Acid Loads (PRALs) of Selected Foods – Figure 5.3

Food	PRAL	Food	PRAL
Dairy		Nuts	
Parmesan cheese	34.2	Pecan	8.3
Hard cheese (average)	19.2	Walnut	6.8
Fresh cheese (quark)	11.3	Fats	
Cottage cheese	8.7	Butter	0.6
Yogurt, full-fat	1.5	Olive oil	0.0
Whole milk	0.7	Vegetables	
Buttermilk	0.5	Cucumber	-0.8
Eggs		Broccoli	-1.2
Egg yolks	23.4	Tomato	-3.1
Egg whites	1.1	Eggplant	-3.4
Eggs, whole	8.2	Celery	-5.2
Meats		Spinach	-14.0
Corned beef	13.2	Fruits	
Turkey	9.9	Apple	-2.2
Veal	9.0	Apricot	-4.8
Lean beef	7.8	Banana	-5.5
Fish		Black currant	-6.5
Trout	10.8	Raisins	-21.0
Cod	7.1	Beverages	
Cereals and legumes		Beer, pale	0.9
Brown rice	12.5	Coca-Cola	0.4
Rolled oats	10.7	Beer, draft	-0.2
White rice	4.6	Wine, white	-1.2
Lentils, green and brown	3.5	Coffee, infusion	-1.4

Protein Source Summary

Protein can come from animal sources or plant sources. Some people may thrive on wholly vegetarian diets, but most do better, especially long-term, with at least some animal foods. To obtain all essential amino acids, certain vitamins, including A, B_{12}, D, and K, and certain essential fatty acids (DHA and EPA), wholly vegetarian, and especially wholly vegan diets, are typically inadequate. Vegetarian diets usually deliver suboptimal fat and excessive carbohydrates, especially from refined cereals and simple sugars. The best sources of highly digestible protein include:

- Eggs (free range, organic)
- Fatty cold-water fish (sardines, anchovies, mackerel, herring, trout, tuna)
- Salmon (only wild, not farm raised)
- Seafood (clams, prawns, shrimp, scallops, etc.)
- Lean white fish (wild pike, snapper, cod, sole, etc.)
- Grass-fed beef and lamb
- Free-range chicken
- Pork, game, and other meats
- Fermented dairy, especially goat/sheep products (feta, yogurt)

The primary consideration for fish and seafood is its source. Choose only wild, not farm raised. The primary considerations for land animals are their diets and their living conditions. As much as possible, select pasture-raised, grass-fed, and hormone-free for ruminants, including cows, goats, and sheep. Poultry should be free range and arsenic-free. Arsenic has been fed to chickens since the 1940s to promote growth, treat disease, and improve meat pigmentation. By 2010, 88 percent of all US chickens were on arsenic-containing drugs.[21] In late 2013, amid sustained pressure from consumer-advocacy groups, the FDA finally rescinded approval for three of the industry's four arsenic drugs.[22] The best plant sources of protein include:

- Nuts, including almonds, hazelnuts, and cashews
- Quinoa, amaranth, and teff
- Lentils, legumes, and tempeh
- Vegetables (cumulative effect)
- Microgreens (spirulina and chlorella)

From a nutritional perspective, cereals and legumes can provide adequate amounts of protein. Cereals and legumes complement each other because cereals are deficient in certain EAAs that legumes are abundant in, and vice versa. Legumes, for example, are high in lysine, whereas cereals are generally lysine deficient (although quantities become much higher via fermentation). Also, cereals are generally rich in sulfurous amino acids (cysteine and methionine), whereas legumes are deficient. While cereals and legumes can provide adequate amounts of protein, the problems with these foods are many, including gluten (discussed below), anti-nutrients (see Chapter 4), and excessive carbohydrates.

Eating a wide variety of protein-rich foods ensures adequate amino acid uptake and distribution. Whole-food sources are generally superior to protein powders and other protein supplements. Many protein powders are soy-based and potentially dangerous, although some are health supportive. Most common protein powders contain excessive amounts of specific EAAs, including leucine, isoleucine, and valine. Collectively, these are known as branched-chain amino acids (BCAAs). The liver bears the brunt of metabolizing them. Elevated concentrations of circulating BCAAs are significantly associated with obesity and may predict insulin resistance, although a causal link has not been firmly established.[23] Manufacturers claim that BCAA protein powders enhance athletic performance and accelerate repair of muscle tissue.[24] The scientific literature, however, does not support this contention. Whereas soy-based protein powders should be strictly avoided, non-denatured whey protein, consumed in moderation, does provide considerable benefits, especially regarding glutathione production (see Chapter 6). In general, whole, natural foods are more balanced and have much better amino acid profiles than those of protein powders.

Protein Scoring

According to the World Health Organization and Food and Drug Administration, the PDCASS (protein digestibility corrected amino acid score) is the best method for determining protein quality with respect to human nutritional requirements. In the early 1990s, PDCAAS replaced several existing methods, including the PER (protein efficiency ratio), NPU (net protein utilization), and BV (biological value), all of which are based on the amino acid requirements of premature rats. PDCAAS, on the other hand, compares a given food's amino acid profile with the amino acid requirements of children (2 to 5 years of age). Although the PDCAAS is based on sound principles, it does have many limitations.

The PDCAAS would be perfect if we consumed only one source of dietary protein (as do infants). Of course, most people consume multiple sources. Whereas certain proteins are limited by certain amino acids, other proteins can compensate, thereby creating complete amino acid profiles. The PDCAAS, however, only considers and scores foods individually. Cereals, for example, generally score between 0.4 and 0.5 due to inferior lysine levels. Most legumes score between 0.6 and 0.7 due to inferior methionine levels. But when consumed together in roughly equal portions (although not necessarily at the same meal), cereals and legumes create complete proteins. The PDCAAS, however, does not account for such combinations.

The PDCAAS also doesn't account for how various processing techniques affect food digestibility. High-heat processing and prolonged storage, for example, decrease lysine bioavailability.[25] Pasteurization negatively affects the digestibility of dairy products. On the other hand, some types of processing, fermentation for example, positively affect digestibility. Cereals have relatively low PDCAAS scores due to low lysine levels. But the fermentation of cereals significantly increases their bioavailable lysine, which should raise PDCASS scores.[26] Finally, PDCAAS does not account for the impact of anti-nutrients (see Chapter 4) on protein digestibility. Consequently, protein quality is typically overestimated for certain foods, unless anti-nutrients are minimized through traditional processing techniques.

Figure 5.4 presents Amino Acid Scores according to Nutrition Data, a useful online nutritional resource based on data from the US Department of Agriculture's National Nutrient Database.[27] The Amino Acid Score is a proprietary calculation of protein quality based on amino acid distributions compared to recommendations by the Institute of Medicine. These scores are also not adjusted for protein digestibility. Amino Acid Scores of 100 or higher indicate complete, high-quality proteins.

Good Soy, Bad Soy

Soy is the most widely consumed plant-based, protein-rich food. Soy, however, poses many nutritional challenges. As discussed in Chapter 4, soy is particularly high in anti-nutrients, including lectins, phytic acid, and trypsin inhibitors.[28] When not properly neutralized through specific food preparation techniques, anti-nutrients can inhibit mineral absorption and the action of digestive enzymes. Soy infant formula, for example, is particularly high in phytates and strongly inhibits zinc absorption.

Amino Acid Scores for Common Foods – Figure 5.4

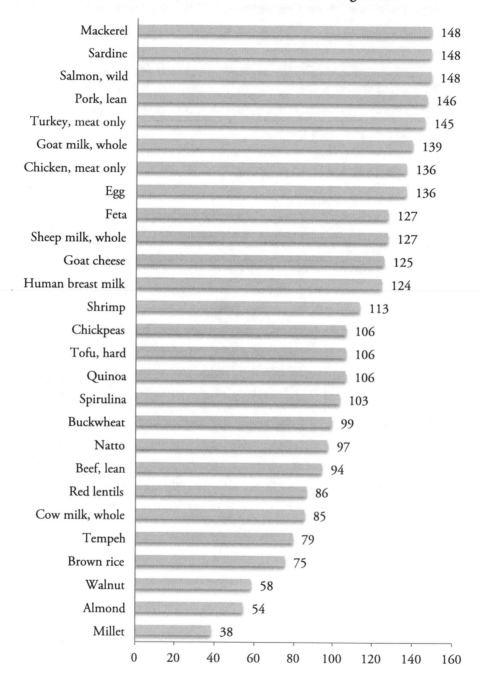

In one study, published in the *American Journal of Clinical Nutrition*, only 14 percent of available zinc from soy formula was absorbable.[29] Being inexpensive and versatile, soy and soy derivatives are extensively used for imitation and other nontraditional products, including soy cheese, soy yogurt, soymilk, soy protein isolate, soy oil, soy lecithin (an emulsifier used in chocolate and many other products), and soy infant formula. All these foods should strictly be avoided. Soy is also the basis of many healthy, traditional foods, including natto, shoyu, tamari, miso, and tempeh.

An essential difference between traditional and nontraditional soy products is the reduction/removal of anti-nutrients via traditional processing techniques. These techniques include soaking, germinating, sprouting, and fermenting. Fermenting soybeans into tempeh, for example, reduces phytic acid by up to one-third.[30] Besides anti-nutrients, soybeans also contain endocrine disruptors and thyroid inhibitors called phytoestrogens, which can be significantly reduced through fermentation.[31] Traditionally, soy was always fermented. The only exception was tofu.

Traditional tofu processing begins by introducing a coagulator, called nigari, into soymilk. Nigari is a bitter white powder made from evaporated seawater. Traditional nigari consists primarily of magnesium chloride, along with dozens of trace mineral salts.[32] Most tofu is unfermented, though travelers to China and Taiwan might be familiar with "stinky tofu," an aptly named dish sold at night markets and roadside stands. This preparation ferments for weeks or months in a special fish and vegetable brine. Many cultures have safely consumed tofu for many centuries, but traditionally they only ate small portions. Modern vegetarians typically consume far too much. Although the research is inconclusive, tofu's phytoestrogen content might promote adverse effects. If you eat tofu, follow the historical precedent and eat small portions, no more than once or twice per week. All other soy foods should be fermented or strictly avoided.

Soy protein isolate (SPI) is perhaps the worst form of soy. Also known as textured vegetable protein, SPI is a byproduct of high-heat soy oil extraction involving hexane solvents. The residual "soy meal" undergoes an extrusion process involving more heat and pressure. Hexane is a neurotoxic, petrochemical solvent used to efficiently and cost-effectively remove oil from grains, seeds, and legumes. The FDA doesn't require manufacturers to test for hexane residues, nor do they set upper limits.[33] Independent testing has determined that soy oil generally contains hexane residues at 10 ppm, whereas soy meal has 21 ppm.[34] The primary ingredient of most meat analogues, cheese analogues, infant formulas, and many other soy products is SPI.

Natto and tempeh are highly nutritious fermented soy foods and are appropriate for regular consumption. Depending on where you live, however, they might be hard to procure. Miso, shoyu, and tamari are other high-quality, fermented soy foods also appropriate for everyday consumption. Shoyu and tamari are traditional versions of soy sauce. The only difference between them is shoyu is made with wheat and can therefore irritate those with gluten sensitivities.

All About Milk

Like soy, milk can be highly nutritious or nutritionally devastating, depending on many factors. Although many people have allergies and sensitivities to lactose, milk proteins are actually far more allergenic.[35] Cow milk, for example, has twenty known protein allergens.[36] Two to six percent of all infants are allergic to these proteins.[37] Milk has two general types of proteins—casein and whey. Most milk protein allergies are attributable only to casein. The whey to casein ratio of human breast milk is 90:10 for early lactation, 60:40 for mature lactation, and 50:50 for late lactation.[38] Cow and goat milk are casein-based and both have 20:80 ratios.[39] In cow milk studies, modified whey/casein ratios (60:40) were far less allergenic compared to standard cow milk.[40] Although casein is generally more problematic than whey, there are many varieties of casein and some are much better than others.

Casein differs according to fraction number, amino acid composition, and peptide mappings. In terms of casein, goat milk and human milk are remarkably similar, whereas cow milk is quite different.[41] During digestion, goat milk forms soft, easily digestible curds. Human milk also forms soft curds, unlike cow and buffalo milks, which form hard curds. Cow milk is preferred for making cheese because of these hard curds. Hard curds promote allergies and intolerances more so than soft curds.

Regarding protein fraction, β-casein is the primary component of goat casein, which is similar to human casein. Cow casein, on the other hand, has proportionally more α-s casein. The ratio of β-casein to α-s casein is 43:57 for cow milk and 70:30 for goat milk.[42] Cow casein is sometimes as low as 30 percent β-casein.[43] Like goat milk, human milk is 69 percent β-casein (other caseins comprise the remainder).[44] The similarities between human and goat milk casein compositions may explain the higher digestibility of goat milk compared to cow milk.[45]

In determining the healthfulness of various milks, another extremely important consideration is the difference between two types of β-casein, A1 and A2. β-casein is an amino acid chain with 229 positions, including a proline amino acid at the 67th position. A peptide called beta-casomorphin-7 (βCM-7) is attached to the 67-position proline. βCM-7 is an opioid with a wide variety of potentially harmful effects, such as immune suppressant activity. Roughly 5,000 years ago, a mutation occurred in cows, which changed the 67-position amino acid from proline to histidine.

The mutated cows, known as A1 cows, produce β-casein A1, whereas the ancient cows, known as A2 cows, produce β-casein A2. The essential difference is the strength of the bonds between their respective 67-position amino acids and βCM-7. The proline bonds are strong, whereas the histidine bonds are weak, thus enabling βCM-7 to pass from the digestive system into the circulatory system.[46] Animals and humans drinking A1 milk test positive for βCM-7 in their GI tracts, blood, and urine, whereas those drinking A2 milk do not.[47] Human, goat, and sheep milk are all A2-like, regarding the 67-position proline.[48]

Many epidemiological studies have demonstrated strong associations between A1 milk consumption and heart disease as well as type 1 diabetes.[49] Also, βCM-7 has been suspected for decades to be a risk factor for sudden infant death syndrome (SIDS). This is because casomorphins have been found within the brainstems of SIDS victims.[50] The digestion of A2 milk is easier than that of A1 milk, despite the fact that both contain lactose. With A1 milk, lactose intolerance is likely accentuated due to the βCM-7 opioid, which slows down the digestion, thus providing more time for lactose fermentation and, consequently, more gas and bloating. The dairy industry and many health institutions have challenged the notion that milk consumption promotes mucus and phlegm.[51] βCM-7, however, has indeed been shown to induce mucins (sticky proteins in mucus), which could explain why some people who drink A1 milk experience mucus.[52]

The US, Australia, New Zealand, and most of Europe produce A1 milk from black-and-white cow breeds, primarily Holsteins. Asia, Africa, and some parts of southern Europe produce A2 milk from older breeds, including Jersey and Guernsey. Holsteins account for over 90 percent of US dairy herds, whereas Jersey cows account for only 7 percent.[53] If sufficient consumer demand could force the issue, the dairy industry could replace A1 cows with A2 cows within ten years at minimal costs.[54]

Goat Milk

Goat milk is highly nutritious. Numerous studies have shown that goat milk, compared to cow milk, offers improved calcium, phosphorous, and zinc metabolism, as well as greater bioavailability of iron.[55] Both goat milk and sheep milk have better amino acid profiles and better fat profiles than cow milk (see Figure 5.4). Goat milk also has respectable amounts of highly digestible SCFAs and MCFAs, as opposed to LCFA-dominant cow milk. As discussed in Chapter 3, SCFAs and MCFAs digest quicker and more efficiently than LCFAs. Milk homogenization involves mixing large quantities of milk and forcing it through small holes using high pressure, which denatures the product. Goat milk has much smaller fat globules than cow milk, which negates the need for homogenization. Accordingly, fat absorption for goat milk is significantly better than for cow milk.[56]

Real Milk

Industrial factory farms are notorious for having deplorable, unsanitary, disease-promoting conditions.[57] Known as concentrated animal feeding operations (CAFOs), industrial animal production heightens the risks of food-borne illnesses. According to the CDC, nearly 48 million people in the US (roughly 1 in 6) get sick every year via contaminated food. Plant foods, particularly from conventional, nonorganic farming, account for 66 percent of all viral contaminations, whereas CAFO animal foods (dairy, eggs, meat) account for nearly 64 percent of all bacterial contaminations.[58]

Confined to very small spaces, animals subjected to CAFOs are often caked in their own feces, thus promoting E. coli and salmonella outbreaks. A recent report by the Pew Commission concluded that CAFOs, as opposed to small-scale, traditional animal husbandry, "can significantly affect pathogen contamination of consumer food products."[59] The risk of pathogen contamination necessitates the widespread use of antibiotics and other medications. Antibiotics are also used because CAFO animals eat unnatural, grain-based diets. These diets weaken their immune systems, thereby promoting sickness and disease. The imprudent use of antibiotics, both in humans and animals, promotes dangerous antibiotic-resistant bacteria.

Udder infection, also known as mastitis, is the most common disease afflicting commercial dairy cows. Since 1970, milk production per cow has nearly doubled, from 4,400 to 8,600 liters/year.[60] Forcing cows to produce milk beyond their natural, physiological limits and extracting milk via industrial milking machines promotes mastitis, which is another reason these cows must consume antibiotics. Inevitably, large-scale, industrial milk is contaminated with drug residues. A recent study found trace amounts of twenty drugs, including growth hormones and antibiotics, in cow milk.[61] Although the quantities were small, the cumulative effects from long-term consumption could be significant.

Industrial milk must also be pasteurized to kill bacteria, viruses, and parasites.[62] Udder infections, cow feces, bacteria, and unhygienic equipment all promote such contamination. Pasteurization is the process of rapidly heating milk to 72°C (162°F) for twenty seconds, then rapidly cooling it below 7°C (45°F). A much more intensive form of pasteurization is ultra-heat treatment (UHT), in which milk is rapidly heated to 138°C (280°F) for two seconds, then rapidly cooled. Pasteurized milk has a three-week shelf life, whereas UHT milk can sit on shelves, unrefrigerated, up to nine months. Pasteurization (especially UHT) denatures milk proteins, decreases vitamin concentrations, negates raw milk's protective association with allergy development, and kills beneficial microorganisms (as well as harmful microorganisms).[63] According to the FDA, pasteurization does not affect milk digestibility, but anecdotally, many people report experiencing much better digestion with raw milk.

In the United States, the FDA and CDC have for years been targeting producers and consumers of raw milk. Small-scale organic farms, where hygiene standards are generally much better than those of large-scale CAFOs, are more conducive to safe raw milk production. Whereas large-scale CAFOs necessitate pasteurization, small-scale organic farms, according to three quantitative microbial risk assessments (QMRA) recently published in the *Journal of Food Protection*, can produce raw milk safely.[64] Ultimately, raw milk consumption comes down to personal choice. From a health perspective, raw is better than pasteurized, but fermented milk products (cheese, yogurt, kefir) are nutritionally superior and even less susceptible to bacterial contamination. So why drink raw milk when you can instead enjoy fermented milk products (made from either raw or pasteurized milk)?

Fermentation dramatically increases lactose digestibility.[65] Probiotic bacteria like lactobacilli and bifidobacteria are known as lactic acid bacteria. While glucose is their preferred energy source, lactic acid bacteria can also metabolize fructose, pentose, and lactose. They can metabolize lactose because they produce the enzyme β-galactosidase (also known as lactase), which breaks down lactose into β-galactose and glucose. From a health perspective, this process makes fermented milk an immune system enhancer. Studies at Japan's Juntendo University School of Medicine, for example, have observed significantly increased natural killer (NK) cells in people consuming fermented milk, especially for people with already low NK levels.[66]

Another fermentation benefit is increased mineral uptake. Calcium, for example, is more bioavailable from yogurt and other fermented dairy products than from milk.[67] Fermented milk consumption is also associated with improved LDL and HDL levels, as compared to non-fermented milk.[68] Clearly, fermented dairy, assuming it comes from healthy, grass-grazing animals, is highly nutritious. Fermented dairy is typically made from pasteurized milk, but sometimes from raw milk, thus offering even more health benefits. Goat and sheep milk are usually more digestible and more nutritious than cow milk. Feta and other varieties of soft goat and sheep cheeses are excellent for regular consumption. You can crumble feta onto your salads or onto steamed vegetables. Yogurt and kefir, especially when made from goat or sheep milk, are also highly nutritious and highly recommended.

All About Gluten

According to the USDA, cereal consumption in the US has increased 45 percent since the 1970s, and 73 percent of all US cereal consumption comes from wheat flour.[69] During the past fifty years, according to Mayo Clinic research, celiac disease has increased fourfold.[70] In the US, and Europe as well, about 1 in 141 people have the disease. Gluten sensitivity is a broad term referring both to celiac disease and non-celiac gluten sensitivities. According to Dr. Kenneth Fine, a pioneer in intestinal research, upwards of 30 percent of Americans are gluten-sensitive.[71]

Celiac disease is a severe autoimmune disorder of the small intestines. The consumption of gluten by celiac patients triggers an immune-mediated toxic reaction that damages the small intestines and prevents proper food absorption. Celiac disease is characterized by alpha-gliadin (a particular variety of gluten) and transglutaminase (an intestinal enzyme) sensitivities. In general, the following transglutaminase (tTG) abnormalities afflict all gluten-sensitive individuals:

1. tTG provokes autoantibodies, which are antibodies against the body's own cells. Prolonged autoantibody activity can cause autoimmune diseases.

2. tTG converts gliadin into deamidated gliadin (discussed below), which can elicit even stronger immune reactions.[72]

Fewer than 1 in 8 people with gluten sensitivities are aware of their conditions.[73] The majority of gluten-sensitivity cases consist of silent celiac disease (undiagnosed) and latent celiac disease (potential to develop the disease).[74] Conventional gluten tests only check for alpha-gliadin and tTG sensitivities. False negative test results happen commonly because other gluten epitopes, besides just alpha-gliadin, can also provoke immune reactions. In other words, you can test negative for alpha-gliadin and tTG sensitivities, but still be gluten-sensitive.

Gliadin and glutenin are the primary gluten fractions of gluten-containing cereals. As shown in Figure 5.5, gliadin has four primary epitopes (alpha, beta, gamma, and omega). All gliadin epitopes, and glutenin as well, can provoke immune reactions. Moreover, gliadin can interact with tTG, resulting in deamidated gliadin (discussed below). The digestion of gliadin can also create gluteomorphins (sometimes known as gliadorphins). Like casomorphins, gluteomorphins have sedative, addictive, and morphine-like properties. Wheat germ agglutinin (WGA), a lectin, can also increase gut permeability, damage the gut lining, and promote autoimmune diseases.

Celiac disease and gluten intolerance are serious conditions impairing not only the gut but also the brain, endocrine system, and liver, with positive correlations to many diseases, including type 1 diabetes, thyroid disorders, osteoporosis, obesity, ADHD, neurodegenerative conditions (Alzheimer's, Parkinson's, and dementia), psychiatric illnesses, rheumatoid arthritis, migraines, and more.[75] What happened to wheat to cause such dramatic reactions? For the past several centuries, humans have selectively bred wheat for increased protein. During the Green Revolution of the 1950s and 1960s, scientists boosted wheat harvests worldwide by crossbreeding and selecting for hardier, better-growing varieties. A study of thirty-six varieties of modern wheat and fifty ancient landrace varieties revealed that modern wheat has significantly more celiac disease epitopes, probably due to modern breeding practices.[76]

Industrial processing techniques resulting in deamidated gliadin (DG) are another serious problem with modern wheat. As mentioned above, tTG is an endogenous enzyme capable of converting gliadin into DG. Immune reactions to DG are typically more severe than reactions to native gluten. Even people without wheat intolerances can have severe reactions.[77] This is significant because deamidation happens not only inside the intestines, but also inside laboratories. To improve the textures of certain processed foods, manufactures add artificially created DG. According to a 2008 study published in the *European Journal of Inflammation*,

> *"This extensive use of wheat isolates in the food industry may be the major cause of hidden food allergies ... Because food isolates or deamidated gluten are new food ingredients, when allergy to wheat is suspected, immune reaction to wheat isolates should be tested."*[78]

Modern wheat has changed dramatically, but so have food processing techniques. Traditional bread, for example, was leavened through sourdough fermentation. Modern bread, cakes, crackers, and other wheat products are typically not fermented.

The WHO and the FDA define gluten-free as less than 20 ppm gluten.[79] Lacto-fermentation has been shown to reduce wheat bread gluten levels from 75,000 ppm to merely 12 ppm.[80] Although such dramatic reductions are possible only through prolonged, specialized fermentation techniques, shorter, traditional fermentations are also highly beneficial. If you choose to eat gluten-containing cereals, traditionally leavened sourdough bread is by far your best option.

Immunoreactive Components of Gluten-Containing Cereals – Figure 5.5

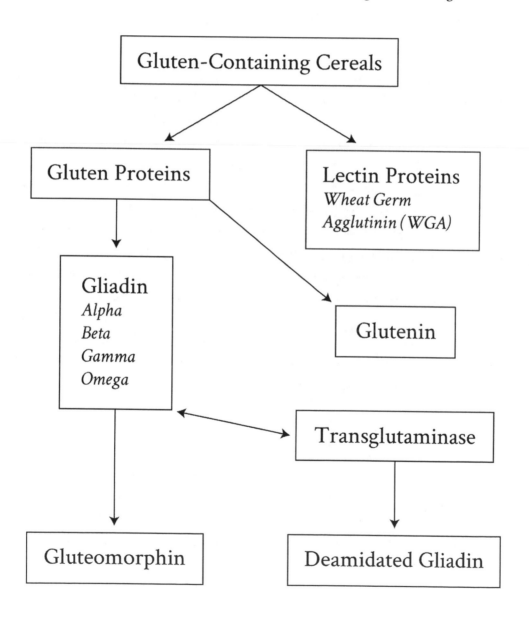

What About Beef?

Beef consumption in the US has declined 13 percent during the past decade and 25 percent since 1980.[81] Nevertheless, Americans still consume more beef per capita than any other nation. Despite claims to the contrary by Colin Campbell through his highly influential book, *The China Study*, there is no scientific evidence that beef and other animal foods are inherently dangerous. Nevertheless, the quality of animal foods varies significantly, based on the diets and living conditions of the animals. Cows, sheep, goats, and other grazing animals have multi-compartment stomachs. One compartment is the rumen, in which bacterial fermentation transforms grass into metabolically accessible protein.

Grass is the natural diet of these animals and the one that makes them most healthy. A diet of cereal grains, however, is more economically viable. Whereas grass-grazing calves typically require three years to grow from 80 to 1,200 pounds, corn-fed calves reach this weight in just fourteen to sixteen months.[82] To achieve such accelerated growth while avoiding disease, industrial cows must consume growth hormones, protein supplements, and antibiotics, all of which compromise their health, thus yielding nutritionally compromised beef.

One reason for declining beef consumption is growing awareness about CAFOs. Grass-fed beef accounts for only 3 percent of total beef consumption, but demand is currently growing at 20 percent per year.[83] Research spanning three decades suggests that grass-fed beef has a better fatty acid profile than grain-fed beef, and has more antioxidants.[84] Grass-fed meat has significantly more omega-3 (up to four times) and therefore a much better 6:3 omega ratio than does grain-fed beef.[85] Regular inclusion of grass-fed beef, as well as naturally raised lamb, chicken, and pork, is an excellent way to consume nutrient-dense protein.

Nitrates Explained

Many people avoid cured and processed meat products because they contain added nitrites (NO_2) and nitrates (NO_3). These are naturally occurring molecules, which prevent bacterial growth while giving cured meats their characteristic flavor and pink color. The traditional process of curing meats, which extends back thousands of years, long before refrigeration, is both safe and effective. Always read the labels on processed meats. Avoid products with synthetic additives and preservatives, but don't worry about nitrites and nitrates.

Sodium nitrite and sodium nitrate are both commonly used to cure meats. Nitrites and nitrates are very much related. Many vegetables and also some fruits are rich in sodium nitrate. During digestion, sodium nitrate converts into sodium nitrite.[86] In the early 1970s, an MIT study suggested that nitrites could be carcinogenic.[87] Later research disconfirmed this, but not before an urban myth grew up linking nitrite consumption to cancer. Today, misinterpreted epidemiological studies are sustaining this myth.

In 2013, *BMC Medicine* published a large epidemiological study, which analyzed the diet, lifestyle, and disease trends of nearly 450,000 people.[88] The study observed "a moderate positive association between processed meat consumption and mortality, in particular due to cardiovascular diseases, but also to cancer." This association was widely reported as positive confirmation that processed meats cause cancer. There are many problems, however, with this interpretation.

The *BMC* study did not differentiate between high quality, naturally cured meat products and low-quality, industrial products. Industrially processed meats contain many synthetic and potentially carcinogenic additives. Were the cancers associated with industrially processed meats, traditionally processed meats, or both? Also, as with all epidemiological studies, was the observed association caused by something else altogether? Correlation is not causation. For example, do people who eat higher amounts of processed meats also eat higher amounts of sugar?

What does the scientific literature actually say about nitrites and nitrates? Dietary nitrites and nitrates are actually beneficial because they modulate nitric oxide. Many diseases, including cardiovascular disease, are characterized by insufficient levels of nitric oxide. Traditionally cured meats, and nitrate-rich vegetables such as leafy greens, have been shown to regulate nitric oxide levels.[89] Research conducted during the past fifteen years thoroughly dispels the nitrite-cancer myth while confirming the safety of dietary nitrites and nitrates.[90] In short, traditionally cured meats are healthy. There is no reason to avoid them. Look for them in organic food supermarkets.

What About Fish?

Fish ranks among the most nutritious, most highly digestible protein-rich foods on the planet. Fish is also the best source of essential fatty acids, especially the critical long-chain omega-3 fatty acids—DHA and EPA. Unfortunately, for many decades, appalling amounts of toxic waste have been dumped into the oceans, resulting in mercury contamination, which inevitably affects aquatic life. Mercury levels tend to concentrate progressively up the food chain. Consequently, swordfish and other large fish have much higher mercury levels than sardines and other small fish (147 micrograms per 100 grams compared to 2 micrograms).[91] But is this necessarily reason for concern? Should we avoid this otherwise incredibly nutritious food source?

The issue of mercury contamination is controversial and not entirely conclusive. Mercury is indeed highly toxic, but some research shows that consuming ocean fish does not promote mercury toxicity. Ocean fish are remarkably rich in selenium, which according to this research, protects against mercury absorption. Mercury has an exceptional binding affinity for selenium—1 million times its binding affinity for sulfur, which is mercury's second-best binding partner.[92] According to this research, discussed below, when a food contains relatively more selenium than mercury, these elements bind together, rendering the mercury benign. Almost all seafood consumed by humans has selenium (Se) to mercury (Hg) ratios greater than 1:1. A 2013 study of seafood from southeastern Brazil looked at Se:Hg ratios for 652 different species of fish, mussels, squid, shrimp, and crab. Almost all had beneficial Se:Hg ratios, with many ratios exceeding 20:1.[93]

Nicholas Ralston, a research scientist and mercury toxicity expert, along with his colleagues at the University of North Dakota, developed the Selenium Health Benefit Value. This formula "incorporates consideration of both the absolute and the relative amounts of Se and Hg in the diet to provide an index that is easily interpreted."[94] Based on Ralston's extensive research, shark and whale meat should be avoided, and lake fish are unpredictable regarding mercury. But nearly all other seafood is safe, with the possible exception of swordfish. Many people discourage pregnant women from eating seafood, based on mercury concerns. This recommendation, however, originated from studies involving pilot whale meat, which has a low Se:Hg ratio (more mercury than selenium).[95] The developing brain of the fetus needs omega-3 fatty acids, particularly DHA and EPA, the best sources of which are fish. "Ocean fish consumption should be encouraged during pregnancy," Ralston explains, because "eating ocean fish is associated with major IQ benefits in children instead of harm."[96]

Based on all the available evidence, I strongly encourage the regular consumption of fish and seafood. If you are worried about mercury, despite the selenium binding research, then choose small fish, like sardines, anchovies, and mackerel, which are lower in mercury. These small, oily fish are also rich in omega-3 (DHA and EPA), protein, vitamin D, and calcium. Choose your fish based on freshness and quality. One major deal-breaker is wild versus farmed. Most commercially sold salmon, trout, sea bass, tilapia, and shrimp are farmed. The differences between wild and farmed fish are considerable. Farmed fish consume antibiotics and unnatural diets. Tuna and small, oily fish are generally always wild. Another issue is radiation. The *Proceedings of the National Academy of Sciences* recently published a study concerning radioactive isotopes originating from the Fukushima disaster, which have been found in Pacific fish, but at extremely low doses. The study concludes, "Such doses are comparable to, or less than the dose all humans routinely obtain from naturally occurring radionuclides in many food items, medical treatments, air travel, or other background sources."[97] This issue will be studied more closely in upcoming years, but for now it seems reasonable to continue consuming Pacific fish.

Conclusions

Finding your optimal protein-fat-carb ratio demands some experimentation and observation. Most people do best with 15 to 25 percent of total calories as protein. The maximum 35 percent recommended by US health agencies is probably too much. Remember, excess protein cannot be stored, as can carbs and fat. Both animal and vegetable protein sources are highly beneficial, although animal protein has several advantages. Industrial animal food, however, is typically denatured via antibiotics, steroids, and other drugs, and should therefore be minimized.

Besides fish, the best sources of animal protein are free-range chicken, grass-fed beef, wild game, organic lamb, eggs, and fermented dairy (especially goat and sheep milk products), including yogurt, kefir, and feta. As one of the most nutrient-dense foods on the planet, eggs deserve special attention. Eggs contain all essential amino acids, excellent-quality fat, and are highly concentrated with vitamins and minerals. Furthermore, eggs are rich in choline, an essential nutrient, important for brain health, which must be attained through food.[98] Research conducted at Iowa State University shows that 90 percent of the US population is choline deficient.[99]

Regarding vegetable protein, gluten is highly problematic and most people should stop consuming gluten entirely, except perhaps occasional consumption of naturally fermented sourdough bread. Quinoa, lentils, beans, and nuts are good vegetarian sources of protein. Fermented soy is also beneficial, particularly tempeh and natto. Regarding protein powders, I recommend high-quality, non-denatured whey protein for moderate consumption, especially for its glutathione-increasing capacity. But in general, whole foods are much better sources of both micro- and macronutrients than are supplements.

Notes

[1] VR Young and PL Pellet, "Plant proteins in relation to human protein and amino acid nutrition," *American Journal of Clinical Nutrition*, May 1994, vol. 59, no. 5, pg. S12035–S1212; American Dietetic Association, "Position of the American Dietetic Association and Dietitians of Canada: Vegetarian diets," *Journal of the American Dietetic Association*, June 2003, vol. 103, no. 6, pg. 748–768

[2] US Department of Agriculture and US Department of Health and Human Services, *Dietary Guidelines for Americans*, 2010, 7th Edition, US Government Printing Office, December 2010, pg. 15

[3] Cornelia Metges, "Metabolic Consequences of a High Dietary-Protein Intake in Adulthood: Assessment of the Available Evidence," *The Journal of Nutrition*, April 1, 2000, vol. 130, no. 4, pg. 886–889

[4] Shane Bilsborough and Neil Mann, "A Review of Issues of Dietary Protein Intake in Humans," *International Journal of Sports Nutrition and Exercise Metabolism*, April 2006, vol. 16, no. 2

[5] Anssi Manninen, "High-Protein Weight Loss Diets and Purported Adverse Effects: Where is the Evidence?" *Journal of the International Society of Sports Nutrition*, 2004, vol. 1, no. 1, pg. 45–51

[6] Kathryn Doyle, "No science behind blood-type diets," *Reuters*, May 30, 2013

[7] Martin Nachbar, "Lectins in the United States diet: a survey of lectins in commonly consumed foods and a review of the literature," *American Journal of Clinical Nutrition*, November 1980, vol. 33, no. 11, pg. 2338–2345

[8] Luiz Mattos and Haroldo Moreira, "Genetic of the ABO blood system and its link with the immune system," *Revista Brasileira de Hematologia e Hemoterapia*, Jan/Mar 2004, vol. 26, no. 1

[9] N Saitou, "Evolution of primate ABO blood group genes and their homologous genes," *Molecular Biology and Evolution*, 1997, vol. 14, no. 4, pg. 399–411

[10] Leila Cusack et al., "Blood type diets lack supporting evidence: a systematic review," *American Journal of Clinical Nutrition*, July 2013, vol. 98, no. 1, pg. 99–104

[11] Colin Campbell, *The China Study: Startling Implications for Diet, Weight Loss, and Long-Term Health*, published by BenBella Books, 2004, pg. 132

[12] Schulsinger DA et al., "Effect of dietary protein quality on development of aflatoxin B1-induced hepatic preneoplastic lesions," *Journal of the National Cancer Institute*, August 16, 1989, vol. 81, no. 16, pg. 1241–1245

[13] Lynda Frassetto et al., "Estimation of net endogenous noncarbonic acid production in humans from diet potassium and protein contents," *American Journal of Clinical Nutrition*, September 1998, vol. 68, no. 3, pg. 576–583

[14] Jeffrey Krau and Nicolaos Madias, "Metabolic Acidosis: Pathophysiology, Diagnosis and Management: Adverse Effects of Metabolic Acidosis," *Medscape Education*, March 23, 2010

[15] University of Maryland Medical Center, Metabolic Acidosis, Umm.edu/Health/Medical/Ency/Articles/Metabolic-acidosis

[16] Bonjour JP, "Dietary protein: an essential nutrient for bone health," *Journal of the American College of Nutrition*, December 2005, vol. 24, pg. 526S–536S

[17] Kerstetter JE et al., "Dietary protein and skeletal health: a review of recent human research," *Current Opinion in Lipidology*, February 2011, vol. 22, no. 1, pg. 16–20

[18] Remer T and Manz F, "Potential renal acid load of foods and its influence on urine pH," *Journal of the American Dietetic Association*, July 1995, vol. 95, no. 7, pg. 791–797

[19] Gerry Schwalfenberg, "The Alkaline Diet: Is There Evidence That an Alkaline pH Diet Benefits Health?" *Journal of Environmental and Public Health*, 2012: 727630

[20] Sebastian A et al., "Estimation of the net acid load of the diet of ancestral preagricultural Homo sapiens and their hominid ancestors," *American Journal of Clinical Nutrition*, December 2002, vol. 76, no. 6, pg. 1308–1316; Thomas Remer and Friedrich Manz, "Paleolithic diet, sweet potato eaters, and potential renal acid load," *American Journal of Clinical Nutrition*, October 2003, vol. 78, no. 4, pg. 802–803

[21] KE Nachman et al., "Roxarsone, Inorganic Arsenic, and Other Arsenic Species in Chicken: A U.S.-Based Market Basket Sample," *Environmental Health Perspectives*, 2013, DOI:10.1289/ehp.1206245

[22] Stephanie Strom, "F.D.A. Bans Three Arsenic Drugs Used in Poultry and Pig Feeds," *New York Times*, October 1, 2013

[23] McCormack SE et al., "Circulating branched-chain amino acid concentrations are associated obesity and future insulin resistance in children and adolescents," *Pediatric Obesity*, February 2013, vol. 8, no. 1, pg. 52–61

[24] Michael Gleeson, "Interrelationship between Physical Activity and Branched-Chain Amino Acids," *Journal of Nutrition*, June 1, 2005, vol. 135, no. 6, pg. 1591S–1595S

[25] Gertjan Schaafsma, "The Protein Digestibility-Corrected Amino Acid Score (PDCAAS), a concept for describing protein quality in foods and food ingredients: a critical review," *Journal of AOAC International*, May–June 2005, vol. 88, no. 3, pg. 988–994

[26] Ahmed Hamad et al., "Evaluation of the protein quantity and available lysine of germinated and fermented cereals," *Journal of Food Science*, March 1979, vol. 44, no. 2, pg. 456–459

[27] Nutrition Data, Nutritiondata.com

[28] Chunmei Gu et al., "Effect of Soybean Variety on Anti-Nutritional Factors Content, and Growth Performance and Nutrients Metabolism in Rat," *International Journal of Molecular Sciences*, 2010, vol. 11, no. 3, pg. 1048–1056; Robert Anderson et al., "Compositional Changes in Trypsin Inhibitors, Phytic Acid, Saponins and Isoflavones Related to Soybean Processing," *Journal of Nutrition*, March 1995, vol. 125, no. 35, pg. 581S–588S

[29] B Lönnerdal et al., "The effect of individual components of soy formula and cows' milk formula on zinc bioavailability," *American Journal of Clinical Nutrition*, November 1984, vol. 40, no. 5, pg. 1064–1070

[30] Slamet Sudarmadji and Pericles Markakis, "The phytate and phytase of soybean tempeh," *Journal of the Science of Food and Agriculture*, April 1977, vol. 28, no. 4, pg. 381–383

[31] Divi RL et al., "Anti-thyroid isoflavones from soybean: isolation, characterization, and mechanisms of action," *Biochemical Pharmacology*, November 15, 1997, vol. 54, no. 10, pg. 1087–1096

[32] Kameyamado Nigari, Kameyamado.com/

[33] Charlotte Vallaeys et al., "Behind the Bean: The Heroes and Charlatans of the Natural and Organic Soy Foods Industry," *The Cornucopia Institute*, 2009

[34] Ibid.

[35] Pelto L et al., "Milk hypersensitivity in young adults," *European Journal of Clinical Nutrition*, August 1999, vol. 53, no. 8, pg. 620–624

[36] EI El-Agamy, "The challenge of cow milk protein allergy," *Small Ruminant Research*, 2007, vol. 68, pg. 64–72

[37] Lara-Villoslada F et al., "Goat milk is less immunogenic than cow milk in a murine model of atopy," *Pediatric Gastroenterology and Nutrition*, October 2004, vol. 39, no. 4, pg. 354–360

[38] Kunz C et al., "Re-evaluation of the whey protein/casein ratio of human milk," *Acta Paediatrica (Oslo, Norway)*, February 1992, vol. 81, no. 2, pg. 107–112

[39] EFSA Panel on Dietetic Products, Nutrition and Allergies, "Scientific Opinion on the suitability of goat milk protein as a source of protein in infant formulae and in follow-on formulae," *European Food Safety Authority Journal*, 2012, vol. 10, no. 3, pg. 2603

[40] Lara-Villoslada F el al., "The balance between caseins and whey proteins in cow's milk determines its allergenicity," *Journal of Dairy Science*, May 2005, vol. 88, no. 5, pg. 1654–1660

[41] EI El-Agamy, "The challenge of cow milk protein allergy," *Small Ruminant Research*, March 2007, vol. 68, no. 1–2, pg. 64–72

[42] Samir Salem et al., "Isolation, Molecular and Biochemical Characterization of Goat Milk Casein and its Fractions," *Tropical and Subtropical Agroecosytems*, 2009, vol. 11, pg. 29–35

[43] Cavallo MG et al., "Cell-mediated immune response to beta casein in recent-onset insulin-dependent diabetes: implications for disease pathogenesis," *Lancet,* October 5, 1996, vol. 348, no. 9032, pg. 926–928

[44] Samir Salem et al., "Isolation, Molecular and Biochemical Characterization of Goat Milk Casein and its Fractions," *Tropical and Subtropical Agroecosytems,* 2009, vol. 11, pg. 29–35

[45] EI El-Agamy, "The challenge of cow milk protein allergy," *Small Ruminant Research,* 2007, vol. 68, pg. 64–72

[46] Elliott RB et al., "Type I (insulin-dependent) diabetes mellitus and cow milk: casein variant consumption," *Diabetologia,* March 1999, vol. 42, no. 3, pg. 292–296

[47] Ivano De Noni, "Release of beta-casomorphins 5 and 7 during simulated gastro-intestinal digestion of bovine beta-casein variants and milk-based infant formulas," *Food Chemistry,* October 2008, vol. 110, no. 4, pg. 897–903

[48] Provot C et al., "Complete nucleotide sequence of ovine beta-casein cDNA: inter-species comparison," *Biochimie (France),* July 1989, vol. 71, no. 7, pg. 827–832; Lönnerdal B et al., "Cloning and sequencing of a cDNA encoding human milk beta-casein," *FEBS Letters,* August 20, 1990, vol. 269, no. 1, pg. 153–156

[49] Laugesen M et al., "Ischaemic heart disease, Type 1 diabetes, and cow milk A1 beta-casein," *New Zealand Medical Journal,* January 24, 2003, vol. 116, no. 1168, pg. U295; McLachlan CN, "beta-casein A1, ischaemic heart disease mortality, and other illnesses," *Medical Hypotheses,* February 2001, vol. 56, no. 2, pg. 262–272

[50] Hedner J et al., "beta-Casomorphins induce apnea and irregular breathing in adult rats and newborn rabbits," *Life Sciences,* November 16, 1987, vol. 41, no. 20, pg. 2303–2312; Pasi A et al., "beta-Casomorphin-immunoreactivity in the brain stem of the human infant," *Research Communications in Chemical Pathology and Pharmacology,* June 1993, vol. 80, no. 3, pg. 305–322

[51] Brunello Wüthrich et al., "Milk Consumption Does Not Lead to Mucus Production or Occurrence of Asthma," *Journal of the American College of Nutrition,* December 2005, vol. 24, no. 6, pg. 547S–555S; Pinnock CB et al., "Relationship between milk intake and mucus production in adult volunteers challenged with rhinovirus-2," *American Review of Respiratory Disease,* February 1990, vol. 141, no. 2, pg. 352–356

[52] Claustre J et al., "Effects of peptides derived from dietary proteins on mucus secretion in rat jejunum," *American Journal of Physiology: Gastrointestinal and Liver Physiology,* September 2002, vol. 283, no. 3, G521–G528; Trompette A et al., "Milk bioactive peptides and beta-casomorphins induce mucus release in rat jejunum," *Journal of Nutrition,* November 2003, vol. 133, no. 11, pg. 3499–3503; Zoghbi S et al., "beta-Casomorphin-7 regulates the secretion and expression of gastrointestinal mucins through a mu-opioid pathway," *American Journal of Physiology: Gastrointestinal and Liver Physiology,* June 2006, vol. 290, no. 6, pg. G1105–G1113

[53] US Environmental Protection Agency, "Dairy Production," Agriculture 101, Epa.gov/agriculture/ag101/printdairy.html

[54] O'Reilly S et al., "A2 Milk, Farmer Decisions, and Risk Management," Proceedings of the 16th International Farm Management Association Congress, Peer Reviewed Papers, Cork University College, July 2007, pg. 641–648

[55] Margarita Campos et al., "Consumption of caprine milk improves metabolism of calcium and phosphorus in rats with nutritional ferropenic anaemia," *International Dairy Journal*, April 2007, vol. 17, no. 4, pg. 412–419; Alferez MJM et al., "Dietary goat milk improves iron bioavailability in rats with induced ferropenic anaemia in comparison with cow milk," *International Dairy Journal*, 2006, vol. 16, no. 7, pg. 813–821; Díaz-Castro J et al., "Effect of calcium-supplemented goat or cow milk on zinc status in rats with nutritional ferropenic anaemia," *International Dairy Journal*, 2009, vol. 19, no. 2, pg. 116–121

[56] W Hachelafa et al., "Comparative digestibility of goat's versus cow's milk fats in children with digestive malnutrition," *Dairy Science and Technology*, 1993, vol. 73, no. 5–6, pg. 593–599

[57] Michael Pollan, The Omnivore's Dilemma: A Natural History of Four Meals, published by Large Print Pr, 2007

[58] John Painter et al., "Attribution of Foodborne Illnesses, Hospitalizations, and Deaths to Food Commodities by using Outbreak Data, United States, 1998–2008," *Emerging Infectious Diseases*, vol. 19, no. 3, March 2013

[59] Pew Commission on Industrial Farm Animal Production, *Putting Meat on the Table: Industrial Farm Animal Production in America*, Pew Charitable Trusts and Johns Hopkins Bloomberg School of Public Health, 2008, pg. 13

[60] US Department of Agriculture, Economic Research Service, Farm Milk Production, Ers.usda.gov/topics/animal-products/dairy/background.aspx

[61] A Azzouz et al., "Simultaneous determination of 20 pharmacologically active substances in cow's milk, goat's milk, and human breast milk by gas chromatography-mass spectrometry," *Journal of Agricultural and Food Chemistry*, May 11, 2011, vol. 59, no. 9, pg. 5125–5132

[62] Centers for Disease Control, Cdc.gov/features/rawmilk/

[63] Frederic Douglas et al., "Effects of Ultra-High-Temperature Pasteurization on Milk Proteins," *Journal of Agriculture and Food Chemistry*, January 1981, vol. 29, no. 1, pg. 11–15; Lauren MacDonald et al., "A Systematic Review and Meta-Analysis of the Effects of Pasteurization on Milk Vitamins, and Evidence for Raw Milk Consumption and Other Health-Related Outcomes," *Journal of Food Protection*, November 2011, no. 11, pg. 1788–1989

[64] Giacometti F et al., "Quantitative risk assessment of verocytotoxin-producing Escherichia coli O157 and Campylobacter jejuni related to consumption of raw milk in a province in Northern Italy," *Journal of Food Protection*, November 2012, vol. 75, no. 11, pg. 2031–2038; Latorre AA et al., "Quantitative risk assessment of listeriosis due to consumption of raw milk," *Journal of Food Protection*, August 2011, vol. 74, no. 8, pg. 1268–1281; Heidinger JC et al., "Quantitative microbial risk assessment for Staphylococcus aureus and Staphylococcus enterotoxin A in raw milk," *Journal of Food Protection*, August 2009, vol. 72, no. 8, pg. 1641–1653

[65] MC Martini et al., "Strains and species of lactic acid bacteria in fermented milks (yogurts): effect on in vivo lactose digestion," *American Journal of Clinical Nutrition*, December 1991, vol. 54, no. 6, pg. 1041–1046

[66] Fumiko Nagao et al., "Effects of a Fermented Milk Drink Containing Lactobacillus casei Strain Shirota on the Immune System in Healthy Human Subjects," *Bioscience, Biotechnology, and Biochemistry*, 2000, vol. 64, no. 12, pg. 2706–2708

[67] Dolores Parra et al., "Acute Calcium Assimilation from Fresh or Pasteurized Yoghurt Depending on the Lactose Digestibility Status," *Journal of the American College of Nutrition*, June 2007, vol. 26, no. 3, pg. 288–294

[68] Marie-Pierre St-Onge et al., "Consumption of fermented and nonfermented dairy products: effects on cholesterol concentrations and metabolism," *American Journal of Clinical Nutrition*, March 2000, vol. 71, no. 3, pg. 674–681; Kiessling G et al., "Long-term consumption of fermented dairy products over 6 months increases HDL cholesterol," *European Journal of Clinical Nutrition*, September 2002, vol. 56, no. 9, pg. 843–849

[69] United States Department of Agriculture, *Agriculture Fact Book 2001-2002*, March 2003, Office of Communications, Usda.gov

[70] "Gluten-free diet fad: Are celiac disease rates actually rising?" *CBS News*, July 31, 2012

[71] Kenneth Fine, Enterolab.com/Default.aspx

[72] Antonio Di Sabatino, "The function of tissue transglutaminase in celiac disease," *Autoimmunity Review*, August 2012, vol. 11, no. 10, pg. 746–753

[73] VM Wolters et al., "Genetic background of celiac disease and its clinical implications," *American Journal of Gastroenterology*, January 2008, vol. 103, no. 1, pg. 190–195

[74] Conleth Feighery, "Fortnightly review: Coeliac disease," *British Medical Journal*, July 24, 1999, vol. 319, no. 7204, pg. 236–239

[75] Ibid.

[76] HC van den Broeck et al., "Presence of celiac disease epitopes in modern and old hexaploid wheat varieties: wheat breeding may have contributed to increased prevalence of celiac disease," *Theoretical and Applied Genetics*, November 2010, vol. 121, no. 8, pg. 1527–1539

[77] Denery-Papini S et al., "Allergy to deamidated gluten in patients tolerant to wheat: specific epitopes linked to deamidation," *Allergy*, August 2012, vol. 67, no. 8, pg. 1023–1032

[78] A Vojdani, "The Immunology of Immediate and Delayed Hypersensitivity Reaction to Gluten," *European Journal of Inflammation*, January 2008, vol. 6, no. 1, pg. 1–10

[79] US Food and Drug Administration, "Questions and Answers Regarding Gluten-Free Labeling of Foods," August 2, 2011

[80] Carlo Rizzello et al., "Highly Efficient Gluten Degradation by Lactobacilli and Fungal Proteases during Food Processing: New Perspectives for Celiac Disease," *Applied Environmental Microbiology*, July 2007, vol. 73, no. 14, pg. 4499–4507

[81] Meredith Davis, "Where's the Beef? U.S. beef consumption in decline," *Reuters*, December 27, 2011

[82] Michael Pollan, "Power Steer," *New York Times Magazine*, March 31, 2002

[83] Georgina Gustin, "Demand for grass-fed beef is growing," *Los Angeles Times*, November 23, 2012

[84] Cynthia Daley et al., "A review of fatty acid profiles and antioxidant content in grass-fed and grain-fed beef," *Nutrition Journal*, March 2010, vol. 9, no. 10

[85] McAfee AJ et al., "Red meat from animals offered a grass diet increases plasma and platelet n-3 PUFA in healthy consumers," *British Journal of Nutrition*, January 2011, vol. 105, no. 1, pg. 80–89

[86] McKnight GM et al., "Dietary nitrate in man: friend or foe?" *British Journal of Nutrition*, 1999, vol. 81, no. 5, pg. 349–358

[87] McCutcheon JW, "Nitrosamines in bacon: a case study of balancing risks," *Public Health Reports*, July–August, 1984, vol. 99, no. 4, pg. 360–364

[88] Rohrmann S et al., "Meat consumption and mortality—results from the European Prospective Investigation into Cancer and Nutrition," *BMC Medicine*, March 7, 2013, vol. 11, no. 63

[89] Milkowski A et al., "Nutritional epidemiology in the context of nitric oxide biology: a risk-benefit evaluation for dietary nitrite and nitrate," *Nitric Oxide: Biology and Chemistry*, February 15, 2010, vol. 22, no. 2, pg. 110–119

[90] Bryan NS et al., "Ingested nitrate and nitrite and stomach cancer risk: an updated review," *Food Chemical Toxicology*, October 2012, vol. 50, no. 10, pg. 3645–3665

[91] US Department of Agriculture and US Health and Human Services, *Dietary Guidelines for Americans*, 2010, 7th Edition, US Government Printing Office, December 2010, pg. 85

[92] Ralston NV et al., "Dietary selenium's protective effects against methylmercury toxicity," *Toxicology*, November 28, 2010, vol. 278, no. 1, pg. 112–123

[93] Kehrig HA et al., "Selenium and mercury in widely consumed seafood from South Atlantic Ocean," *Ecotoxicology and Environmental Safety*, July 2013, vol. 93, pg. 156–162

[94] Nicholas Ralston, "Selenium Health Benefit Values as Seafood Safety Criteria," *Ecohealth*, December 2008, vol. 5, no. 4, pg. 442–455

[95] Pál Weihe et al., "Dietary recommendations regarding pilot whale meat and blubber in the Faroe Islands," *International Journal of Circumpolar Health*, July 2012, vol. 71, PMC3417701

[96] Nicholas Ralston, "Selenium Health Benefit Values as Seafood Safety Criteria," *Ecohealth*, December 2008, vol. 5, no. 4, pg. 442–455

[97] Nicholas Fisher et al., "Evaluation of radiation doses and associated risk from the Fukushima nuclear accident to marine biota and human consumers of seafood," *Proceedings of the National Academy of Sciences*, June 3, 2013, DOI: 10.1073/pnas.1221834110

[98] Blusztajn JK, "Choline, a vital amine," *Science*, August 7, 1998, vol. 283, no. 5378, pg. 794–795

[99] H Jensen et al., "Choline in the diets of the US population: NHANES, 2003–2004," *The Journal of the Federation of American Societies for Experimental Biology*, March 2007, vol. 21, pg. LB46

CHAPTER SIX

Detoxification

Chronic, low-dose exposure to environmental toxins is quite possibly today's most pernicious health threat. The Industrial and technological revolutions, despite bringing prosperity and many modern conveniences, have seriously compromised our once-pristine food, water, and air. Whether ingested, inhaled, or absorbed through the skin, toxins are continually entering and bioaccumulating within our bodies. Some toxins disrupt the endocrine system; others damage the reproductive system, thus promoting infertility. Some toxins are carcinogenic; others weaken the liver and kidneys. As your cumulative toxic load increases, you absorb and assimilate nutrients less efficiently. Being healthy therefore requires ongoing detoxification, especially in today's modern urban environments.

The liver is the primary detoxification organ, but other organs also play critical roles. The liver converts fat-soluble toxins into water-soluble compounds, which can then be excreted. Detoxification generally involves the metabolism and elimination of foreign compounds, known as xenobiotics, as well as endogenous compounds, known as endobiotics. Pesticides, dioxins, polychlorinated biphenyls (PCBs), food-processing residues, prescription drugs, and industrial waste are some examples of common xenobiotics. Respiratory exposure to volatile organic compounds is another major concern, which commonly occurs indoors, where building materials such as carpet, particleboard, adhesives, and paint are constantly outgassing toxic fumes. The endobiotics of primary concern include certain hormones, inflammatory molecules, and certain signaling compounds.

Cancer mortality has steadily increased since the twentieth century.[1] According to the WHO, cancer is the leading cause of death worldwide, accounting for 13 percent of all deaths in 2008.[2] Since the 1980s, prominent institutions tasked with assessing disease causation have consistently attributed only 4 percent of total cancer deaths to occupational toxins, and only 2 percent to environmental toxins. These estimates originate from a 1981 study by two British scientists, published in the *Journal of the National Cancer Institute.*[3] According to the 2009 annual report for the President's Cancer Panel, however, these estimates "are woefully out of date, given our current understanding of cancer initiation as a complex, multifactorial, multistage process."[4] The report concludes that "the true burden of environmentally induced cancers has been grossly underestimated," and calls for significant, proactive healthcare reforms.[5] Environmental toxins are greatly contributing to ever-increasing global cancer rates. Accordingly, natural detoxification products and procedures are becoming more and more popular.

Effective detoxification requires long-term, health-supportive diet and lifestyle choices. External treatments such as footbaths, body wraps, and skin scrubs are what Dr. Frank Lipman, an integrative medicine specialist, refers to as "third-level detox."[6] Second-level detoxification includes short-term juicing and cleansing regimes. Many people embrace sporadic second- and third-level detoxification between long spells of careless diet and lifestyle choices. While they sometimes achieve rapid weight loss, such results are generally temporary and unsustainable. Short-term, intensive detoxes (second-level) are best for people already engaged in first-level detoxification (long-term healthy diet and lifestyle). Those with unhealthy diets and lifestyles often have higher toxic loads (the level of toxicity within the body), which cause considerable physiological stress during second-level cleansing and detoxing.

First-level detoxification is an ongoing process involving every cell in the body. The approach is gentle, effective, and sustainable. The primary goal is establishing dietary habits that strengthen and support the critical detoxification organs, primarily the liver, kidneys, and intestines, but also the blood, lymph, and lungs. Foods and herbs that support these organs should be consumed regularly, not periodically. When the primary detoxification organs are strong and unburdened, they function much more efficiently. There are three general phases of detoxification. In Phase 1: *Enzymatic Transformation*, various enzymes convert fat-soluble toxins into water-soluble toxins. In Phase 2: *Enzymatic Conjugation*, various enzymes neutralize free radicals and other destructive compounds formed during Phase 1. Also other toxins not addressed during Phase 1 are addressed during Phase 2. In Phase 3: *Transport and Elimination*, transporter cells shuttle away and eliminate water-soluble compounds created in Phases 1 and 2. Effective ongoing detoxification strategies should include the following:

1. Minimize toxic inputs.

2. Increase antioxidants while minimizing free radicals.

3. Support glutathione production.

4. Consume foods/herbs that support the detoxification organs.

5. Consume foods/herbs that chelate heavy metals.

Minimizing Toxic Inputs

Through contaminated food, water, and air, personal hygiene products, and many other sources, we are continually exposed to toxins that gradually bioaccumulate within our cells. If unaddressed, the increasing toxic burden can eventually manifest as disease. Suggestions for minimizing toxic inputs include the following:

- Invest in an effective water filtration system and use filtered water for both drinking and cooking. Reverse osmosis filters are excellent, as are high-quality carbon filters (see Chapter 7). Also invest in a good shower filter (KDF technology). Skin pores expand under hot water, thus creating direct pathways for toxins to enter the body.

- Take steps to maintain clean, fresh indoor air quality. Carpet, furniture, and household cleaning products outgas toxic fumes, making indoor air quality generally worse than outdoor air. Buy nontoxic cleaning products (available at most organic food stores) and open your windows daily for air circulation. Also keep green plants inside your home and office. According to studies conducted by NASA scientists, many common houseplants have excellent air purification properties.[7]

- Buy nontoxic personal hygiene products. Toxicity standards are much more lenient for personal hygiene products than for food because regulatory agencies presume we don't "eat" personal hygiene products. Nevertheless, the skin is porous and what you apply topically generally enters your body, thereby stressing your liver and kidneys. Check your deodorant label. Most deodorants contain highly toxic aluminum and/or aluminum derivatives. Sodium lauryl sulfate (or sodium laureth sulfate) is another harmful chemical commonly found in soaps, shampoos, and many other products. Most health food stores sell clean, nontoxic personal hygiene products.

- Limit your exposure to mobile phones, wireless technology, and microwave ovens. This will profoundly improve your long-term health. Electromagnetic pollution is a serious issue that even the mainstream health establishment is finally acknowledging. In 2011, for example, the WHO formally recognized mobile phone radiation as "possibly carcinogenic to humans."[8] Practical mobile phone solutions include using speaker mode and/or purchasing special earphones with hollow tubes (not wires) that transmit the sound.

- Buy all food (or as much as possible) organic quality.

- Reduce your exposure to BPA (see Chapter 7).

Assisting Antioxidants, Pacifying Free Radicals

Understanding the relationship between antioxidants and free radicals requires a brief recap of basic high school chemistry. An atom consists of a nucleus (which has protons and neutrons) and several orbiting electrons. Electrons occupy progressive layers, or shells, which surround the nucleus. Only two electrons can occupy the first shell. Any additional electrons must occupy the second shell, which holds a maximum of six electrons. Atoms with a full outer shell are stable and therefore are unlikely to interact chemically with other atoms. Atoms naturally seek maximum stability by gaining/losing electrons to fill/empty their outer shells, or by sharing electrons with other atoms.

When weak chemical bonds break, free radicals with odd, unpaired electrons are formed. Free radicals are inherently unstable and highly reactive. They can only gain stability by "stealing" electrons from nearby stable molecules. When this happens, a) the original free radical becomes stable, and b) the formerly stable molecule becomes an unstable free radical. A debilitating chain reaction quickly ensues as the new free radical steals an electron from another nearby stable molecule, which then creates yet another new free radical. A single free radical has the potential to cause considerable damage.[9] To visualize this, imagine a single man entering a dancehall occupied only by couples. The single man breaks into one couple and steals the woman, thereby creating a) a new couple, and b) a new single man. The newly single man then breaks into another couple and steals that woman. This volatile pattern quickly spreads across the dance floor, causing confusion, resentment, and perhaps violence.

Whereas "free radicals" on the dance floor can inflame interpersonal relationships, free radicals within the body are among the primary factors contributing to chronic, systemic inflammation.[10] Chronic, systemic inflammation affects blood vessel linings and many internal organs and systems, and is a primary marker for cardiovascular disease, stroke, and many other degenerative diseases. In a landmark 2003 scientific statement, the AHA and CDC concluded,

> *"Basic science and epidemiological studies have developed an impressive case that atherogenesis is essentially an inflammatory response to a variety of risk factors and the consequences of this response lead to the development of acute coronary and cerebrovascular syndromes."* [11]

Free radicals also denature DNA strands, degrade fat cells by attacking the cell membranes, and damage protein cells by inactivating certain enzymes.[12] Cancer, heart disease, acute respiratory distress syndrome, and rheumatoid arthritis are just some of the conditions caused by free radicals.[13] Additionally, the free radical theory of aging (supported by many studies yet refuted by others) contends that aging is primarily caused, and accelerated, by free radical reactions.

Both normal metabolic reactions and external influences regularly trigger free radical chain reactions. External influences include pharmaceutical drugs, cigarette smoke (including second-hand smoke), environmental pollution, electromagnetic pollution (from cell phones, computers, televisions, power lines, microwaves), household chemicals, denatured food, artificial preservatives, herbicides, pesticides, emotional and physical stress, excessive exercise, and excessive sun exposure. Normal metabolic reactions commonly create oxygen-derived radicals, also known as reactive oxygen species. With two unpaired electrons, oxygen is very prone to causing free radical reactions.

Antioxidants are the body's primary defense against free radicals. Antioxidants, as the name suggests, inhibit free radical oxidation reactions. As discussed above, when stable molecules interact with free radicals, they become free radicals themselves. A chain reaction ensues, which is capable of damaging many cells. Because antioxidants are extremely stable, they can donate electrons to free radicals without becoming free radicals themselves. But when this happens, the antioxidant becomes inactive, thus necessitating more antioxidants to neutralize other free radicals. We can curb free radicals in two basic ways: 1) by implementing healthy dietary and lifestyle changes, and 2) by increasing our consumption of dietary antioxidants. The body synthesizes some antioxidants, but we can help ourselves considerably by consuming foods rich in antioxidants. Foods rich in vitamin E, vitamin C, carotenoids, and polyphenols are all important dietary sources of antioxidants.

Many phytochemicals, vitamins, enzymes, and other nutrients either behave as antioxidants or assist antioxidants. When antioxidant enzymes and/or antioxidant nutrient levels are insufficient, the body cannot properly prevent free radical chain reactions. The end result is oxidative stress, which damages cellular proteins, cell membranes, and genes. When cell membranes are damaged, the cells are vulnerable. If left unchecked, long-term oxidative stress leads to chronic, systemic inflammation, which is a major contributor to many diseases. Chronic, systemic inflammation, however, is quite different from temporary, local inflammation (an essential defense mechanism). For example, by triggering a temporary inflammatory response, the body can effectively ward off infections and rehabilitate physical injuries.

Prolonged inflammation due to oxidative stress disrupts both the immune system and certain metabolic processes. Prolonged inflammation promotes asthma, arthritis, appendicitis, gastritis, peptic ulcers, premature aging, and wrinkling. The next step is chronic, systemic inflammation of the blood vessel linings, which ultimately impairs numerous internal organs and systems. Cancer, heart disease, diabetes, lymphoma, leukemia, and various kidney and liver diseases are all connected to chronic systemic inflammation (caused by oxidative stress and free radical damage).

Phytochemicals, though generally not considered essential nutrients, are bioactive plant compounds that promote an array of extraordinary therapeutic effects. The most important classes of phytochemicals are polyphenols and flavonoids (which is a subcategory of polyphenols). Polyphenols are the most abundant source of dietary antioxidants. A typical healthy diet provides around 1 gram per day of polyphenols, which is ten times the vitamin C and one hundred times the carotenoids and vitamin E that such a diet would provide.[14]

Polyphenols are abundant in fruits, especially blueberries, cherries, blackberries, strawberries, raspberries, apples, peaches, pomegranates, apricots, nectarines, and grapes; vegetables, especially artichokes, onions, spinach, broccoli, asparagus, and potatoes; and herbs and spices, especially cloves, peppermint, anise, oregano, sage, thyme, rosemary, parsley, cumin, and cinnamon. Also tea, red wine, olive oil, olives, capers, cacao powder, dark chocolate, and coffee are potent sources.[15] According to Joe Vison, a University of Scranton chemist with sixteen published papers on antioxidants, "Americans get more of their antioxidants from coffee than any other dietary source. Nothing else comes close."[16] Phytochemicals work synergistically to prevent oxidative damage by modulating detoxification enzymes, scavenging for oxidative agents (free radicals), stimulating the immune system, regulating gene expression, and through various antibacterial and antiviral actions.[17]

Promoting Glutathione Production

Antioxidants have an amazing propensity to function synergistically. As discussed above, when an exogenous antioxidant like vitamin C or vitamin E neutralizes a free radical, the antioxidant becomes an inactive molecule. An extraordinary antioxidant called glutathione, however, can recycle these inactive molecules, thereby making them potent antioxidants once again. Glutathione is commonly known as the master antioxidant due to its unique interaction with other antioxidants.

Strictly speaking, glutathione is a tri-peptide, a protein comprised of three amino acids: glutamic acid, cysteine, and glycine. Besides maintaining and regenerating antioxidants, glutathione facilitates many metabolic reactions, including DNA synthesis and repair, protein synthesis, mitochondria regeneration, and enzyme activation. Glutathione is also the body's principal detoxifier. Phase 2 detoxification, as discussed above, is called conjugation. Glutathione is critical to Phase 2, conjugating drugs, hormones, pesticides, heavy metals, and other toxins, thereby neutralizing them and making them water-soluble. These water-soluble, glutathione-bound toxins are then transported to the liver or kidneys to be excreted via watery fluids (bile or urine). Glutathione is essential for detoxifying from alcohol, nicotine, drugs, environmental pollutants, and heavy metals (especially mercury, arsenic, and lead).

How To Increase Glutathione

Glutathione is an endogenous protein synthesized from glutamic acid, cysteine, and glycine. This means we cannot obtain glutathione directly from food. We must instead empower the body to make glutathione by a) eating foods rich in these three amino acids (glutathione precursors), and b) eating foods rich in other molecules that facilitate glutathione production. Most people consume sufficient levels of glutamic acid and glycine, both of which are non-sulfur amino acids. Cysteine, a sulfurous amino acid, tends to be the limiting factor.

Cysteine is a nonessential amino acid, meaning the body can synthesize it when methionine, another sulfurous amino acid, is sufficient. Methionine is an essential amino acid, meaning it must be obtained from food. Therefore, the best glutathione-increasing strategy is eating plenty of foods rich in sulfurous amino acids (methionine and cysteine). The best sources are eggs, red peppers, garlic, onions, and cruciferous vegetables (cauliflower, broccoli, Brussels sprouts, kale, and collard greens). Poultry and dairy also contain high amounts of these amino acids. Additionally, a molecule common in cruciferous vegetables called cyanohydroxybutene has been shown in numerous studies to significantly elevate glutathione levels.[18] Cruciferous vegetables, oranges, grapefruit, strawberries, tomatoes, and avocados are the best sources of this glutathione-stimulating molecule. Also, daily consumption of 25 ml of high-quality olive oil has been shown to improve glutathione status.[19]

Endogenous production of cysteine via methionine requires sufficient quantities of specific nutrients, including vitamins B_1, B_2, B_6, B_{12}, and folic acid (B_9). Eating foods high in these nutrients is therefore of utmost importance. B_{12} levels are particularly important, especially for those on vegetarian and vegan diets. In 2013, the *British Journal of Nutrition* published the first-ever meta-analysis comparing homocysteine and vitamin B_{12} levels for vegetarians and omnivores.[20] Homocysteine is a homologue of cysteine, which can be recycled into methionine or converted into cysteine with the aid of B-vitamins. A major biomarker of many chronic conditions, including cardiovascular disease, is elevated homocysteine (suggesting insufficient B vitamin levels). The study concluded that vitamin B_{12} and homocysteine are inversely related and that B_{12} deficiency and elevated homocysteine levels are common for vegetarians, and especially for vegans.

The best food for stimulating glutathione production is whey. Because whey is dairy, always source it from grass-fed, non-industrial cows, free from hormones and antibiotics. Also, whey should never be heated or pasteurized. Whey contains all three of the amino acid precursors of glutathione. It also contains a highly bioactive molecule called glutamylcysteine, which converts into glutathione. Furthermore, whey is rich in various critical co-factors, which help create the optimal metabolic environment for glutathione production.

Selenium

Glutathione peroxidase (GPx) is a family of enzymes, which behave as free radical scavengers. Glutathione and GPx are not the same, although they do support and complement each other. Selenium is a key GPx co-factor. Many selenium-dependent enzymes are hugely supportive of antioxidants, which means selenium is essential for effectively preventing oxidative damage. Dr. Nicholas Ralston, a research scientist and expert on selenium's protective effects against mercury toxicity, explains,

"Selenium-dependent enzymes are probably the most functionally elite enzymes there are for preventing oxidative damage."[21]

Selenium also supports glutathione by supporting certain detoxification pathways. Selenium, for example, counteracts cadmium and mercury toxicity.[22] This is because mercury has an incredible binding affinity for selenium, 1 million times its binding affinity for sulfur, which is mercury's second-best binding partner.[23] As discussed in Chapter 5, foods with higher amounts of selenium relative to mercury (including most ocean fish consumed by humans), probably pose no mercury toxicity threats. The mercury and selenium bind together, thus preventing assimilation and allowing for easy elimination. Dietary selenium is therefore extremely important.

Though toxic in large amounts, selenium is an essential micronutrient, which functions as an antioxidant and works synergistically with vitamin E. According to the Institute of Medicine, the tolerable upper level for adults is 400 micrograms (mcg) per day.[24] The FDA recommends 70 mcg per day, but this is probably insufficient. Research conducted at the University of Buffalo's Roswell Park Cancer Institute, for example, has established 200 mcg per day as the safest, most therapeutic amount for cancer prevention (specifically prostate, colon, and lung cancers).[25] The notion that selenium effectively prevents prostate cancer is an ongoing debate. The mainstream of allopathic medicine typically rejects this claim, but certain factions are beginning to acknowledge selenium's therapeutic benefits.

A famous 1996 study by Dr. Larry Clark of the University of Arizona observed a 63 percent reduction in incidents of terminal prostate cancer among men consuming 200 mcg per day of selenium compared to those consuming placebos. His study of roughly 1,300 volunteers prompted a Harvard follow-up study of nearly 34,000 men. The Harvard team confirmed the inverse correlation between selenium and prostate cancer, concluding that 159 mcg per day is optimal.[26] The National Cancer Institute (NCI), on the other hand, categorically rejects the notion that selenium can prevent prostate cancer.[27] The NCI, however, has historically rejected effective, inexpensive, herbal and nutritional cancer treatments.

The best dietary sources of selenium include mushrooms, eggs, seafood, poultry, garlic, onions, broccoli, asparagus, tomatoes, cereal grains, seeds, and nuts. Brazil nuts are the most potent known source. A mere 10 grams has 192 mcg of selenium. Anecdotally, Cornell scientist Donald Lisk and his colleagues once experimented on themselves, eating six Brazil nuts per day for three weeks. Their subsequent blood serum selenium levels rose between 100 to 350 percent.[28] Don't waste your money on expensive selenium supplements. One or two Brazil nuts per day provide plenty of bioavailable selenium on the cheap.

Supporting The Detoxification Organs

The liver, kidneys, and intestines are the primary detoxification organs. Excessive sugar consumption, especially fructose, burdens the liver considerably. Reasonable amounts of fructose (around 25 grams per day) consumed as whole fruit are healthy and encouraged, but most people consume far too much fructose through soda, fruit juice, and processed foods containing high fructose corn syrup (HFCS). The average American consumes 97 pounds of sugar per year, half of which is HFCS.[29] According to Harvard Medical School, 30 percent of US adults (and presumably those of other developed nations) have nonalcoholic fatty liver disease, a virtually unknown disease before 1980.[30] Additionally, a 2012 study funded by the National Institutes of Health found that nearly 10 percent of US teens have this disease.[31] Research presented at the 2011 International Liver Congress made headlines with the suggestion that half the US population could have nonalcoholic fatty liver disease by 2030.[32]

Nonalcoholic fatty liver disease is directly related to excessive consumption of fructose (sugar). Besides drastically reducing (or eliminating) sugar, the best way to support the liver is by eating foods that promote detoxification, and foods high in antioxidants. Garlic, onions, and cruciferous vegetables are highly beneficial. Also, according to traditional Chinese medicine, sour foods, including lemons and limes, support the liver.[33] An excellent herb for liver support is milk thistle.

Milk thistle is an inexpensive yet very beneficial herb that supports liver function while preventing glutathione depletion. Milk thistle is the most well-researched plant for the treatment of liver disease.[34] Silymarin, the active component of milk thistle, acts as an antioxidant by reducing free radicals and lipid peroxidation. Silymarin has been used effectively to treat alcoholic liver disease, acute and chronic viral hepatitis, and various toxin-induced liver diseases.[35] Milk thistle seeds contain 4 to 6 percent silymarin, whereas extracts contain upwards of 65 to 80 percent.

Clinical research suggests that milk thistle effectively combats nonalcoholic fatty liver disease.[36] Traditionally, milk thistle has been used for centuries to support and protect the liver. It consistently ranks among the best-selling herbal supplements in the US. The US Department of Health and Human Services recognizes milk thistle's liver protective properties through the mechanisms of "antioxidant activity, toxin blockade at the membrane level, enhanced protein synthesis, anti-fibrotic activity, and possible anti-inflammatory or immunomodulating effects."[37]

Besides supporting the liver, we must also support the kidneys and intestines for proper and effective detoxification. Optimal kidney function requires plenty of pure water. Generally speaking, many of the same foods that support the liver also support the kidneys. Cruciferous vegetables and fruits/vegetables high in antioxidants are particularly beneficial as are the following herbs: dandelion, meadowsweet, nettle, and parsley. Strengthening the intestines requires thorough chewing, and eating foods containing probiotics and adequate amounts of fiber.

Strengthening The Digestion

The intestines house a vibrant, dynamic ecosystem of some 500 different bacterial species. Approximately thirty to forty species account for 99 percent of this bacterial community.[38] Humans coexist in symbiotic relationships with these microorganisms, which are collectively known as intestinal flora (or gut flora). The intestinal flora perform many useful functions, including assisting digestion, warding off pathogenic bacteria, training the immune system to respond only to pathogens, regulating gut development, and synthesizing essential vitamins. Not all gut bacteria, however, are necessarily beneficial.

Dysbiosis is an imbalance of bad bacteria caused by antibiotics, pesticides, and many other factors. To build and maintain strong intestinal flora, one must avoid antibiotics as much as possible, while consuming plenty of probiotics and prebiotics. Although antibiotics are indeed effective against life-threatening bacterial infections, they are notoriously overprescribed. One prescription can sufficiently compromise an entire colony of gut bacteria. Antibiotics are pervasive throughout the food supply because industrial farming and fishing practices necessitate their use. Chlorinated water also damages intestinal flora. While chlorination of public water supplies may indeed be prudent, individuals should use home water filters to remove chlorine and harmful chlorine byproducts.

Food choices profoundly influence the intestinal flora. Excessive sugar intake, for example, feeds bad bacteria (anaerobic bacteria, fungi, and yeast) to the detriment of good bacteria. Pesticides, herbicides, insecticides and fungicides also damage good bacteria. The best way to populate the intestinal flora is eating fermented foods rich in probiotics. Fermentation occurs when airborne microorganisms (or microorganisms from a starter culture) colonize foods within a certain temperature range for a certain period of time. Raw, unpasteurized, fermented foods have microorganisms capable of surviving the digestion, thereby populating our intestinal flora. The best sources include yogurt, kefir, lacto-fermented vegetables, kombucha, miso, and natto. Probiotics are also available as supplements, but natural foods are generally superior. Prebiotics are indigestible fibers that promote the growth of beneficial gut bacteria. Prebiotics are abundant in garlic, onions, bananas, and foods rich in soluble fiber.

Fiber

Dietary fiber occurs in plant foods, but not animal foods. Fiber is indigestible, though it aids digestion by pulling food through the gastrointestinal tract. The two basic varieties of fiber are insoluble and soluble. Insoluble fiber, found in many fruits and vegetables, cannot be dissolved in water. Cellulose, the substance that provides rigidity to plants, is the most common form of insoluble fiber. Insoluble fiber is a natural laxative. It gives bulk to stools and promotes efficient movement through the gastrointestinal tract. Soluble fiber attracts water, thereby forming a gel, which slows the digestion and gives the feeling of fullness. Dr. Robert Lustig, a prominent expert on sugar and metabolic disease, explains the interaction of soluble and insoluble fiber:

> *"Metabolically, the two together are an unbeatable pair. The insoluble fiber forms a latticework for the soluble fiber to sit on, while the soluble fiber bridges the gaps in the latticework to maintain its integrity."*[39]

How much fiber is enough? The Institute of Medicine recommends 35 grams per day for a 2,500-calorie diet.[40] Mean intakes of dietary fiber, however, typically range from 10 to 18 grams per day in the US, with 90 percent of the US population failing to meet the recommended levels.[41] From an evolutionary perspective, prior to the introduction of agriculture and animal husbandry, our distant hunting and foraging ancestors consumed much higher amounts of fiber than do modern humans.

An anthropological study published in the *European Journal of Nutrition*, based on DNA analysis, determined that our distant ancestors ate upwards of 100 grams per day of dietary fiber.[42] Jeff Leach, the study's author, is a prominent anthropologist and founder of both the Human Food Project and the American Gut Project. Leach explains that decreased fiber in modern diets "has resulted in decreased metabolic and physiological activity in the distal colon, thus opening the pathogenic door to cancer in this region."[43]

Fiber slows down the digestion of sugar, thereby increasing glucose tolerance and mitigating the harmful effects of fructose (see Chapter 4). Fiber is essentially what makes whole fruit healthy and fruit juice unhealthy. Although fruit juice does have beneficial vitamins, it also has too much concentrated fructose. Excessive fructose consumption, especially free fructose (devoid of fiber) taxes the liver and promotes metabolic disease, obesity, and numerous degenerative diseases. The fiber content of whole fruit significantly slows down the absorption of fructose.[44] Also, whole fruit has less absolute fructose than fruit juice does. To make one glass of fruit juice, for example, requires several servings of whole fruit.

Nutritional smoothies are a practical, delicious format for whole fruit. The intense action of the blender, however, can compromise the integrity of the insoluble fiber. According to Dr. David Katz, a highly acclaimed nutrition expert, smoothies made with whole fruit still have fiber and are almost as good as whole, chewed fruit.[45] Katz acknowledges, however, that scientific research is lacking on this subject. A 1977 study published in *The Lancet* tested the plasma-glucose and serum-insulin effects of apples (whole), apple juice, and puréed apples. The authors explained,

> *"Fibre-free juice could be consumed eleven times faster than intact apples and four times faster than fibre-disrupted purée ... The removal of fibre from food, and also its physical disruption, can result in faster and easier ingestion, decreased satiety, and disturbed glucose homoeostasis which is probably due to inappropriate insulin release."*[46]

According to Lustig,

> *"The shearing action of the blender blades completely destroys the insoluble fiber of the fruit. The cellulose is torn to smithereens. While the soluble fiber is still there, and can help move food through the intestine faster, it now does not have the 'latticework' of the insoluble fiber to help form that intestinal barrier."*[47]

The bottom line: smoothies are great, but whole, chewed fruit is probably better.

Daily fiber requirements are largely individualistic. Those with strong intestinal flora may require somewhat less fiber, whereas those transitioning to a healthier diet and working on strengthening their digestion may require somewhat more. Eating mostly vegetables, as opposed to cereals, is perhaps the best strategy. A long-term observational study published in the *British Journal of Nutrition* found that diets high in cereals, despite being high in fiber, lead to increased consumption of phytates.[48] Some fruits and vegetables also contain phytates, but at relatively insignificant levels. As discussed in Chapter 4, phytates bind to zinc and other minerals, thus preventing absorption. Occasional consumption of quinoa, buckwheat, and nuts can provide beneficial fiber, but vegetables are the best source.

Chewing

Good chewing habits are essential for efficient digestion. The digestion of fats, for example, begins in the mouth with the secretion of lipase from the lingual serous glands. Lipase enzymes help the stomach convert triglycerides into free fatty acids. Carbohydrate digestion also begins in the mouth with the secretion of amylase, an essential digestive enzyme secreted by the salivary glands. The pancreas and small intestines also secrete amylase, thus ensuring proper digestion even when chewing is meager. Proper chewing, however, significantly reduces stress on these organs, thus making the digestive process more efficient. So how much chewing is enough?

Some health experts advise twenty-five, fifty, or some other arbitrary amounts of chewing per bite. Good intentions notwithstanding, this approach is far too robotic. Rather than counting, try to develop an increased awareness and sensitivity regarding chewing. Some foods require more chewing than others. Also, your own unique chewing technique will influence the process. The best advice is simply to chew until you can swallow your food comfortably. Food should be as liquid as possible before swallowing. If you can identify a food by its texture, you should probably continue chewing. According to Mahatma Gandhi, you should "drink your food." In other words, chew until your food is liquid, then swallow.

Boosting The Immune System

The digestive system and the immune system are closely interrelated. In fact, much of the immune system is physically located within the gastrointestinal tract. Strong digestion and strong intestinal flora greatly support the immune system. Also, the removal of toxins through normal detoxification processes sometimes burdens and overwhelms the immune system. For these reasons, eating foods that support the immune system is essential for optimal detoxification.

Medicinal mushrooms are among the best immune-supporting foods. Shiitakes, for example, have sublime culinary properties and impressive therapeutic effects, making them one of the world's most treasured mushrooms. Shiitakes have proven antibiotic, antiviral, and anticancer properties, and they enhance detoxification by supporting liver function.[49] Shiitakes also have immune-boosting properties. They contain active hexose correlated compound (AHCC), a potent molecule that increases natural killer (NK) cell activity and, in mice studies, has been shown to mitigate the severity of influenza.[50] Shiitakes ameliorate many conditions, including depressed immune function (including AIDS), frequent colds and flu, environmental allergies, bronchial inflammation, heart disease, hypertension, infectious disease, diabetes, hepatitis, and cancer.[51] According to Paul Stamets and George Hudler, two of the world's most renowned mycologists, cooking mushrooms enhances their immune-boosting properties and also destroys certain toxins they sometimes harbor.[52]

Agaricus bisporus, also known as the common button mushroom, is perhaps the most widely consumed mushroom species worldwide. Cultivated in over seventy countries, button mushrooms have many culinary uses. And while they do have some medicinal properties, button mushrooms pale in comparison to shiitake, enokitake, maitake, reishi, and oyster mushrooms. In studies, white button mushrooms have been shown to enhance NK activity, suggesting they could protect against tumors and viruses, but not as effectively as the aforementioned mushrooms.[53]

Button mushrooms should be cooked to minimize agaritine, a naturally occurring mycotoxin and potential carcinogen. Shiitake mushrooms, for example, also contain agaritine, but button mushrooms contain 278 times more.[54] Cooking, drying, and freezing can dramatically reduce agaritine levels (up to 75 percent).[55] Maitake, reishi, cordyceps, mannentake, and chaga are other powerful medicinal mushrooms worth researching and incorporating into your nutrition program.

Miso

A traditional Japanese variety of fermented soy, miso has remarkable healing properties and sophisticated culinary qualities. Miso consists of cooked soy (and sometimes barley, rice, and/or other cereals/legumes), inoculated with koji (a special mold that initiates the fermentation process), and sea salt. Miso typically ferments between three months and three years. Miso is a living food containing beneficial microorganisms, including tetragenococcus halophilus, a form of lactic acid. For this reason, miso is better unheated or heated only very gently.

In Japan, miso has been used effectively to treat radiation poisoning. The atomic bombings of Nagasaki and Hiroshima paved the way for miso's rise to international prominence. Following the attacks, Dr. Tatuichiro Akizuki, director of Nagasaki's St. Francis Hospital (only 1.4 kilometers from the epicenter), famously instructed his twenty employees and seventy tuberculosis patients to consume miso soup daily. None of them suffered from acute radiation disease.[56] Akizuki was the first person to suggest that miso has radioprotective properties, which was subsequently confirmed, repeatedly, in numerous experimental studies.[57]

Miso contains a powerful chelating compound called dipicolinic acid, which binds to heavy metals and draws them from the body. According to research conducted at Hiroshima University, dipicolinic acid gives miso radioprotective and anticancer properties. In experimental research, miso has proven to be effective in reducing breast, lung, liver, and gastric tumors.[58]

Cayenne

Cultures around the world have used cayenne medicinally for centuries, especially for weight loss and detoxification. Research conducted at the Yale University Medical School shows that cayenne also helps regulate blood pressure.[59] Capsaicin, the active, heat-producing component of cayenne, has anti-inflammatory properties, which can relieve pain from arthritis and sore muscles. Capsaicin also has anticancer properties and is especially effective against prostate and breast cancer.[60] Furthermore, capsaicin promotes increased metabolism, which is one reason people consume cayenne for weight loss.[61] Capsaicin, as well as caffeine and catechins (found in green tea), are thermogenic compounds, meaning they create heat. When ingested, the body burns excess fat. In one study conducted at Maastricht University, fat oxidation increased 10 to 16 percent through such dietary adjustments.[62] Cayenne is excellent as a beverage mixed with water and lime juice, and great for guacamole, salads, sauces, and soups.

Chelating Heavy Metals

Chelation is the process of removing heavy metals from the body, especially lead, mercury, cadmium, and arsenic. Certain foods and herbs have chelating properties, which can assist with this natural detoxification process. Exposure to heavy metals is an unavoidable reality of twenty-first-century life, which makes proactive chelation very important. Dr. Garry Gordon, a world-renowned expert on chelation therapy, summarizes the situation as follows:

> *"No one on planet earth is operating at optimal levels without doing something about the toxic metals. Thus the conclusion I draw is that chelation appears a lifetime necessity for all."*[63]

Chelation using synthetic chemicals is controversial and has potentially dangerous side effects. Natural chelation using specific foods and herbs, however, is effective, safe, and relatively inexpensive.

Dr. Mark Sircus, the director of the Federation for Safe and Effective Medicine, is a pioneer of holistic medicine and a prolific writer, researcher, and educator. In his book *Winning the War on Cancer*, Sircus describes "the Golden Triangle of Natural Chelation" as the combined use of alpha-lipoic acid (ALA), cilantro, and chlorella, along with sufficient dietary minerals, which is "the ultimate in safe chelation for a broad array of heavy metals."[64] Sircus credits this detox modality to "the genius of Dr. Alan Greenberg who brought these three agents together for the first time and tested extensively to prove their effectiveness and safety."

Alpha-Lipoic Acid

ALA (not to be confused with alpha-linolenic acid, the omega-3 fatty acid) is an endogenous antioxidant responsible for converting glucose into energy. ALA also stimulates glutathione production and helps regenerate other antioxidants, including vitamin C and ubiquinol (coenzyme Q_{10}). Additionally, ALA is a powerful chelating agent. According to a review published by the *British Journal of Radiology*, ALA also effectively and non-toxically (within standard dose ranges) protects against radiation poisoning.[65] A 1993 study conducted by the Russian Institute for Haematology found, for example, that children living near Chernobyl and suffering from chronic exposure to low-dose radiation benefited considerably from ALA treatments.[66]

ALA also crosses the blood-brain barrier, which is significant because lead and mercury readily accumulate within the brain. ALA scavenges and traps heavy metals, thereby preventing cellular damage. Sources of ALA include various organ meats, broccoli, tomatoes, spinach, collard greens, Brussels sprouts, peas, and brewer's yeast. According to the Memorial Sloan-Kettering Cancer Center, therapeutic doses of ALA are best derived via supplements rather than food.[67]

Cilantro

Cilantro has been clinically demonstrated to accelerate the excretion of mercury, lead, and aluminum.[68] A study published in the *Journal of Ethnopharmacology* found that cilantro is particularly good at chelating lead.[69] Besides its chelating properties, cilantro also has powerful antimicrobial properties,[70] anti-inflammatory properties,[71] and blood-sugar-lowering properties.[72] With respect to its chelating properties, both Dr. George Georgiou and Dr. Andrew Hall Cutler, world-leading experts on mercury detoxification, have noted that cilantro works much better in conjunction with other chelating agents, like chlorella. Georgiou notes,

"It is very probable that cilantro, which is known as an intracellular chelator, takes metals from the interior of the cell and brings them out into the mesenchyme or extracellular space. As there is nothing to mop them up here, as the osmotic gradient increases, then you get a rush of metals from the extracellular environment into the intracellular environment. Personally, I have seen patients who were given only cilantro by other practitioners get worse while on this protocol."[73]

While normal dietary quantities of cilantro absent chlorella are safe and beneficial, chlorella should accompany therapeutic doses to obtain the full chelating potential of both these plants.

Chlorella

Chlorella is a single-celled, freshwater algae species containing high amounts of chlorophyll, the highest per-gram quantity of any known edible plant. Chlorella is a powerhouse of vitamins, minerals, protein, and micronutrients. Besides containing upwards of 60 percent highly digestible protein, chlorella also contains significant amounts of zinc, iron, calcium, magnesium, potassium, trace minerals, and essential fatty acids. Additionally, chlorella has strong antiviral, antibacterial, and detoxifying properties. Dr. Sircus explains,

"Chlorella algae contain phytochemicals that support detoxification while the cell walls function as an ion exchange resin to absorb and retain toxic metals which can then be excreted. Chlorella is a food-like all-purpose mild detoxifier (not chelator) of heavy metals. The detoxification capability of Chlorella is due to its unique cell wall and the material associated with it."[74]

Chlorella also has remarkable immune-system-boosting properties. In studies of mice infected by listeria monocytogenes, a virulent food-borne pathogen, chlorella boosted immune responses by significantly increasing natural killer (NK) cell activity, thus promoting swifter recovery times.[75] Many studies have also proven chlorella's capacity to stimulate interferon production, which is an important function of the non-specific immune system. The non-specific immune system staves off viral and bacterial infections early on, before the specific immune system must respond.[76] Moreover, scientists in South Korea have recently demonstrated chlorella's powerful anticancer properties. Carotenoid extracts from two varieties of chlorella were shown to inhibit the growth of cancer cells.[77]

Characteristically, the American Cancer Society (ACS) denies that chlorella has any anticancer potential: "Available scientific evidence does not support claims that chlorella is effective against cancer or other diseases in humans."[78] Despite the ACS's assertion, chlorella is indeed potent natural medicine capable of preventing numerous diseases, fully supported by clinical evidence and scientific research.

Other strong chelators include miso and various algae species. Magnesium plays a strong role in chelation, which is one reason why magnesium-rich foods (like algae) are effective. Garlic, though not known for its chelating properties, has been shown to bind with lead, thus facilitating its excretion.[79] To obtain it's full potential, garlic should be crushed and eaten raw. Allicin, one of garlic's most powerful components, becomes unlocked and bioavailable when you crush the garlic and wait ten minutes.[80] Crushing catalyzes an enzymatic reaction whereby alliinase combines with alliin to produce allicin.

Detoxification Conclusions

Many people approach detoxification through second- and third-level strategies while neglecting the all-important first level. Instead of thinking of detox as a series of temporary cleanses or one-off treatments, think of detox as an everyday process, assisted by proper nutrition, specifically foods that support the liver, kidneys, and intestines. Eat plenty of glutathione precursors. These include poultry, dairy, whey, eggs, red peppers, garlic, onions, cruciferous vegetables, avocados, and olive oil. Eat plenty of chelating foods, including cilantro, chlorella, and miso. Strive to minimize toxic inputs. When the body's toxic load is minimized, the entire organism works more efficiently. This translates into higher energy, deeper sleep, and overall better quality of life.

Notes

[1] Sherry Murphy et al., Division of Vital Statistics, "Deaths: Final Data for 2010," *National Vital Statistics Reports*, May 8, 2013, vol. 61, no. 4; Centers for Disease Control, "Leading Causes of Death, 1900–1998," Cdc.gov/nchs/data/dvs/lead1900_98.pd

[2] World Health Organization, Media Centre, Who.int/mediacentre/factsheets/fs297/en/

[3] Doll and Peto, "The causes of cancer: quantitative estimates of avoidable risks of cancer in the United States today," *Journal of the National Cancer Institute*, June 1981, vol. 66, no. 6, pg. 1191–1308

[4] Suzanne Reuben et al., "Reducing Environmental Cancer Risk: What We Can Do Now," President's Cancer Panel, 2008–2009 Annual Report, pg. 2

[5] Ibid.

[6] Abby Ellin, "Flush Those Toxins! Eh, Not So Fast," *New York Times*, January 21, 2009

[7] BC Wolverton, "Foliage Plants for Improving Indoor Air Quality," *Nation Foliage Foundation Interiorscape Seminar*, Hollywood, Florida, July 19, 1988; Ssc.nasa.gov/environmental/docforms/water_research/water_research.html

[8] Danielle Dellorto, "WHO: Cell phone use can increase possible cancer risk," *CNN*, March 31, 2011

[9] Bagachi and Puri, "Free radicals and antioxidants in health and disease," *Eastern Mediterranean Health Journal*, 1998, vol. 4, no. 2, pg. 350–360

[10] Daniel Closa and Emma Folch-Puy, "Oxygen Free Radicals and the Systemic Inflammatory Response," *IUBMB Life*, April 2004, vol. 56, no. 4, pg. 185–191

[11] Thomas Pearson et al., "AHA/CDC Scientific Statement: Markers of Inflammation and Cardiovascular Disease," *Circulation*, 2003, vol. 107, pg. 499–511

[12] Robert Floyd and John Carney, "Free radical damage to protein and DNA: Mechanisms involved and relevant observations on brain undergoing oxidative stress," *Annals of Neurology*, 1992, vol. 32, pg. S22–S27

[13] Bagachi and Puri, "Free radicals and antioxidants in health and disease," *Eastern Mediterranean Health Journal*, 1998, vol. 4, no. 2, pg. 350–360

[14] Augustin Scalbert et al., "Polyphenols: antioxidants and beyond," *American Journal of Clinical Nutrition*, January 2005, vol. 81, no. 1, pg. 215S–217S

[15] J Pérez-Jiménez et al., "Identification of the 100 richest dietary sources of polyphenols: an application of the Phenol-Explorer database," *European Journal of Clinical Nutrition*, 2010, vol. 64, pg. S112–S120

[16] Patrick Barkham, "Coffee a good source of antioxidants," *The Guardian*, August 29, 2005

[17] LO Dragsted et al., "Cancer-protective factors in fruits and vegetables: biochemical and biological background," *Pharmacology & Toxicology*, February 1993, vol. 72, no. S1, pg. 116–135; R Waladkhani et al., "Effect of dietary phytochemicals on cancer development (review)," *International Journal of Molecular Medicine*, April 1998, vol. 1, no. 4, pg. 747–753

[18] MA Davis et al., "Differential effect of cyanohydroxybutene on glutathione synthesis in liver and pancreas of male rats," *Toxicology and Applied Pharmacology*, December 1993, vol. 123, no. 2, pg. 257–264; Matthew Wallig and Elizabeth Jeffry, "Enhancement of pancreatic and hepatic glutathione levels in rats during cyanohydroxybutene intoxication," *Fundamental and Applied Toxicology*, January 1990, vol. 14, no. 1, pg. 144–159

[19] María-Isabel Covas, et al., "The Effect of Polyphenols in Olive Oil on Heart Disease Risk Factors," *Annals of Internal Medicine*, September 5, 2006, vol. 145, no. 5, pg. 333–341

[20] Derek Obersby et al., "Plasma total homocysteine status of vegetarians compared with omnivores: a systematic review and meta-analysis," *British Journal of Nutrition*, March 14, 2013, vol. 109, no. 5, pg. 785–794

[21] Chris Kresser, "RHR: The Truth About Toxic Mercury in Fish," Interview with Dr. Nicholas Ralston, October 17, 2012

[22] Phil Whanger, "Selenium in the treatment of heavy metal poisoning and chemical carcinogenesis," *Journal of Trace Elements and Electrolytes in Health and Disease*, December 1992, vol. 6, no. 4, pg. 209–221

[23] Ralston NV et al., "Dietary selenium's protective effects against methylmercury toxicity," *Toxicology*, November 28, 2010, vol. 278, no. 1, pg. 112–123

[24] Dietary Supplement Fact Sheet: Selenium, Office of Dietary Supplements, National Institutes of Health, Ods.od.nih.gov/factsheets/selenium/

[25] Reid ME et al., "The nutritional prevention of cancer: 400 mcg per day selenium treatment," *Nutrition and Cancer*, March 2008, vol. 60, no. 2, pg. 155–163

[26] "Selenium and prostate cancer," Harvard University website, Health.harvard.edu/fhg/updates/Selenium-and-prostate-cancer.shtml

[27] Press Release, "Review of Prostate Cancer Prevention Study Shows No Benefit for Use of Selenium and Vitamin E Supplements," National Cancer Institute, October 27, 2008

[28] Ralph Moss, "Cancer Therapy: The Independent Consumer's Guide to Non-Toxic Treatment and Prevention," *Equinox Press*, March 1993, pg. 122

[29] Stephanie Strom, "U.S. Cuts Estimate of Sugar Intake," *New York Times*, October 26, 2012

[30] "Abundance of fructose not good for the liver, heart," *Harvard Heart Letter*, September 2011

[31] Kristina Fiore, "Fatty Liver Disease on Rise in Teens," *Med Page Today*, May 25, 2012

[32] Press release, "New 10 year data shows non-alcoholic fatty liver disease will reach epidemic status in the US," European Association for the Study of the Liver, 2011 International Liver Congress, Berlin, Germany, March 2011

[33] Tom Monte, *The Complete Guide to Natural Healing*, published by Perigee, 1997, pg. 554

[34] L Abenavoli et al., "Milk thistle in liver diseases: past, present, future," *Phytotherapy Research*, October 2010, vol. 24, no. 10, pg. 1423–1432

[35] Ibid.

[36] Hajaghamohammadi et al., "The Efficacy of Silymarin in Decreasing Transaminase Activities in Non-Alcoholic Fatty Liver Disease: A Randomized Controlled Clinical Trial," *Hepatitis Monthly*, Summer 2008, vol. 8, no. 3, pg. 191–195

[37] US Department of Health and Human Services, "Milk Thistle: Effects on Liver Disease and Cirrhosis and Clinical Adverse Effects Summary," Evidence Report/Technology Assessment Number 21, AHRQ Publication 01-E025

[38] Laurent Beaugerie and Jean-Claude Petit, "Antibiotic-associated diarrhoea," *Best Practice & Research Clinical Gastroenterology*, April 2004, vol. 18, no. 2, pg. 337–352

[39] Robert H. Lustig, *Fat Chance: Beating the Odds Against Sugar, Processed Food, Obesity, and Disease*, published by Hudson Street Press, December 2012, pg. 145

[40] National Research Council, *Dietary Reference Intakes for Energy, Carbohydrate, Fiber, Fat, Fatty Acids, Cholesterol, Protein, and Amino Acids (Macronutrients)*, published by The National Academies Press, 2005

[41] Roger Clemens et al., "Filling America's Fiber Intake Gap: Summary of a Roundtable to Probe Realistic Solutions with a Focus on Grain-Based Foods," *Journal of Nutrition*, July 1, 2012, vol. 142, no. 7, pg. 1390S–1401S

[42] JD Leach, "Evolutionary perspective on dietary intake of fibre and colorectal cancer," *European Journal of Clinical Nutrition*, January 2007, vol. 61, no. 1, pg. 140–142

[43] Ibid.

[44] Rachmiel Levine, "Monosaccharides in Health and Disease," *Annual Review of Nutritional Medicine*, July 1986, vol. 6, pg. 211–224

[45] David Katz, "Does Blending Fruit Reduce Its Fiber Content?" *O, The Oprah Magazine*, May 2008

[46] Haber GB et al., "Depletion and disruption of dietary fibre. Effects on satiety, plasma-glucose, and serum-insulin," *The Lancet*, October 1, 1977, vol. 2, no. 8040, pg. 679–682

[47] Robert H. Lustig, *Fat Chance: Beating the Odds Against Sugar, Processed Food, Obesity, and Disease*, published by Hudson Street Press, December 2012, pg. 147

[48] Celia Prynne et al., "Dietary fibre and phytate; a balancing act. Results from 3 time points in a British Birth Cohort," *British Journal of Nutrition*, January 2000, vol. 103, no. 2, pg. 274–280

[49] PS Bisen et al., "Lentinus edodes: a macrofungus with pharmacological activities," *Current Medicinal Chemistry*, 2010, vol. 17, no. 22, pg. 2419–2430; Itoh et al., "Hepatoprotective effect of syringic acid and vanillic acid on concanavalin a-induced liver injury," *Biological and Pharmaceutical Bulletin*, July 2009, vol. 32, no. 7, pg. 1215–1219

[50] Barry Ritz et al., "Supplementation with Active Hexose Correlated Compound Increases the Innate Immune Response of Young Mice to Primary Influenza Infection," *Journal of Nutrition*, November 2006, vol. 136, no. 11, pg. 2868–2873

[51] Bisen PS et al., "Lentinus edodes: a macrofungus with pharmacological activities," *Current Medicinal Chemistry*, 2010, vol. 17, no. 22, pg. 2419–2430

[52] Elizabeth Landau, "The 'forbidden fruit' of medicinal mushrooms," *CNN.com*, February 3, 2012

[53] Wu D et al., "Dietary supplementation with white button mushroom enhances natural killer cell activity in C57BL/6 mice," *The Journal of Nutrition*, June 2007, no. 137, vol. 6, pg. 1472–1477

[54] Hashida C et al., "Quantities of agaritine in mushrooms (Agaricus bisporus) and the carcinogenicity of mushroom methanol extracts on the mouse bladder epithelium," *Japanese Journal of Public Health*, June 1990, vol. 37, no. 6, pg. 400–405

[55] Schulzová V et al., "Influence of storage and household processing on the agaritine content of the cultivated Agaricus mushroom," *Food Additives and Contaminants*, September 2002, vol. 19, no. 9, pg. 853–862

[56] Hiromitsu Watanabe, "Beneficial Biological Effects of Miso with Reference to Radiation Injury, Cancer and Hypertension," *Journal of Toxicologic Pathology*, June 2013, vol. 26, no. 2, pg. 91–103

[57] Ohara M et al., "Radioprotective effects of miso (fermented soy bean paste) against radiation in B6C3F1 mice: increased small intestinal crypt survival, crypt lengths and prolongation of average time to death," *Hiroshima Journal of Medical Sciences,* December 2001, vol. 50, no. 4, pg. 83–86; Hiromitsu Watanabe, "Beneficial Biological Effects of Miso with Reference to Radiation Injury, Cancer and Hypertension," *Journal of Toxicologic Pathology*, June 2013, vol. 26, no. 2, pg. 91–103

[58] Gotoh T et al., "Chemoprevention of N-nitroso-N-methylurea-induced rat mammary cancer by miso and tamoxifen, alone and in combination," *Japanese Journal of Cancer Research*, May 1998, vol. 89, no. 5, pg. 487–495; Shiraki K et al., "Inhibition by long-term fermented miso of induction of pulmonary adenocarcinoma by diisopropanolnitrosamine in Wistar rats," *Hiroshima Journal of Medical Sciences*, March 2003, vol. 52, no. 1, pg. 9–13; Ito A et al., "Effects of soy products in reducing risk of spontaneous and neutron-induced liver-tumors in mice," *International Journal of Oncology*, May 1993, vol. 2, no. 5, pg. 773–776; Watanabe H et al., "Influence of concomitant miso or NaCl treatment on induction of gastric tumors by N-methyl-N'-nitro-N-nitrosoguanidine in rats," *Oncology Reports*, Sep–Oct 1999, vol. 6, no. 5, pg. 989–993

[59] Sessa WC, "A new way to lower blood pressure: pass the chili peppers please," *Cell Metabolism*, August 4, 2010, vol. 12, no. 2, pg. 109–110

[60] Akio Mori et al., "Capsaicin, a Component of Red Peppers, Inhibits the Growth of Androgen-Independent, p53 Mutant Prostate Cancer Cells," *Cancer Research*, March 15, 2006, vol. 66, pg. 3222; NH Thoennissen et al., "Capsaicin causes cell-cycle arrest and apoptosis in ER-positive and -negative breast cancer cells by modulating the EGFR/HER-2 pathway," *Oncogene*, January 14, 2010, vol. 29, no. 2, pg. 285–296

[61] P Chaiyata et al., "Effect of chili pepper (Capsicum frutescens) ingestion on plasma glucose response and metabolic rate in Thai women," *Journal of the Medical Association of Thailand*, September 2003, vol. 86, no. 9, pg. 854–860

[62] R Hursel et al., "Thermogenic ingredients and body weight regulation," *International Journal of Obesity*, April 2010, vol. 34, no. 4, pg. 659–669

[63] Mark Sircus, Transdermal Magnesium Therapy: A New Modality for the Maintenance of Health, published by iUniverse, July 2011

[64] Mark Sircus, *Winning the War on Cancer*, published by International Medical Veritas Association Publishing, 2008

[65] KN Prasad et al., "Radiation protection in humans: extending the concept of as low as reasonably achievable (ALARA) from dose to biological damage," *British Journal of Radiology*, February 1, 2004, vol. 77, no. 914, pg. 97–99

[66] LG Korkina et al., "Antioxidant therapy in children affected by irradiation from the Chernobyl nuclear accident," *Biochemical Society Transactions*, August 1993, vol. 21, no. 3, pg. 314

[67] Memorial Sloan-Kettering Cancer Center website, Mskcc.org/cancer-care/herb/alpha-lipoic-acid

[68] Y Omura et al., "Role of mercury (Hg) in resistant infections & effective treatment of Chlamydia trachomatis and Herpes family viral infections (and potential treatment for cancer) by removing localized Hg deposits with Chinese parsley and delivering effective antibiotics using various drug uptake enhancement methods," *Acupuncture and Electro-Therapeutics Research*, 1995, vol. 20, no. 3–4, pg. 195–229

[69] M Aga et al., "Preventive effect of Coriandrum sativum (Chinese parsley) on localized lead deposition in ICR mice," *Journal of Ethnopharmacology*, October 2001, vol. 77, no. 2–3, pg. 203–208

[70] P Delaquis et al., "Antimicrobial activity of individual and mixed fractions of dill, cilantro, coriander and eucalyptus essential oils," *International Journal of Food Microbiology*, March 2002, vol. 74, no. 1–2, pg. 101–109

[71] V Chithra et al., "Coriandrum sativum changes the levels of lipid peroxides and activity of antioxidant enzymes in experimental animals," *Indian Journal of Biochemistry and Biophysics*, February 1999, vol. 36, no. 1, pg. 59–61

[72] Alison Gray et al., "Insulin-releasing and insulin-like activity of the traditional anti-diabetic plant Coriandrum sativum (coriander)," *British Journal of Nutrition*, March 1999, vol. 81, no. 3, pg. 203–209

[73] Mark Sircus, *Winning the War on Cancer*, published by International Medical Veritas Association Publishing, 2008

[74] Ibid.

[75] Mary Queiroz et al., "Effects of chlorella vulgaris extract on cytokines production in listeria monocytogenes infected mice," *Immunopharmacology and Immunotoxicology*, 2002, vol. 24, no. 3, pg. 483–496; Denise Dantas et al., "The Effects of Chlorella Vulgaris in The Protection of Mice Infected With Listeria Monocytogenes. Role of Natural Killer Cells," *Immunopharmacology and Immunotoxicology*, 1999, vol. 21, no. 3, pg. 609–619

[76] R Merchant et al., "Dietary Chlorella pyrenoidosa for patients with malignant glioma: Effects on immunocompetence, quality of life, and survival," *Phytotherapy Research*, December 1990, vol. 4, no. 6, pg. 220–231

[77] KH Cha et al., "Antiproliferative effects of carotenoids extracted from Chlorella ellipsoidea and Chlorella vulgaris on human colon cancer cells," *Journal of Agriculture and Food Chemistry*, November 2008, vol. 56, no. 22, pg. 10521–10526

[78] American Cancer Society website, Cancer.org/Treatment/TreatmentsandSideEffects/ComplementaryandAlternativeMedicine/HerbsVitaminsandMinerals/chlorella

[79] SK Senapati et al., "Effect of garlic (Allium sativum L.) extract on tissue lead level in rats," *Journal of Ethnopharmacology*, August 2001, vol. 76, no. 3, pg. 229–232; MS Hanafy et al., "Effect of garlic on lead contents in chicken tissues," *Deutsche Tierärztliche Wochenschrift*, April 1994, vol. 101, no. 4, pg. 157–158

[80] PF Cavagnaro et al., "Effect of cooking on garlic (Allium sativum L.) antiplatelet activity and thiosulfinates content," *Journal of Agricultural and Food Science*, February 2007, vol. 55, no. 4, pg. 1280–1288

CHAPTER SEVEN

Water

ater is the most abundant molecule within the human body. An adult woman is roughly 55 percent water, an adult man 60 percent, and a baby 78 percent.[1] The brain is roughly 70 percent water, lean muscle tissue 75 percent, the blood 83 percent, and the lungs 90 percent. Each day we must replace approximately 2.4 liters of water—some through drinking, some through food. Water is obviously essential, yet many people overlook water quality. In Europe and North America, most people presume tap water is clean and safe. But is this really the case?

Arsenic, pharmaceutical drug residues, pesticides, and uranium are just some of the many contaminants commonly found in the public water supplies of developed nations. These toxins pollute the water either by accident or oversight. Other toxins such as fluoride and chlorine are added to public water supplies intentionally, for a variety of reasons. Travelers to underdeveloped countries are usually aware of water contamination issues, but many don't realize that developed nations also face serious water quality issues. Gradually and subtly, large populations are being poisoned. This chapter explains what's in our water, how it got there, and what you can do to ensure that you and your family are drinking clean, healthy water.

What's In Our Water?

The Environmental Working Group (EWG) maintains the largest database of US drinking water quality analyses, consisting of more than 20 million tests performed by water utilities since 2004. A three-year study of this data revealed the presence of 316 contaminants in US drinking water, including industrial solvents, factory farm waste, weed killers, refrigerants, and rocket fuel.[2] The US Environmental Protection

Agency (EPA) sets enforceable, maximal levels for only 114 of these contaminants. The other 202 are unregulated, thus posing potentially serious public health risks. Jane Houlihan, EWG's senior vice president for research, observed,

> *"It is not uncommon for people to drink tap water laced with 20 or 30 chemical contaminants. This water may be legal, but it raises serious health concerns."*[3]

Pharmaceuticals

In 2008, the Associated Press (AP) conducted a five-month study concerning pharmaceutical drugs in the US water supply. At least 46 million Americans, they concluded, were drinking water contaminated with drugs, including antibiotics, mood stabilizers, and sex hormones.[4] These drugs enter public water supplies both through the disposal of unused products and human excretion. The AP estimates that hospitals and long-term healthcare facilities dump 250 million pounds of expired or otherwise unwanted pharmaceuticals into the water annually. The US government does not impose safety limits for pharmaceuticals in public water.

Pharmaceutical contamination of public water supplies is also pervasive in Asia, Australia, Canada, Europe, and the UK. In Europe, tests of major population centers in France, Germany, Norway, and Switzerland have linked drug-tainted drinking water to genetic mutations and the spread of antibiotic-resistant germs.[5] In 2008, the UK's Drinking Water Inspectorate released a one hundred-page study, thoroughly detailing the contamination of British public water supplies by chemotherapy and psychiatric drugs.[6] Although the drugs were found at trace levels, researchers were concerned about the risks posed to pregnant women and newborn babies. Also, the cumulative effect of long-term exposure to these drugs is unknown.

Waterborne pharmaceuticals are already causing gender mutations in fish. Female fish are developing male genitalia and male fish are producing egg yolk proteins. Sex ratios are becoming skewed, and scientists have even discovered bass that produce both sperm and eggs.[7] In a landmark seven-year study published in 2007, scientists deliberately laced a pristine Canadian lake with birth control pills in concentrations similar to those found contaminating public water supplies. After just seven weeks, male fathead minnows started producing egg protein, their gonads shrank, and they demonstrated feminized behavior—becoming passive and fighting less. They also stopped reproducing, leading to a near-extinction situation.[8]

Arsenic and Other Contaminants

In 2000, the Natural Resources Defense Council (NRDC), after studying EPA data, determined that at least 56 million Americans were drinking water with unsafe levels of arsenic.[9] The actual number, they noted, was probably much higher because only 25 states were reporting arsenic data at that time. In 1999, the National Academies of Sciences (NAS) also studied the arsenic-tainted water issue, concluding that arsenic in drinking water causes bladder, lung, and skin cancers, and possibly kidney and liver cancers.[10] According to the NAS, arsenic also damages the central and peripheral nervous systems, the heart and blood vessels, and causes serious skin problems.

In 2009, *The New York Times* conducted a similar analysis of federal drinking water data. According to their investigation, more than 20 percent of the nation's water treatment systems violated the US Safe Drinking Water Act over the preceding five years.[11] Water provided to over 49 million people contained illegal levels of arsenic, radioactive substances like uranium, and dangerous sewage bacteria. Regulators were informed of these violations, but the law went unenforced 94 percent of the time. Clearly, even the most advanced industrial nations are facing serious problems with accidental water contamination. But many of these same nations also *intentionally* add known toxins to public water supplies.

Fluoride

Supposedly to prevent dental caries, the US and many other nations add fluoride to public water supplies. Most scientists agree that fluoride works topically, but does it also work systemically? In other words, applying fluoride directly to the teeth helps prevent dental caries, but does ingested fluoride also provide protective benefits? Let's suppose for a moment that it does.

Assuming that ingested fluoride does actually promote dental health, which would you rather drink: a) water containing pure, pharmaceutical-grade sodium fluoride (NaF), or b) water containing an industrial-grade, chemical-waste byproduct of the phosphate fertilizer industry? Toothpaste contains NaF, but your drinking water contains industrial-grade hydrofluorosilicic acid (HFSA), or the sodium salt of that acid (NaSF). These chemicals are not refined for purity and thus contain significant amounts of various chemical contaminants and heavy metals, particularly arsenic.[12] In 2013, *Environmental Science & Policy* published a study comparing treatment costs for lung and bladder cancers associated with HFSA-treated water with the costs of switching to pure, pharmaceutical grade NaF-treated water. The authors concluded that $1 billion to $5 billion dollars per year could be saved, "while simultaneously mitigating the pain and suffering of citizens that result from use of the technical grade fluoridating agents."[13]

How Widespread Is Fluoridation?

Most nations do not fluoridate their drinking water. Fluoridation occurs primarily in the US and certain Commonwealth countries, including the UK, Canada, New Zealand, and Australia. Seventy-four percent of US communities, accounting for 204 million people, have water fluoridation programs.[14] The CDC calls fluoridation "one of the ten greatest public health achievements of the twentieth century," supposedly because it prevents dental caries.[15] With such accolades, one might presume that the countries with the most established and most widespread fluoridation programs, like the US, Australia, and New Zealand, have the best dental health.

The US has been fluoridating drinking water since 1951. Fluoridation began in 1953 in Australia and 1954 in New Zealand, today reaching 80 and 61 percent of those populations, respectively. According to the WHO Global Oral Health Database, the US ranks 55th among 193 countries maintaining DMFT (decayed, missing, filled teeth) records. Australia and New Zealand rank 41st and 76th, respectively.[16] Many nations without water fluoridation programs, like Denmark, Finland, Germany, Switzerland, and the Netherlands, rank much higher. Figure 7.1 shows fluoridation rates by country alongside DMFT rankings.[17] There appears to be no correlation whatsoever between fluoridation coverage and dental health.

Does Fluoride Protect Teeth?

The American Dental Association (ADA) claims that ingested fluoride gradually becomes incorporated into the teeth, subsequently providing "systemic benefits."[18] The entire concept of water fluoridation is built around this premise. If fluoride doesn't work systemically, then adding it to public drinking water makes no sense. According to a 2004 study published in *Caries Research*,

> *"A dogma has existed for many decades, that fluoride has to be ingested and acts mainly pre-eruptively. However, recent studies concerning the systemic effect of fluoride supplementation concluded that the caries-preventive effect of fluoride is almost exclusively posteruptive."*[19]

Decayed, Missing, and Filled Teeth Compared to Fluoridation Rates by Country – Figure 7.1

Country	% Population with Fluoridated Water	Mean DMFT	DMFT Global Ranking
Denmark	0	0.7	21
Finland	0	0.7	22
Germany	0	0.7	23
United Kingdom	10	0.7	24
Hong Kong	100	0.8	26
Switzerland	0	0.8	28
Netherlands	0	0.9	29
Belgium	0	0.9	32
Sweden	0	0.9	38
Australia	80	1.0	41
Singapore	100	1.0	46
Italy	0	1.1	50
South Africa	0	1.1	53
Spain	11	1.1	54
USA	74	1.2	55
France	0	1.2	58
Greece	0	1.4	70
Austria	0	1.4	72
New Zealand	61	1.4	76
Israel*	70	1.7	89
Japan	1	1.7	93
Norway	0	1.7	95
Ireland	73	1.8	98
Chile	71	1.9	105
Canada	44	2.1	116
Brazil	41	2.8	142

* In 2013, the Israeli Supreme Court voted to ban fluoridation, effective 2014.[20]

In other words, topical fluoride applications are effective but ingested fluoride has no benefits. Even the ADA, the most adamant supporter of water fluoridation, has acknowledged this well-established scientific fact. In their own study, published in 2000 in the *Journal of the American Dental Association*, they concluded:

"Fluoride, the key agent in battling caries, works primarily via topical mechanisms ... Fluoride incorporated during tooth development is insufficient to play a significant role in caries protection." [21]

So the ADA's own study says fluoride provides no systemic benefits, but officially, they still claim it does. The CDC is another unwavering adherent of fluoridation. Just like the ADA, the CDC has twice in its own publications acknowledged the overwhelming scientific evidence against systemic efficacy. According to the CDC,

"The laboratory and epidemiologic research suggests that fluoride prevents dental caries predominately after eruption of the tooth into the mouth, and its actions primarily are topical for both adults and children." [22]

Systemic efficacy is the foundational premise justifying the fluoridation of public water. As the science against ingested fluoride becomes increasingly unambiguous, prominent fluoride enthusiasts are increasingly defending the indefensible. And yet, paradoxically, they are acknowledging the science against systemic efficacy while maintaining their steadfast support for water fluoridation. As Dr. Arvid Carlsson, a recipient of the Nobel Prize in Medicine and Physiology, observed,

"In pharmacology, if the effect is local [topical], it's awkward to use it in any other way than as a local treatment. I mean this is obvious. You have the teeth there, they're available for you, why drink the stuff?" [23]

The inclusion of fluoride in toothpaste, mouthwash and other topical applications makes sense, assuming these products are not accidentally swallowed. But ingesting fluoride is misguided and dangerous, especially considering its side effects.

What Are The Effects Of Fluoride?

The acute toxicity of fluoride is slightly higher than that of lead and slightly lower than that of arsenic. This is one reason why pesticides and rat poisoning products are largely comprised of fluoride. This is also why fluoridated toothpaste and mouthwash products carry poison control warnings. By FDA mandate, these products must bear the following warning: "If you accidentally swallow more than used for brushing, seek professional help or contact a poison control center immediately."[24] Fluoride is a chronic and cumulative toxin. Small doses gradually accumulate within the body, eventually threatening many organs. The primary health concerns are detailed below.

Musculoskeletal system

Fluoride has been shown to directly cause osteoarthritis at levels as low as 6 mg/day.[25] A 2003 large-scale Chinese study demonstrated this convincingly.[26] The EPA has set a maximum contaminant level goal (MCLG) for fluoride of 4 milligrams per liter or 4 ppm. The MCLG is "the level of contaminants in drinking water at which no adverse health effects are likely to occur."[27] The EPA notes, "Some people who drink water containing fluoride in excess of the MCL over many years could get bone disease (including pain and tenderness of the bones); children may get mottled teeth." Obviously different people consume different amounts of water. In the US, tap water contains fluoride ranging from 0.7 to 1.2 ppm.[28] According to the Department of Health and Human Services, adults in fluoridated communities ingest between 1.6 and 6.6 mg of fluoride daily, easily enough to promote osteoarthritis.[29] Furthermore, according to the National Research Council (NRC), "Life-long exposure to fluoride at the MCLG of 4 mg/L may have the potential to induce stage II or stage III skeletal fluorosis and may increase the risk of fracture."[30]

Brain function

According to the EPA, fluoride is a developmental neurotoxin.[31] Also the NRC, in its comprehensive review of the scientific literature on fluoride, noted, "On the basis of information largely derived from histological, chemical, and molecular studies, it is apparent that fluorides have the ability to interfere with the functions of the brain and the body by direct and indirect means."[32] The NRC acknowledges the possibility that fluoride decreases intellectual capacity including IQ, problem solving, and short and long-term memory.

By 2012, forty-two studies had been conducted concerning fluoride and human intelligence, and seventeen studies on fluoride and learning/memory in animals. Thirty-six of the forty-two human studies linked fluoride to reduced IQ and sixteen of the seventeen animal studies demonstrated impaired learning and memory.[33] In 2012, researchers from the Harvard School of Public Health and the China Medical University in Shenyang published a first-of-its-kind meta-analysis of twenty-seven studies concerning fluoride and cognitive development.[34] Fluoride, they determined, can impair neurodevelopment, including IQ reductions of seven points. Anna Choi, the study's lead research commented, "Fluoride exposure to the developing brain, which is much more susceptible to injury caused by toxicants than is the mature brain, may possibly lead to damage of a permanent nature."[35] Senior author Philippe

Grandjean remarked, "Fluoride seems to fit in with lead, mercury, and other poisons that cause chemical brain drain. The effect of each toxicant may seem small, but the combined damage on a population scale can be serious, especially because the brain power of the next generation is crucial to all of us."[36]

Endocrine system

Fluoride damages many hormone-producing glands and organs, including the pancreas, pineal gland, thyroid gland, and parathyroid gland. According to the NRC, fluoride is "an endocrine disruptor in the broad sense of altering normal endocrine function or response."[37] The principal regulator of thyroid function is thyroid-stimulating hormone (TSH). The NRC specifically acknowledges fluoride's capacity to elevate TSH, increase calcitonin activity, increase parathyroid hormone activity, cause secondary hyperparathyroidism, impair glucose tolerance, and alter the timing of sexual maturity.[38] Regarding the pineal gland, which produces melatonin and is associated with mysticism and spiritual development, the NRC notes, "Fluoride is likely to cause decreased melatonin production and to have other effects on normal pineal function, which in turn could contribute to a variety of effects in humans."[39]

Carcinogenicity

In 2005, a highly publicized case of scientific misconduct elicited fresh attention and awareness regarding the link between fluoridated water and a rare bone cancer called osteosarcoma. The EWG accused Dr. Chester Douglass, a prominent Harvard School of Dental Medicine researcher, of misrepresenting a then-unpublished paper concerning bone cancer and fluoridated water in his written testimony to the NRC.[40] Douglass ignored research conducted by his doctoral student Elise Bassin showing a fivefold increase in osteosarcoma among boys drinking fluoridated water compared to boys drinking non-fluoridated water. According to Bassin's study, later published in the journal *Cancer Causes and Control*, this association is greatest among boys six to eight years of age, but does not apply to girls.[41]

Bassin's observed, gender-specific effect is consistent with other fluoride studies. In 1977, the US Congress commissioned the National Toxicology Program (NTP) to study the carcinogenicity of fluoride. The NTP conducted extensive animal testing during the 1980s before publishing their results in 1990. They observed a statistically significant, dose-dependent increase in bone cancer rates among male rats ingesting fluoride. Nevertheless, the NTP report characterized fluoride carcinogenicity as only "biologically plausible," and supported by "equivocal evidence."[42] Many scientists, such as William Marcus, a senior science advisor in the office of drinking water at the EPA, protested the NTP's conclusions while questioning their methodology.[43]

In response to the NTP report, the National Cancer Institute (NCI) published a study acknowledging that osteosarcoma rates among young males are indeed higher in fluoridated communities than in non-fluoridated communities. But according to the NCI, this correlation is "not linked to the fluoridation of water supplies."[44] The New Jersey Department of Health later conducted its own osteosarcoma study. Though small and limited, their study observed a statistically significant relationship between fluoridated water consumption and osteosarcoma among males under 20. According to the authors, the findings did not support halting fluoridation programs, "but do support the importance of investigating the possible link between osteosarcoma and overall ingestion of fluoride."[45] During the ensuing years, government agencies and pro-fluoridation advocates have continually downplayed the evidence linking osteosarcoma with fluoride consumption among young males. The NRC, to its credit, has at least acknowledged fluoride's carcinogenic potential. In their latest assessment, from 2006, the NRC concluded, "Fluoride appears to have the potential to initiate or promote cancers, particularly of the bone, but the evidence to date is tentative and mixed."[46]

Chlorine

Ninety-eight percent of US water utilities chlorinate drinking water.[47] Chlorine effectively kills microbial waterborne pathogens, including cholera, typhoid fever, dysentery, and Legionnaires' disease. Despite its merits, chlorine has many risks. Many studies show, for example, that chlorinated water promotes bladder cancer.[48] The risks of chlorinated water come not from chlorine itself, but from disinfection byproducts—chemical compounds formed when disinfectants like chlorine react with naturally occurring organic matter within water. A meta-analysis published in 1992 by the *American Journal of Public Health* demonstrated a positive association between chlorination byproducts in water and bladder and rectal cancers in humans.[49]

Chlorine poses many other health risks besides just cancer. Although relatively few toxicological/epidemiological studies have been conducted concerning its effects on reproductive health, the scant literature does show a positive association with low birth weights, spontaneous abortions, stillbirths, and certain types of birth defects.[50] A study published in 2003 by *Occupational Environmental Medicine* identified chlorine exposure via swimming pools as a potential cause of childhood asthma and allergies.[51] The risks of chlorination, according to many studies, are highest from showering, bathing, and swimming in chlorinated water.[52]

Showering involves inhalation and dermal exposure. Showering in chlorinated water results in higher chlorine exposure than drinking chlorinated water. A Rutgers University study, for example, calculated that one ten-minute shower is equivalent to drinking nearly two liters of chlorinated water, in terms of chlorine exposure.[53] Safe alternatives to chlorine include UV disinfection and ozone.[54] These alternatives, however, have their own limitations and are generally less effective than chlorine at neutralizing pathogens. Chlorination, therefore, makes sense because its benefits outweigh its risks. Nevertheless, we should always use filters to reduce our chlorine exposure for cooking, drinking, and showering water.

Lithium: The Next Great Hope?

Chatter has increased during the past several years regarding lithium, a psychiatric drug prescribed for depression, mania, and bipolar disorder. A dangerous trend has emerged, as numerous experts and public health officials are calling for lithium to be added to public water supplies. Allegedly, such measures would help prevent suicides. Lithium advocates cite several key studies to support their mass-drugging ambitions. For example, a 1990 study of twenty-seven counties in Texas determined,

> *"The incidence rates of suicide, homicide, and rape are significantly higher in counties whose drinking water supplies contain little or no lithium than in counties with water lithium levels ranging from 70–170 micrograms/L."*[55]

A 2009 study published in the *British Journal of Psychiatry* analyzing suicide rates in 18 Japanese communities with low levels of naturally occurring lithium concluded,

> *"These findings suggest that even very low levels of lithium in drinking water may play a role in reducing suicide risk within the general population."*[56]

And a 2011 study examining all 99 districts of Austria drew the same conclusions:

> *"In replicating and extending previous results, this study provides strong evidence that geographic regions with higher natural lithium concentrations in drinking water are associated with lower suicide mortality rates."*[57]

Scores of psychiatrists and bioethicists are lobbying politicians to take action on lithium. All health-conscious people and civil rights activists should remain vigilant. Public water supplies tend to inspire dangerous social engineering fantasies. Even the Obama administration's top science and technology advisor, John Holdren, once wrote about the possibility of "adding a sterilant to drinking water or staple foods" to help regulate population levels, provided it could be "uniformly effective, despite widely varying doses received by individuals, and despite varying degrees of fertility and sensitivity among individuals."[58] Clearly the challenges of obtaining clean and healthy water are complex and multifaceted. So what is the solution?

BPA and Bottled Water

Tap water is contaminated and generally unfit for daily, long-term consumption. As an alternative, many people turn to bottled water, which is a practical short-term solution and indeed generally much better than tap water. Bottled water, however, also has serious drawbacks. For example, many people switch to bottled water for drinking water while still using tap water for cooking. Conceivably, you could buy enough bottled water for all your drinking and cooking purposes, but this would quickly become expensive, logistically impractical, and environmentally straining. Another major concern regarding bottled water is the chemicals contained in plastic bottles, which leach into the water. You could of course purchase glass bottles, but this again would quickly become very expensive, impractical, and wasteful. Effective, high-quality home water filters are the best solutions. And while drinking water from plastic bottles occasionally is harmless, you should understand the associated risks.

What Is BPA?

Bisphenol A (BPA) is an industrial chemical used to manufacture polycarbonate plastics and epoxy resins. Polycarbonate plastic applications include water bottles, other food and drink containers, food storage containers, and baby bottles. Epoxy resins are lacquers used to coat metallic food cans and bottle tops. With 2.2 million tons produced annually, BPA is one of the world's most prolific chemicals.[59] BPA was first synthesized in 1891 by a Russian chemist. Since the 1930s, scientists have known that BPA exhibits estrogen-like properties and interferes with numerous hormonal processes. Nevertheless, during the 1940s the chemical industry started using BPA to make plastic food containers stronger and more resilient. By the 1960s, BPA was widespread and completely unregulated.

In 1976 the US passed the Toxic Substances Control Act, the country's first-ever attempt to regulate industrial chemicals. Though tasked with protecting the public from dangerous and potentially carcinogenic substances, the act excluded some 62,000 existing chemicals, including BPA. Since 1976, an additional 22,000 chemicals have legally entered the marketplace without testing for health and public safety.[60] Many of these chemicals have since been linked to various types of cancer as well as hormonal, reproductive, and immune system damage. According to the NRDC,

"The law is widely considered to be a failure and, most recently, the EPA's own Inspector General found it inadequate to ensure that new chemicals are safe."[61]

Finally in 1982, after studying BPA toxicity, the National Toxicology Program set the lowest adverse effect level (LOAEL) to 50 micrograms per kilogram of body weight per day (50 mcg/kg/d).[62] In 1988, the EPA (and by extension, the FDA) adopted this safety standard. Despite a steady flow of scientific studies demonstrating harm caused by low-dose BPA exposure, the EPA and FDA have remained loyal to the chemical industry at the expense of public health.

What Are The Effects Of BPA?

By 2005, over 150 studies had been published regarding the effects of low-dose BPA exposure. Of the twelve studies published by the chemical industry, none showed BPA risks. Of the 139 government-funded studies, 128 showed many adverse effects including breast and prostate cancers, reduced sperm count, obesity, diabetes, early onset of puberty, and other serious medical problems.[63] Fluoride, as discussed above, particularly threatens young boys, whereas BPA seems to be more aggressive towards girls. But both chemicals pose serious health threats to both sexes.

According to a 2011 study published in *Pediatrics*, higher gestational BPA exposure can cause increased rates of hyperactivity, anxiety, and depression. The researchers identified this association for girls but not for boys. While acknowledging that more research is required, the study advises "concerned patients to reduce their exposure to certain consumer products."[64]

BPA has also been linked to female infertility. A 2009 study conducted by Yale University researchers found that BPA damages a specific gene responsible for female fertility in mice. The uterine linings of BPA-exposed mice fail to develop properly, thus decreasing their ability to carry pregnancies to term. The gene in question, HOXA10, is the same in mice and humans.[65] Hugh Taylor, the study's co-author and chief of reproductive endocrinology at the Yale School of Medicine, asserted, "We've discovered the exact mechanism by which BPA affects this gene."[66] Although the study tested mice at exposure levels higher than those typically affecting humans, Taylor lamented,

> *"It's troubling that the changes are permanent and irreversible. I don't want to say that at typical human exposure, there's clear and present danger, but there's enough concern that there might be to warrant further investigation."*[67]

Plenty of scientific research has in fact already been conducted. The following is a brief encapsulation of BPA's risks according to published research:

- BPA disrupts/inverts sexual differentiation, induces hyperactivity, and increases aggression.[68]

- At exposure levels forty times lower than the EPA's 1993 safe levels, BPA causes altered maternal behavior in mice, including reduced nursing time.[69]

- Low-dose, chronic exposure to BPA causes insulin resistance in adult mice, leading to type 2 diabetes, hypertension, and cardiovascular disease.[70]

- Low-dose BPA exposure promotes the early onset of puberty.[71]

- Even at extremely low doses, BPA causes aneuploidy, a cell division error that causes 10 to 20 percent of all birth defects, including Down syndrome.[72]

- Low-dose BPA exposure decreases testosterone levels, fertility, and daily sperm production in both developmental and adult male mice.[73]

- Low-dose BPA exposure stimulates mammary gland development, a likely precursor to breast cancer.[74]

- Low-dose BPA exposure increases prostate size, promoting prostate cancer.[75]

- BPA damages the immune system.[76]

BPA Research and Chicanery

The chemical industry has always maintained that BPA is completely safe. And yes, according to their research, it is. But industry-funded studies use toxicological testing procedures established five decades ago. The fallacy of their methodology is the presumption that high-dose effects accurately predict low-dose effects. Regarding hormones (as well as synthetic hormone mimickers), however, this is not always the case. Low doses of synthetic hormones can indeed cause damage not caused at higher doses. In 1997, a team of researchers led by biologist Frederick vom Saal published the first study confirming the dangers of low-dose BPA exposure (twenty-five times lower than the EPA's established *safe* level).[77]

In the late 1990s, when vom Saal was beginning his research, several revelations concerning BPA exposure for babies were drawing considerable public attention. In 1997, for example, an FDA study found widespread contamination of canned baby formula, with BPA levels exceeding those already shown to cause developmental harm.[78] Two years later, a *Consumer Reports* study demonstrated that baby bottles, when heated, were leaching unsafe levels of BPA. The FDA was forced to respond. Their response, however, was a prompt reconfirmation of BPA safety. FDA product policy director George Pauli stated,

> *"Our conclusion is we should go with the track record. We have evaluated in a thorough manner, and concluded its use is safe. We haven't seen anything that would persuade us to change that."[79]*

This patronizing attitude, attempting to pacify the public, even presuming that ordinary people cannot read scientific journals, would foreshadow the FDA's entire regulatory history of BPA. The FDA has been extremely nonchalant towards BPA research. Perhaps they are simply buying time for the chemical industry, enabling them to develop alternative plastics ahead of an inevitable BPA ban. But according to the FDA mandate, "FDA is responsible for protecting the public health by assuring that foods are safe, wholesome, sanitary and properly labeled."[80] BPA's regulatory history, however, suggests that industry profits take precedence over public health.

By 2003, the US government finally began its first official low-dose BPA study. The National Institutes of Health (NIH), after nominating BPA for evaluation as a potential reproductive and developmental toxin, proceeded to hire chemical industry contractor Sciences International Inc. (SII) to lead the assessment. SII, along with the Center for the Evaluation of Risk to Human Reproduction (CERHR), handpicked fifteen scientists to serve on the government's expert advisory panel. These scientists would review SII's assessments and recommendations. SII and CERHR deliberately excluded all scientists with BPA expertise, claiming this would prevent the review process from becoming biased. In 2006, CERHR finally published the government's conclusions. Not surprisingly, they concluded that BPA is completely safe and should not be regulated.

In 2007, a *Los Angeles Times* investigation revealed SII's dirty laundry concerning their ostensibly independent investigation. Of particular concern was the fact that SII was being funded by over fifty chemical companies, including Dow Chemical and BASF, both major manufacturers of BPA.[81] This revelation sparked investigations regarding the obvious conflicts of interest. The NIH later fired SII, but continued recognizing their study as sound.[82] This prompted a chorus of protests from many independent scientists and advocacy groups. Leading BPA experts soon identified 297 errors and inconsistencies within the government's BPA report.[83]

Following the SII debacle, the government commissioned a new BPA study. The NIH funded thirty-eight of the world's leading BPA experts to assess its overall risk potential. In 2007, these scientists concluded that the average BPA levels detected in humans are above those known to cause significant damage in animals. The scientists expressed concern that BPA had been contributing to the following disease trends:

> *"...increase in prostate and breast cancer, uro-genital abnormalities in male babies, a decline in semen quality in men, early onset of puberty in girls, metabolic disorders including insulin resistant (type 2) diabetes and obesity, and neurobehavioral problems such as attention deficit hyperactivity disorder (ADHD)."*[84]

In 2008, following the NIH study, the US House Committee on Energy and Commerce launched a major BPA investigation, culminating in demands that the FDA reveal the basis of its BPA safety assertions. The FDA finally acknowledged its safety standards had been based on two studies, both sponsored by the American Plastics Council, one of which was unpublished and unavailable to the public. The other study was highly criticized by independent BPA experts. Shortly thereafter, the National Toxicology Program released their own assessment statement, aligning themselves with the overwhelming evidence linking low-dose BPA exposure to early puberty, breast cancer, prostate problems, and behavioral problems. This, along with a concurrent statement by the Canadian government classifying BPA as a "dangerous substance," prompted the US Congress to once again demand that the FDA reassess its safety standards.

Just days later, major manufacturers and retailers (including Toy "R" Us and Walmart) announced they would voluntarily begin phasing out baby bottles made with BPA. Several months later, the FDA released a draft statement reconfirming BPA safety. But the FDA's Science Board Subcommittee would have to approve this draft before it could be considered a definitive statement. Ultimately the Science

Board rejected the FDA's draft assessment and demanded a new assessment, one that would fully consider infant exposure and low-dose exposure studies. During the next several years, while the FDA casually reconsidered its position, numerous state and city legislatures passed BPA bans, despite furious industry protests.

Governments Acting Against BPA

Japan has perhaps been the most proactive nation regarding BPA. In 1998, Japan's canning industry voluntarily began phasing out BPA epoxy resin linings. Today, BPA is virtually nonexistent in canned foods manufactured in Japan. The results have been impressive. BPA urine concentrations have decreased dramatically compared to 1992 levels.[85] Europe and North America have acted much more lackadaisically. In these nations, early regulatory action has focused solely on BPA exposure to babies.

In 2008, Canada became the first country to ban BPA from baby bottles. Based on a meta-analysis of 150 studies, Canada's National Toxicology Program determined that BPA mimics estrogen and can cause cancer.[86] Canada's regulatory decision drew fierce challenges from the American Chemistry Council (ACC), a group that to this day still insists on BPA's safety, despite voluminous evidence to the contrary. It was primarily the ACC's formal complaint filed in June 2009 that delayed further BPA regulatory action. Finally in October 2010, Canada officially declared BPA a toxic chemical. In response, both the ACC and the European Union's food safety watchdog issued statements insisting BPA is safe.[87] Finally in late 2010, the EU bowed to public outcry over the mounting body of scientific evidence against BPA and subsequently outlawed the chemical in baby bottles effective June 2011.[88]

In characteristic fashion, the US preserved big-business interests as long as they possibly could. In 2008, following Canada's BPA baby bottle ban, the FDA convened a special subcommittee to reassess BPA safety. They concluded that BPA is entirely safe for babies and the Canadian government was merely acting "out of an abundance of caution."[89] By July 2012, the EU, Canada, China, Malaysia, and South Africa all had implemented BPA baby bottle bans. The US sat on the sidelines year after year, as if subserviently waiting for the chemical industry to voluntarily change its course. In October 2011, the ACC finally announced that manufacturers would voluntarily stop using BPA for baby bottles and infant cups. The ACC later requested a formal BPA ban, which the FDA dutifully implemented in July 2012.

According to both the industry and the FDA, this ban was only to quell concerns and confusion, not because BPA poses any actual threats. The ACC's Steven Hentges explained,

> *"Although governments around the world continue to support the safety of BPA in food contact materials, confusion about whether BPA is used in baby bottles and sippy cups had become an unnecessary distraction to consumers, legislators and state regulators."*[90]

FDA spokesperson Curtis Allen wholeheartedly concurred,

> *"We agree that BPA has been abandoned by industry in baby bottles and sippy cups, and as such we have moved to ban it going forward in those two products, but we still believe that overall BPA is a safe product."*[91]

Despite Canada's progressive actions in identifying BPA health risks for babies, the Canadian government has not yet implemented an outright ban. They claim, "Current dietary exposure to BPA through food packaging is not expected to pose a health risk to the general population."[92] Most European governments have taken a similar position. The tide however, is slowly turning. In 2012, Sweden announced a BPA ban for all canned food intended for children three years of age and younger.[93] And most significantly, in December 2012, France approved an outright ban on all BPA food packaging effective 2015.[94]

How to Avoid BPA

BPA is extremely pervasive. According to a Canadian government study, 91 percent of Canadians test positive for BPA in their urine.[95] A similar study conducted by the CDC showed 93 percent of Americans testing positive.[96] BPA exposure is not limited to food packaging. In 2010, the Washington Toxics Coalition, a prominent nonprofit organization, issued a report titled *On the Money: BPA on Dollar Bills and Receipts*. According to the report, about half of all retail receipts contain BPA in large quantities (about 2.2 percent of total weight). BPA is not chemically bound to receipts and thus transfers quickly and easily to hands and other objects.[97] The report also tested dollar bills and found that 95 percent of those sampled tested positive for BPA, though at levels much lower than cash register receipts.

To limit BPA exposure, avoid buying water and all other foods and beverages contained in plastic. Canned tomatoes are particularly high in BPA, as the acidity of the tomatoes causes increased BPA leaching.[98] With increasing consumer demand for

BPA-free products, more and more companies are introducing BPA-free containers. Coconut milk and sardines, two products traditionally sold in BPA-epoxy-resin-lined metallic cans, are increasingly available in health-conscious containers, free of BPA. Also, the Eden company now sells preservative-free beans in BPA-free cans. If you don't see "BPA-free" on your canned food and plastic bottle labels, you can reasonably assume they do contain BPA. Luckily, consumers in France will soon be alleviated of this burden. Hopefully the US and other nations will promptly follow suit. Until then, we can avoid BPA as much as possible, lobby our governments to outlaw it, and proactively inform ourselves about its likely replacements.

Unfortunately, BPA alternatives are not necessarily safe. The industry and the government bureaucracies that brought us BPA are now promoting bisphenol S (BPS) as an ideal alternative. A recent study, however, exposed rats to very low levels of BPS and found it also disrupts hormones.[99] Rene Vinas, one of the University of Texas researchers involved with the study, commented, "We didn't think it would have those effects, but it's essentially the same as BPA."[100]

Recourse Through Filtration

Since most people don't have access to pure mountain spring water, municipal tap water and bottled water are their two primary water options. By now, it should be abundantly clear that neither source is viable since both promote long-term disease. The best option is therefore some type of home filtration system. Many people waste their money on cheap filters, which yield ineffective results. While any filter is better than none, some are decidedly better than others. A little research goes a long way when considering which filter to purchase, both for your health and your finances. Most water filters utilize one or more of the following five technologies.

Carbon Filtration

Usually derived from charcoal, activated carbon has an extremely high internal porosity, and thus an amazing absorptive capacity. With innumerable low-volume micropores, activated carbon also has an extremely high internal surface area. The surface area for 1 gram ranges between 500 and 1500 square meters.[101] Carbon filters effectively remove volatile organic compounds and chlorination byproducts, such as trihalomethanes (THMs). Additionally, high-quality carbon filters remove pathogens, bacteria, viruses, and 95 percent or more of heavy metals. Carbon filters typically do not remove salts, minerals, or dissolved inorganic compounds.

Kinetic Degradation Fluxion (KDF)

KDF technology uses a basic chemical process called redox (reduction along with oxidation) to neutralize chlorine, pesticides, organic matter, lead, mercury, iron, and hydrogen sulfide. During a redox reaction, electrons transfer between molecules, thus creating new elements. For example, when free chlorine contacts the filtration media, it changes into benign, water-soluble chloride, which is too large to evaporate or be absorbed by the skin. KDF is typically used in conjunction with carbon filtration. KDF is the primary technology used for shower filters.

Reverse Osmosis (RO)

Originally developed by the US Navy to convert seawater into drinking water for submarine crews, RO technology works by forcing water through an extremely fine, semipermeable membrane. Like a microscopic sieve, the membrane filters out almost all contaminants, including heavy metals, pesticides, volatile organic compounds, and microorganisms. Though RO cannot remove chlorine, modern RO systems combine membrane technology with both carbon and mechanical filtration to produce highly purified, chlorine-free water. RO technology also removes beneficial trace minerals, a source of unresolved controversy in the world of water filtration.

Distillation

The oldest form of water purification, distillation works by boiling water and then collecting the evaporating steam. Distillers remove most contaminants but they fail to remove volatile chemicals with low boiling points. Distilled water is pure, but it usually tastes flat. Like RO, distilled water systems typically work in conjunction with carbon filters. Also like RO, distilled water is stripped of beneficial minerals.

Ionization

According to water ionizer manufacturers, these products create alkaline water through a process called electrolysis. By introducing negatively and positively charged electrodes into water, the atoms give or receive electrons, thereby causing the water to become more acid or more alkaline. This technology is expensive and somewhat dubious, especially considering the absence of scientific research supporting the lofty claims of its adherents.

Demineralized Water

Both distillation and RO produce demineralized water, which is controversial and potentially problematic. Such water has total dissolved solids (TDS) lower than 50 mg/L. Consequently, RO and distilled water can be acidic, meaning the pH is lower than 7. Long-term consumption of RO and otherwise demineralized water may negatively affect homeostasis mechanisms and could compromise mineral and water metabolism in the body.[102] According to human and animal studies conducted by the WHO, demineralized water causes: 1) increased diuresis (increased urine by roughly 20 percent), increased body water volume, and increased serum sodium concentrations, 2) decreased serum potassium concentrations, and 3) increased elimination of sodium, potassium, chloride, calcium, and magnesium ions from the body.[103]

The German Society for Nutrition has drawn similar conclusions. In a position paper from 1993, they asserted that demineralized water requires the intestines to relinquish electrolytes (sodium and potassium, for example) from body reserves. Since the body never eliminates fluids as pure water but always together with salts, adequate intake of electrolytes must be ensured. Ingestion of demineralized water dilutes the body's electrolytes. Symptoms can include headaches and fatigue, and can progress to muscle cramps and impaired heart rate.[104] Other problems arise from cooking with demineralized water. Multiple studies have demonstrated significant mineral losses from food cooked with demineralized water, including upwards of 60 percent losses of magnesium and calcium and even higher losses for microelements like copper, manganese, and cobalt. Conversely, cooking in mineralized water results in far lower mineral losses.[105]

In Support Of RO

The physiological effects of consuming low-TDS water are not definitively known. Very little scientific research has been conducted. The WHO hosts on its website a 2004 draft review of the scientific literature with unofficial guidelines.[106] This review presents low-TDS water as decidedly problematic and unhealthy. The Water Quality Association (WQA), an international trade association representing the residential, commercial, and industrial water treatment industries, has heavily criticized this WHO report, claiming its conclusions are based on dubious studies.[107] Observational data does tend to support the WQA's contention that low-TDS water is safe. The US Navy, for example, has for decades been using distilled water with less than 3 mg/L of TDS for drinking water aboard ships with no reported ill effects. Also many large US cities have water with naturally low TDS levels, less than 100 mg/L. These cities include Boston, Portland, San Francisco, and Seattle. Thus far, there have been no studies demonstrating health problems particular to residents of these cities.

Filter Recommendations

Each filtration system has its own pros and cons. Cost, of course, can be a serious consideration, as RO filters are generally much more expensive than carbon filters. The acidity of RO water due to mineral loss is another issue to consider. Some RO manufacturers are combining RO filtration with other technologies, including carbon filtration and special post-filtration mechanisms, which add minerals back into the water, thus resulting in completely clean, alkalized water. This method for alkalizing water is different from the ionization technology discussed above.

Cheap filters like Brita remove chlorine but cannot handle pathogens, herbicides, pesticides, aluminum, arsenic, fluoride, lead, and volatile organic compounds. My personal preferences are RO and Berkey carbon filters. I recently started using an RO system and am thoroughly satisfied. On the other hand, I used Berkey filters for years and was always satisfied. Berkey filters require no under-counter installation, nor any faucet attachments. You simply pour tap water (or even non-potable water) into the stainless-steel housing and filtered water starts trickling through. Berkey systems have optional additional filters that effectively remove arsenic and fluoride. Berkey also manufactures shower filters using KDF technology, which converts chlorine into harmless chloride. There are certainly other quality filters on the market, including many excellent RO systems. With the information above and some simple research, you can determine which filter best suits your needs and your budget.

Notes

[1] US Department of the Interior, US Geological Survey, *The Water in You*, Ga.water.usgs.gov/edu/propertyyou.html

[2] Taryn Luntz, "U.S. Drinking Water Widely Contaminated," *Scientific American*, December 14, 2009; EWG's Drinking Water Quality Analysis and Tap Water Database, Ewg.org/tap-water/home

[3] Taryn Luntz, "U.S. Drinking Water Contaminated," *Scientific American*, December 14, 2009

[4] Jeff Donn et al., "Health facilities flush estimated 250M pounds of drugs a year," *USA Today* via *Associated Press*, September 14, 2008

[5] Ibid.

[6] Richard Gray, "Cancer drugs found in tap water," *London Telegraph*, January 13, 2008

[7] Jeff Donn and Martha Mendoza, "Drug residue tainting fish," *The Press Democrat* via *Associated Press*, March 11, 2008

[8] Ibid.

[9] Natural Resources Defense Council, Arsenic in Drinking Water; Nrdc.org/water/drinking/qarsenic.asp

[10] National Research Council, *Arsenic in Drinking Water*, published by the National Academy Press, 1999

[11] Charles Duhigg, "Millions in U.S. Drink Dirty Water, Records Show," *New York Times*, December 7, 2009

[12] J Hirzy et al., "Comparison of hydrofluorosilicic acid and pharmaceutical sodium fluoride as fluoridating agents—A cost–benefit analysis," *Environmental Science & Policy*, May 2013, vol. 29, pg. 81–86

[13] Ibid.

[14] Centers for Disease Control, 2010 Water Fluoridation Statistics, Cdc.gov/fluoridation/statistics/2010stats.htm

[15] Centers for Disease Control, "Ten Great Public Health Achievements—United States, 1900–1999," *MMWR Weekly*, April 2, 1999, vol. 48, no. 2, pg. 241–243

[16] WHO Collaborating Centre for Education, Training and Research in Oral Health, Oral Health Country/Area Profile Project, Malmö University, Sweden, Mah.se/CAPP/

[17] British Fluoridation Society, One in a Million: the facts about water fluoridation, 3rd edition, March 2012, Bfsweb.org/onemillion/onemillion2012.html

[18] ADA Division of Communications, "Fluoride: Nature's cavity fighter," *Journal of the American Dental Association*, December 2005, vol. 136, pg. 1783

[19] E Hellwig et al., "Systemic versus topical fluoride," *Caries Research*, May–June 2004, vol. 38, no. 3, pg. 258–262

[20] "Israeli Supreme Court Backs Work of Irish Scientist on Fluoride," *Hot Press*, August 6, 2013

[21] John Featherstone, "The Science and Practice of Caries Prevention," *The Journal of the American Dental Association*, July 2000, vol. 131, no. 7, pg. 887–899

[22] Centers for Disease Control, "Achievements in Public Health, 1900–1999: Fluoridation of Drinking Water to Prevent Dental Caries," *MMWR Weekly*, October 22, 1999, vol. 48, no. 41, pg. 933–940; Centers for Disease Control, "Recommendations for Using Fluoride to Prevent and Control Dental Caries in the United States," *MMWR Recommendations and Reports*, August 17, 2001, vol. 50, no. RR14, pg. 1–42

[23] Paul Connet, The Case Against Fluoride: How Hazardous Waste Ended Up in Our Drinking Water and the Bad Science and Powerful Politics That Keep it There, published by Chelsea Green Publishing, 2010, pg. 14

[24] American Dental Association, "Statement on FDA Toothpaste Warning Labels," July 19, 1997, Ada.org/1761.aspx

[25] Su Wei-min et al., "Total hip arthroplasty for the treatment of severe hip osteoarthritis due to fluorosis," *Chinese Journal of Tissue Engineering Research*, February 26, 2012, vol. 16, no. 9, pg. 1543; S Savas et al., "Endemic fluorosis in Turkish patients: relationship with knee osteoarthritis," *Rheumatology International*, September 2001, vol. 21, no. 1, pg. 30–35; Czerwinski E et al., "Bone and joint pathology in fluoride-exposed workers," *Archives of Environmental Health*, 1988, vol. 43, no. 5, pg. 340–343

[26] Bao W et al., "Report of investigations on adult hand osteoarthritis in Fengjiabao Village, Asuo Village, and Qiancheng Village," *Chinese Journal of Endemiology*, November 2003, vol. 22, no. 6, pg. 517–518

[27] United States Environmental Protection Agency, Basic Information about Fluoride in Drinking Water, Water.epa.gov/drink/contaminants/basicinformation/fluoride.cfm

[28] Centers for Disease Control, My Water's Fluoride, Apps.nccd.cdc.gov/MWF/Index.asp

[29] Paul Connet, The Case Against Fluoride: How Hazardous Waste Ended Up in Our Drinking Water and the Bad Science and Powerful Politics That Keep it There, published by Chelsea Green Publishing, 2010, pg. 159

[30] National Research Council, Committee on Fluoride in Drinking Water, *Fluoride in Drinking Water: A Scientific Review of EPA's Standards*, published by the National Academies Press, 2006, pg. 179

[31] SJ Padilla et al., "Building a Database of Developmental Neurotoxitants: Evidence from Human and Animal Studies," presented at Society of Toxicology Annual Meeting, Baltimore, MD, March 15–19, 2009

[32] National Research Council, Committee on Fluoride in Drinking Water, *Fluoride in Drinking Water: A Scientific Review of EPA's Standards*, published by the National Academies Press, 2006, pg. 223

[33] Michael Connett and Tara Blank, "Fluoride & Intelligence: The 36 Studies," *Fluoride Action Network*, December 9, 2012

[34] Anna Choi et al., "Developmental Fluoride Neurotoxicity: A Systematic Review and Meta-Analysis," *Environmental Health Perspectives*, July 2012, vol. 120, pg. 1362–1368

[35] Reuters PR Newswire, "Harvard Study Finds Fluoride Lowers IQ," July 24, 2012

[36] "Impact of fluoride on neurological development in children," *Harvard School of Public Health News*, July 25, 2012

[37] National Research Council, Committee on Fluoride in Drinking Water, *Fluoride in Drinking Water: A Scientific Review of EPA's Standards*, published by the National Academies Press, 2006, pg. 266

[38] Ibid., pg. 260

[39] Ibid., pg. 256

[40] Sharon Begley, "Fluoridation, cancer: did researchers ask the right questions?" *Wall Street Journal*, July 22, 2005

[41] Bassin EB et al., "Age-specific fluoride exposure in drinking water and osteosarcoma," *Cancer Causes and Controls*, May 2006, vol. 17, no. 4, pg. 421–428

[42] JR Bucher et al., "Toxicology and Carcinogenesis Studies of Sodium Fluoride (CAS NO. 7681-49-4) in F344/N Rats and $B6C3F_1$ Mice," *National Toxicology Program: Technical Report Series*, December 1990, no. 393, pg. 6 and 73

[43] Bette Hileman, "Fluoride Bioassay Study Under Scrutiny," *Chemical & Engineering News*, September 17, 1990

[44] Hoover RN et al., "Time trends for bone and joint cancers and osteosarcomas in the Surveillance, Epidemiology and End Results (SEER) Program," National Cancer Institute, Review of Fluoride: Benefits and Risks Report, 1991, Appendix E and Appendix F

[45] Perry Cohn, "A Brief Report on the Association of Drinking Water Fluoridation and the Incidence of Osteosarcoma Among Young Males," New Jersey Department of Health, November 8, 1992

[46] National Research Council of the National Academies, Committee on Fluoride in Drinking Water, *Fluoride in Drinking Water: A Scientific Review of EPA's Standards*, published by the National Academies Press, 2006, pg. 336

[47] Jon Calomiris, "How does chlorine added to drinking water kill bacteria and other harmful organisms? Why doesn't it harm us?" *Scientific American*, May 4, 1998

[48] Zierler S et al., "Bladder cancer in Massachusetts related to chlorinated and chloraminated drinking water: a case-control study," *Archives of Environmental Health*, March–April 1988, vol. 43, no. 2, pg. 195–200; McGeehin MA et al., "Case-control study of bladder cancer and water disinfection methods in Colorado," *American Journal of Epidemiology*, October 1, 1993, vol. 138, no. 7, pg. 492–501

[49] RD Morris et al., "Chlorination, chlorination by-products, and cancer: a meta-analysis," *American Journal of Public Health*, July 1992, vol. 82, no. 7, pg. 955–963

[50] Mark Nieuwenhuijsen et al., "Chlorination disinfection byproducts in water and their association with adverse reproductive outcomes: a review," *Occupational Environmental Medicine*, 2000, vol. 57, pg. 73–85

[51] A Bernard et al., "Lung hyperpermeability and asthma prevalence in schoolchildren: unexpected associations with the attendance at indoor chlorinated swimming pools," *Occupational Environmental Medicine*, 2003, vol. 60, pg. 385–394

[52] Villanueva CM et al., "Bladder Cancer and Exposure to Water Disinfection By-Products through Ingestion, Bathing, Showering, and Swimming in Pools," *American Journal of Epidemiology*, 2007, vol. 165, no. 2, pg. 148–156; Villanueva CM et al., "Assessment of lifetime exposure to trihalomethanes through different routes," *Occupational Environmental Medicine*, April 2006, vol. 63, no. 4, pg. 273–277

[53] Jo WK et al., "Chloroform exposure and the health risk associated with multiple uses of chlorinated tap water," *Risk Analysis*, December 2010, vol. 10, no. 4, pg. 581–585

[54] AC Anderson et al., "A Brief Review of the Current Status of Alternatives of Chlorine Disinfection of Water," *American Journal of Public Health*, November 1982, vol. 72, no. 11, pg. 1290–1293

[55] Schrauzer GN et al., "Lithium in drinking water and the incidences of crimes, suicides, and arrests related to drug addictions," *Biological Trace Element Research*, May 1990, vol. 25, no. 2, pg. 105–113

[56] Hirochika Ohgami et al., "Lithium levels in drinking water and risk of suicide," *British Journal of Psychiatry*, 2009, vol. 194, pg. 464

[57] Nestor Kapusta et al., "Lithium in drinking water and suicide mortality," *British Journal of Psychiatry*, 2011, vol. 198, pg. 346

[58] Anne Ehrlich, Paul Ehrlich and John Holdren, *Ecoscience: Population, Resources, Environment*, published by W.H. Freeman, 1977, pg. 787–788

[59] Kate Kelland, "Experts demand European action on plastics chemical," *Reuters*, June 22, 2010

[60] "More than 80,000 chemicals permitted in the United States have never been fully assessed for toxic impacts on human health and the environment," *Natural Resources Defense Council*, Nrdc.org/health/toxics.asp; "EarthTalk: Toxic Substances Control Act of 1976? Toilet paper rolls?" *E: The Environmental Magazine*, January 3, 2011

[61] Ibid.

[62] "National Toxicology Program Technical Report on the Carcinogenesis Bioassay of Bisphenol A in F344 Rats and B6C3F$_1$ Mice," National Institutes of Health, Publication no. 82–1771, March 1982

[63] Frederick vom Saal and Claude Hughes, "An Extensive New Literature Concerning Low-Dose Effects of Bisphenol A Shows the Need for a New Risk Assessment," *Environmental Health Perspectives*, vol. 113, no. 8, August 2005, pg. 926; "Toxic BPA detected in 91 percent of Canadians: study," *Agence France Presse*, August 16, 2010

[64] Joe Braun et al., "Impact of Early-Life Bisphenol A Exposure on Behavior and Executive Function in Children," *Pediatrics*, vol. 128, no. 5, November 1, 2011, pg. 873

[65] Jason Bromer et al., "Bisphenol-A exposure in utero leads to epigenetic alterations in the developmental programming of uterine estrogen response," *The FASEB Journal*, vol. 24, no. 7, July 2010, pg. 2273

[66] Elaine Shannon, "Yale Scientists Discover How Exposure to BPA Causes Infertility," *Huffington Post*, June 26, 2009

[67] Ibid.

[68] Masami Ishido et al., "Bisphenol A causes hyperactivity in the rat concomitantly with impairment of tyrosine hydroxylase immunoreactivity," *Journal of Neuroscience Research*, vol. 76, no. 3, May 2004, pg. 423; Keisuke Kawai et al., "Aggressive Behavior and Serum Testosterone Concentration during the Maturation Process of Male Mice: The Effects of Fetal Exposure to Bisphenol A," *Environmental Health Perspectives*, February 2003, vol. 111, no. 2, pg. 175; Kazuhiko Kuboa et al., "Low dose effects of bisphenol A on sexual differentiation of the brain and behavior in rats," *Neuroscience Research*, March 2003, vol. 45, no. 3, pg. 345

[69] Paola Palanza et al., "Exposure to a Low Dose of Bisphenol A during Fetal Life or in Adulthood Alters Maternal Behavior in Mice," *Environmental Health Perspectives*, June 2002, vol. 110, no. 3, pg. 415

[70] Paloma Alonso-Magdalena et al., "The Estrogenic Effect of Bisphenol A Disrupts Pancreatic β-Cell Function In Vivo and Induces Insulin Resistance," *Environmental Health Perspectives*, January 2006, vol. 114, no. 1, pg. 106

[71] K Howdeshell et al., "Environmental toxins: Exposure to bisphenol A advances puberty," *Nature*, October 21, 1999, vol. 401, pg. 763

[72] PA Hunt et al., "Bisphenol A Exposure Causes Meiotic Aneuploidy in the Female Mouse," *Current Biology*, April 1, 2003, vol. 13, pg. 546

[73] A Al-Hiyasat et al., "Effects of bisphenol A on adult male mouse fertility," *European Journal of Oral Sciences*, April 2002, vol. 110, no. 2, pg. 163; Frederick vom Saal et al., "A Physiologically Based Approach To the Study of Bisphenol a and Other Estrogenic Chemicals On the Size of Reproductive Organs, Daily Sperm Production, and Behavior," *Toxicology and Industrial Health*, January 1998, vol. 14, no. 1, pg. 239; Motoharu Sakaue et al., "Bisphenol-A Affects Spermatogenesis in the Adult Rat Even at a Low Dose," *Journal of Occupational Health*, 2001, vol. 43, no. 4, pg. 185–190

[74] Sarah Jenkins et al., "Chronic Oral Exposure to Bisphenol A Results in a Nonmonotonic Dose Response in Mammary Carcinogenesis and Metastasis in MMTV-erbB2 Mice," *Environmental Health Perspectives*, November 2011, vol. 119, no. 11, pg. 1604; Monica Munoz-de-Toro et al., "Perinatal Exposure to Bisphenol-A Alters Peripubertal Mammary Gland Development in Mice," *Endocrinology*, September 2005, vol. 146, no. 9, pg. 4138; Caroline Markey et al., "In Utero Exposure to Bisphenol A Alters the Development and Tissue Organization of the Mouse Mammary Gland," *Biology of Reproduction*, October 1, 2001, vol. 65, no. 4, pg. 1215

[75] Shuk-Mei Ho et al., "Developmental Exposure to Estradiol and Bisphenol A Increases Susceptibility to Prostate Carcinogenesis and Epigenetically Regulates Phosphodiesterase Type 4 Variant 4," *Cancer Research*, June 1, 2006, vol. 66, no. 11, pg. 5624

[76] Catherine Sawai et al., "Effect of bisphenol A on murine immune function: modulation of interferon-gamma, IgG2a, and disease symptoms in NZB X NZW F1 mice," *Environmental Health Perspectives*, December 2003, vol. 111, no. 16, pg. 1883; Shin Yoshino et al., "Effects of bisphenol A on antigen-specific antibody production, proliferative responses of lymphoid cells, and TH1 and TH2 immune responses in mice," *British Journal of Pharmacology*, April 2003, vol. 138, no. 7, pg. 1271; Shin Yoshino et al., "Prenatal exposure to bisphenol A up-regulates immune responses, including T helper 1 and T helper 2 responses, in mice," *Immunology*, July 2004, vol. 112, no. 3, pg. 489

[77] Frederick vom Saal et al., "Prostate enlargement in mice due to fetal exposure to low doses of estradiol or diethylstilbestrol and opposite effects at high doses," *Physiology*, March 1997, vol. 94, no. 5, pg. 2056

[78] Environmental Working Group with Washington Post staff writers, "117 Years of BPA," *Washington Post*, April 27, 2008

[79] Jane Houlihan et al., "Timeline: BPA from Invention to Phase-Out," Environmental Working Group, April 2008 (updated March 2011), Ewg.org/reports/bpatimeline

[80] FDA website, http://www.fda.gov/aboutfda/transparency/basics/ucm194877.htm

[81] Marla Cone, "NIH sidelines contractor in conflict inquiry," *Los Angeles Times*, April 4, 2007

[82] Lindsay Layton, "NIH Drops Contractor For Conflict of Interest," *Washington Post*, April 14, 2007

[83] Press release, "Federal Panel's Report on Food Contaminant Flunks Basic Science," Environmental Working Group, August 6, 2007

[84] Frederick vom Saal et al., "Chapel Hill Bisphenol A Expert Panel Consensus Statement: Integration of Mechanisms, Effects in Animals and Potential to Impact Human Health at Current Levels of Exposure," *Reproductive Toxicology*, August 2007, vol. 24, no. 2, pg. 131

[85] Akiko Matsumoto et al., "Bisphenol A levels in human urine," *Environmental Health Perspectives*, January 2003, vol. 111, no. 1, pg. 101–104

[86] Lyndsey Layton and Christopher Lee, "Canada Bans BPA From Baby Bottles," *Washington Post*, April 19, 2008

[87] Louise Egan, "Canada declares BPA toxic, sets stage for more bans," *Reuters*, October 14, 2010

[88] "EU orders ban on dangerous chemical in baby bottles," *Daily Record*, November 26, 2010

[89] FDA Press Release, "FDA Statement on Release of Bisphenol A (BPA) Subcommittee Report," October 28, 2008

[90] Rebecca Trager, "US bans BPA in baby bottles," *Chemistry World*, July 19, 2012

[91] Ibid.

[92] "Toxic BPA detected in 91 percent of Canadians: study," *Agence France Presse*, August 16, 2010

[93] "Sweden acts on endocrine disruptor Bisphenol A," *International Chemical Secretariat*, April 12, 2012

[94] "France bans contested chemical BPA in food packaging," *Agence France Presse*, December 13, 2012

[95] "Toxic BPA detected in 91 percent of Canadians: study," *Agence France Presse*, August 16, 2010

[96] Steven Reinberg, "Controversial Chemical Lingers Longer in the Body: Study," *Washington Post*, January 28, 2009

[97] Erika Schreder, *On the Money: BPA on Dollar Bills and Receipts*, Washington Toxics Coalition, December 2010

[98] "Concern over canned foods: Our tests find wide range of Bisphenol A in soups, juice, and more," *Consumer Reports*, December 2009

[99] René Viñas and Cheryl Watson, "Bisphenol S Disrupts Estradiol-Induced Nongenomic Signaling in a Rat Pituitary Cell Line: Effects on Cell Functions," *Environmental Health Perspectives*, March 2013, vol. 121, no. 3, pg. 352–358

[100] Sheila Eldred, "Are BPA-Free Plastics Just As Bad?" *Discovery News*, January 28, 2013

[101] "What is Activated Carbon?" Norit, Norit.com/carbon-academy/introduction/

[102] F. Kozisek, *Health Risks from Drinking Demineralized Water*, Rolling Revision of the WHO Guidelines for Drinking-water Quality, World Health Organization, Geneva, 2004

[103] WHO, *Guidelines on health aspects of water desalination*, 1980, ETS/80.4, World Health Organization, Geneva

[104] Deutsche Gesellschaft für Ernährung, "Destilliertes Wasser trinken?" *Medizinische Monatsschrift für Pharmazeuten*, May 1993, vol. 16, pg. 146

[105] BS Haring et al., "Changes in the mineral composition of food as a result of cooking in 'hard' and 'soft' waters," *Archives of Environmental Health*, Jan–Feb 1981, vol. 36, no. 1, pg. 33–35; F. Kozisek, *Health Risks from Drinking Demineralized Water*, Rolling Revision of the WHO Guidelines for Drinking-water Quality, World Health Organization, Geneva, 2004

[106] F. Kozisek, *Health Risks from Drinking Demineralized Water*, Rolling Revision of the WHO Guidelines for Drinking-water Quality, World Health Organization, Geneva, 2004

[107] Water Quality Association Science Advisory Committee, "Consumption of Low TDS Water," WQA Technical Services, March 1993

CHAPTER EIGHT

Implementation

This chapter shows you how to implement the advice from the preceding chapters by readying your kitchen for wholesome, holistic cooking. With the right tools and equipment, cooking is much more enjoyable and efficient. This chapter also covers food preparation techniques, menu planning, and salt.

Cookware

High-quality cookware can significantly improve your culinary creations. Many different varieties are available. Enamel-coated cast-iron and ceramic cookware are optimal, but also cost the most. Stainless-steel cookware is affordable, durable, and performs excellently. The size of your kitchen, the number of people you cook for, and your budget should all influence your cookware choices.

Cast-Iron Cookware

<u>Pros</u> – For nearly a thousand years in Europe and more than two thousand years in Asia, people have been preparing their meals in cast-iron cookware. This versatile, durable material boasts excellent heat retention, making it suitable for slow cooking, both on the stovetop and inside the oven. Traditional cast-iron cookware, as opposed to enamel-coated cast iron, requires seasoning. This is a process whereby a natural sealant is formed through a process called polymerization. This involves heating oil to high temperatures, thereby initiating a chemical reaction (polymerization) that hardens the oil. The most effective oils for seasoning are drying oils, of which the only edible one is flax. Used for centuries for making paint, flax has drying properties, which work well for seasoning cast iron pots.[1] Price-wise, cast iron is very affordable.

Cons – Cast-iron pans are heavy and bulky. Seasoning the pans can be somewhat complicated. Excessive iron uptake could be a possible concern. There may also be hygienic concerns, as cast-iron pans should only be cleaned with water, not soap.

Enamel-Coated Cast-Iron Cookware

Pros – These cast-iron pans have a protective glaze, which eliminates the need for seasoning. The glaze also protects these pans from rusting (although seasoning does the same) and makes them easier to clean. Traditional cast-iron cookware typically absorbs strong flavors and transfers these flavors to subsequent meals. Enamel-coated cast iron solves this problem completely because the coating protects against flavor absorption and transfer. Enamel-coated cast iron also has high aesthetic properties as various pigments used in the enameling process create vibrant, beautiful colors. This cookware not only looks great in your kitchen, but you can also use it for serving meals on the table.

Cons – The enamel coating makes these pans somewhat less durable than their traditional cast iron counterparts. This means you must take some extra precautions. For example, because the enamel can chip, you must avoid banging or dropping this cookware. Also you should avoid using metal utensils, which can scratch the enamel, leading to chipping. This being said, enamel-coated cookware is quite durable, and with proper care, lasts indefinitely. Another potential con is price. Enamel-coated cast iron is typically more expensive than other types of cookware.

Stainless-Steel Cookware

Due both to its durability and reliability, stainless steel is the most popular type of cookware. By definition, stainless steel is an iron alloy containing at least 11 percent chromium. You may have noticed stainless-steel cookware bearing the designation 18/10. The first number refers to the chromium content whereas the second number refers to the nickel content. Therefore, 18/10 stainless steel, the most popular variety, contains 18 percent chromium and 10 percent nickel. Stainless steel is generally a poor conductor of heat. Therefore, most high-quality stainless steel normally has an aluminum or copper core for proper, efficient heat transfer.

Pros – Stainless-steel cookware does not change the taste of food. Stainless steel is very durable, resistant to scratching and denting, generally very affordable, and it lasts indefinitely.

<u>Cons</u> – Stainless steel can be reactive, especially with acidic foods, causing nickel, iron, and chromium to leach during cooking.[2] A Pennsylvania State University study stated, "It is recommended that nickel-sensitive patients switch to a material other than stainless, and that the stainless steel cookware industry seriously consider switching to a non-nickel formulation."[3] While the amount of leaching is certainly small, it may be significant, especially after decades of exposure. If you do choose stainless steel cookware, definitely avoid cheaper versions with plastic handles. Most high-quality stainless-steel cookware can also be used in the oven.

Ceramic Cookware

Ceramic cookware generally has a steel core with a ceramic coating. The coating is antibacterial, taste-neutral, and nickel-free. Ceramic cookware has excellent heat conductivity. The Silargan line of ceramic cookware, made by Silit, is perhaps the best on the market. These pans come with a ten-year warranty. They are also ovenproof, making them particularly versatile.

Aluminum Cookware

Lower-grade, non-anodized, aluminum cookware has no place in the health-conscious kitchen. Numerous studies confirm this cookware leaches aluminum, a dangerous neurotoxin, into food.[4] Anodized aluminum, however, has undergone chemical changes to create a surface layer of aluminum oxide. Manufacturers insist leaching is not possible with anodized aluminum. The only advantage of aluminum cookware is price. Stainless steel, however, is superior and not much more expensive.

Nonstick Cookware

Fluorotelomers are fluoride-carbon-based chemicals used in food packaging, stain-resistant clothing, carpeting, and carpet protection products. Fluorotelomers break down into perfluorooctanoic acid (PFOA), a widespread industrial chemical in use since the 1940s. PFOA is used to make PTFE, the chemical present in Teflon (nonstick cookware) and Gore-Tex consumer products. More than 98 percent of the US population tests positive for perfluoroalkyl chemicals (PFC), including PFOA, in their blood.[5]

Many independent studies confirm that PTFE indeed contains traces of PFOA, though researchers are unsure whether this PFOA transfers during cooking.[6] DuPont, the maker of Teflon, adamantly claims, "Teflon non-stick coatings do not contain PFOA."[7] But this is the same company that paid $10.25 million in fines in 2005 for hiding what they knew about PFOA, including one study describing it as "extremely toxic" at levels measured in human blood samples.[8]

According to research published in the *American Journal of Epidemiology*, PFOA and other PFCs are positively associated with chronic kidney disease.[9] In 2005, the EPA categorized PFOA as "likely to be carcinogenic to humans."[10] Women who have elevated PFC blood serum levels have higher rates of infertility.[11] PFOA is also a liver toxicant, developmental toxicant, and immune system toxicant.[12] It also alters thyroid hormone levels.[13] Furthermore, PFOA causes testicular, liver, and pancreatic cancers in laboratory animals.[14] PFOA does not break down within the body. The chemical gradually accumulates, ultimately leading to various diseases.

If you choose to cook with PTFE pans, never use metallic utensils. They can easily scratch the pans, degrading the PFTE layers and increasing the chance of noxious chemicals contaminating your food. Secondly, never cook over high heat with these pans. DuPont itself only guarantees the integrity of PTFE below 500°F (260°C). Starting at 680°F, PTFE emits toxic fumes, which are carcinogenic to some animals.[15] Depending on the duration and intensity of exposure, these fumes can cause polymer fume fever, an unpleasant pulmonary condition.[16] PTFE pans can reach temperatures of 750°F after heating just eight minutes on a conventional stovetop.[17]

To conclude, PFOA is absolutely dangerous and should never be used for cooking pans. PFOA is used to make PTFE, but PTFE manufacturers claim their products contain no PFOA. The most prominent PTFE manufacturer, however, has a rather dubious history extending far beyond its 2005 criminality settlement. The popularity of Teflon pans is not surprising, as they are very versatile and practical. Every kitchen should have at least one nonstick pan, but you must decide for yourself whether or not to use Teflon. There are indeed many manufactures selling ceramic and other versions of PFOA-free, non-PTFE nonstick pans.

Cookware Recommendations

Good-quality cookware is an investment that lasts many years or even decades. Paying more for better quality makes sense. Even on a limited budget, you can still purchase effective, efficient, health-conscious cookware. I recommend two or three stainless-steel pots with lids. If your budget permits, I also recommend at least one enamel-coated cast-iron pot with a lid. Finally, I also recommend one PFOA-free, non-PTFE pan for frying eggs, searing meat, and other applications.

Essential Utensils and Machines

<u>Bamboo sushi mat</u> – Although not essential for making nori rolls, a basic bamboo mat will help you make consistently tight and attractive rolls.

<u>Cheesecloth</u> – Traditionally made from gauze-like cotton cloth, cheesecloth is used for separating whey from cheese curds during cheese production. I use it for making almond milk and coconut milk. The best varieties are made from nylon/poly fibers because they are very strong and reusable.

<u>Garlic press</u> – I always prefer pressed garlic to chopped garlic. Besides being more convenient, pressing liberates garlic's oils and juices, thus enhancing the flavor of your dish. A basic, heavy-duty, stainless steel garlic press is perfect.

<u>Glass jars</u> – Great for various home-fermentation projects. If you want to make sauerkraut or kombucha, large glass jars are essential.

<u>Mandoline</u> – This very useful kitchen tool is used for making very fine, thin cuts with uniform consistency. It is useful for julienne cuts. The best brand is De Buyer.

<u>Meat thermometer</u> – Used to measure the internal temperature of meats. You will cook roasts, steaks, and chicken to perfection every time.

<u>Mixing bowls</u> – No kitchen can have enough mixing bowls. Stainless-steel bowls, because they are lightweight and durable, are optimal. Buy many in different sizes.

<u>Nonmetallic utensils</u> – If you have enamel-coated, ceramic-coated, or nonstick cookware, then you definitely need nonmetallic cooking utensils. Metallic utensils can chip or scratch cookware surfaces. Wooden utensils are preferable. I'm wary of plastic utensils because they can melt, although some are designed to withstand high temperatures.

<u>Peeler</u> – While it's generally better to retain the nutrient-rich outer layers of your vegetables, a good peeler is still essential. For some applications, you can use a peeler instead of a mandoline. For example, ultrathin fennel is excellent with salads. If you don't have a mandoline, use your peeler to make very thin slices.

<u>Rubber spatula</u> – For all kinds of sauces, smoothies, cake batters, doughs, and sticky, runny creations, a rubber spatula is very handy. Look for one with adequate flexibility and high heat tolerance. Check out the spatulas made by Le Creuset.

Salad spinner – It's always a good idea to rinse salad greens before eating them. Don't just take them out of the package and serve them. It's best to serve them dry, crisp, and clean. A decent salad spinner is therefore very important.

Sprouting trays – Although you can sprout seeds in just about any container, sprouting trays are ideal because they have small holes for ventilation. It's always nice to put some fresh sprouts on your salads.

Steamer – Steaming is probably the most health-conscious cooking method, thus it's essential to have some steaming baskets. These can be stainless steel (preferably designed to exactly fit your cookware) or traditional bamboo baskets. Another good option is an electric steamer.

Storage containers – Plastic containers are of course more practical than glass. They are lightweight, unbreakable, and ideal for taking homemade lunches to work. Most plastic, however, contains an extremely noxious estrogen-mimicking chemical called BPA (see Chapter 7). Some companies are now selling BPA-free containers. If a plastic container is not labeled "BPA-free," you should assume it contains BPA.

Strainers – Essential for rinsing and straining seeds, nuts, grains, and beans. The holes should be at least small enough to strain quinoa. You might occasionally cook even smaller grains like teff or amaranth, so a very fine strainer is also recommended.

Thai vegetable shredder – This handheld, very basic tool allows you to make thin strips of carrots and other vegetables. It's great for sushi and stir-fries.

Water Filters

For many years I used Berkey water filters, which are gravity-driven carbon filters requiring neither electricity nor special plumbing adjustments. An attractive-stainless steel unit consisting of two chambers sits atop your counter. You simply pour tap water into the upper chamber, and it passes through the filter, depositing clean water into the lower chamber. Berkey effectively removes bacteria, parasites, herbicides, pesticides, solvents, and chlorine to non-detectable levels. It also removes fluoride and heavy metals, including lead, mercury, aluminum, cadmium, and chromium.

Recently I switched to reverse osmosis (RO), which is a pressurized filtration method allowing small molecules to pass through a special membrane while blocking larger molecules. Both RO and quality gravity-driven filters are excellent. Chapter 7 contains a detailed discussion about water filters and the necessity of having one.

Food Processors

Food processing machines are extremely versatile and practical. Sometimes known as S-blade processors, these machines are great for homogenizing wet and semi-wet mixtures. I use them for making burgers, hummus, tapenades, piecrusts, and cookies. They can also process onions, mince herbs, and grate carrots. The best commercial-grade processors are made by Robot Coupe. They also make excellent home models under the name Magimix (sold mostly in Europe). In the US, Cuisinart sells the highest-quality home models. A food processor is helpful, but not essential.

Blenders

For me, a high-performance blender is indispensable. Unlike standard blenders, high-performance blenders lend an incredibly smooth texture to smoothies, sauces, and soups. They are also great for making almond milk, coconut milk, and avocado-based salad dressings, among other things. Blendtec and Vitamix are the leading brands. Although they are much more expensive than common household blenders, both are backed by impressive seven-year guarantees.

Juicers

It's wonderful to have the option for fresh vegetable juices. Fruit juices, however, should be avoided (see Chapter 4). Standard juicers use blades to cut vegetable matter while rapidly spinning it through a strainer. This process creates too much heat and introduces too much oxygen, thereby compromising the integrity of the juice and significantly reducing both its nutritional value and its potency. Furthermore, this type of machine is very wasteful and inefficient. I recommend masticating juicers like those made by Green Star or Matstone. These machines gently crush the vegetable matter while pressing its juices through a fine strainer.

Slow Cookers

Using a slow cooker is an amazingly easy way to make incredible soups and stews. Slow cookers are very inexpensive and work by cooking foods at low temperatures for many hours. They require no supervision and can be used for beef, lamb, or chicken stews. You can also make lentil curries and bone broths. A basic slow cooker consists of a lidded round or oval cooking pot made of glazed ceramic or porcelain, surrounded by a housing, which contains an electric heating element.

Ice Cream Machines

While it's certainly not essential, an ice cream machine enables you to make healthy ice cream. Everyone loves ice cream, especially children, but most ice cream, is made with pasteurized milk, sugar, chemical additives, and various other unhealthy ingredients. With an ice cream machine, you can make your own "ice cream" with yogurt, coconut milk, or nut milks, sweetened with stevia, dates, erythritol, and other sweeteners discussed in Chapter 4. Ice cream machines run the gamut from your basic $50 model to those costing over $1,000. The basic models are fine. You just need a machine that slowly stirs your creation while keeping it cold. Even without an ice cream machine, you can still make the ice cream recipes in the upcoming chapter.

Knives

Good knives are essential. Most people have terrible knives. Don't waste your money on "complete sets" of poor-quality knives. It's much better to spend $100 on one good knife than the same amount on twenty losers. The cutlery industry profits handsomely by convincing you that you need many more knives than you actually do. I use one good knife for almost everything. One good chef's knife works for almost all your vegetable, meat, and fish needs. While not essential, it would also be good to have a heavy-duty cleaver for cutting meat with bones and for other tasks (opening coconuts). You can find a quality cleaver by searching online auctions or second-hand stores. Having one serrated-edge knife also comes in handy. Finally, you should have a sharpening rod or sharpening stone to maintain the edges on your knives. Sharpen your knives two times per week. So what constitutes a good knife?

The most important considerations are construction and materials. Look for full tang blades, which means one piece of metal extends continuously from the tip of the blade to the end of the handle. With lower-quality knives, the metal typically stops halfway through the handle. Metal knives are generally carbon steel or stainless steel. Carbon-steel knives are easy to sharpen and retain their edges. Over time, however, they are prone to rusting and staining. High-grade stainless-steel knives maintain very sharp edges and generally outperform their carbon-steel counterparts. Global makes some of the best stainless-steel knives, whereas Wüsthof makes some of the best carbon-steel knives. Ceramic knives are another option. They hold their edges even longer than steel knives but are much more prone to chipping and can easily break if dropped. For most people, high-quality carbon-steel or stainless-steel knives are best, with a cleaver and serrated-edge knife for backup.

Salt

According to research conducted at Harvard University, salt consumption within the US has remained stable for fifty-plus years.[18] Americans consume 3,700 mg per day, more than double the American Heart Association's recommended 1,500 mg.[19] The AHA and other prominent health organizations claim increased consumption of salt promotes hypertension and cardiovascular disease. In 1977, the US Senate Select Committee on Nutrition and Human Needs released a report encouraging Americans cut salt intake by 50 to 85 percent. This recommendation was largely based on studies conducted several years earlier by Lewis Dahl, a scientist working for Brookhaven National Laboratory. Dahl induced hypertension in rats by feeding them the human equivalent of 500 grams of sodium per day (135 times normal consumption rates).[20]

While there is certainly an upper threshold at which salt becomes harmful, there is no evidence that typical consumption levels cause hypertension or cardiovascular disease. A 2008 study published in the *Journal of General Internal Medicine* noted, "Higher sodium is unlikely to be independently associated with higher CVD or all-cause mortality."[21] Modern research suggests higher salt intakes are actually healthy, whereas lower intakes promote disease. A 2010 Harvard Medical School study found that low-salt diets significantly increase insulin resistance in healthy subjects.[22] Low salt consumption also increases plasma triglycerides, bad cholesterol, and certain hormones (renin, adrenaline, aldosterone), the combined effect of which increases insulin resistance, a common risk factor for heart disease. A study published in the *Journal of the American Medical Association* in 2011 found that decreased consumption of salt predicts increased cardiovascular mortality. The authors concluded,

> *"Taken together, our current findings refute the estimates of computer models of lives saved and health care costs reduced with lower salt intake. They do also not support the current recommendations of a generalized and indiscriminate reduction of salt intake at the population level."*[23]

Hypersensitive individuals might need to reduce salt consumption, but for most people, 3,000 to 7,000 mg per day is healthy (higher levels, for example, for those who exercise vigorously). The AHA's recommended level is too low. Sodium is an essential nutrient. It's also a principal component of extracellular fluid and a major determinant of intravascular fluid volume.[24] Sodium plays critical roles in regulating digestion, blood pressure, metabolism, brain function, and adrenal function.

People living in hot climates and people engaging in rigorous daily exercise lose significant amounts of sodium through perspiration. Without adequate replacement, these people have an increased risk of symptomatic hyponatremia, including lethargy and fatigue.[25]

Commercial table salt is highly refined and stripped of valuable trace minerals. Typically only sodium chloride remains, although iodine is sometimes added afterwards. The trace mineral content of sea salt ranges from 1.36 to 2.46 percent.[26] Many people wrongly claim that natural sea salt contains 10 to 15 percent trace minerals. While it's true that sea salt may contain 85 to 90 percent sodium chloride, one should not assume the remainder is trace minerals. In fact, it's mostly water.

Typical Sea Salt Trace Mineral Report – Figure 8.1

Mineral	Amount (%)	Mineral	Amount (%)
Vanadium	0.000321	Gold	<0.00001
Hafnium	0.000285	Antimony	<0.00010
Chromium	0.000172	Lithium	0.000092
Dysprosium	0.000145	Neodymium	0.000089

Another common misconception about sea salt involves its actual number of trace minerals. Some companies claim to sell sea salt containing 85 different trace minerals. Figure 8.1 shows a typical example of sea salt trace mineral reporting. The reported gold and antimony results suggest this particular sample contains miniscule amounts of these elements. It doesn't. Quite simply, the lab's equipment cannot detect amounts of gold less than 0.00001 percent and antimony less than 0.0001 percent. Despite claims to the contrary, natural sea salt generally does not contain more than 60 to 65 trace minerals. It's important to have good-quality salt, but don't pay extra for brands claiming to have 85 trace minerals.

In terms of composition and nutritional value, Himalayan salt is almost the same as sea salt. The primary difference is price; Himalayan salt is much more expensive. There are some concerns about sea salt contamination from industrial toxins. From this perspective, Himalayan salt is potentially more pure. However, some sea salt companies source their salt from ancient seas, as opposed to modern seas, thereby negating the contamination issue. Additionally, some companies also utilize special washing techniques, which ensure more purity. Also, be aware that some companies add chemicals for stability, color, taste, and anti-caking purposes. Always read labels.

In short, choose sea salt, preferably sourced from ancient seas and cleaned using special techniques. If you can't find this, ordinary sea salt without added chemicals is fine. Himalayan salt is an excellent product, but in my opinion, it makes more sense to spend money on food rather than luxury salt, which is functionally almost the same as common sea salt. You can save money by purchasing large, coarse-grain sea salt and processing it into fine powder using a completely dry blender.

Cooking Methods

Steaming is the easiest and most nutritious cooking method. Steaming offers the most vitamin retention and consistently delivers delicious results. Steaming is also quick and easy, perfect for people who cannot spend all day in the kitchen. Steaming works not only for vegetables, but also for fish, meat, and eggs (whole eggs, remove shells after). Other healthy cooking methods include boiling, stewing, light frying, and baking. Most people enjoy the taste of browned foods, but regularly consuming these foods could pose some risks.

High-temperature cooking of meats, cereal grains, and starchy vegetables creates two potent mutagens—benzo[a]pyrene (BaP) and acrylamide.[27] According to the WHO, acrylamide causes nerve damage at high doses in humans and causes cancer in animals.[28] Recent studies, however, suggest acrylamide is carcinogenic only with very high and persistent consumption. Conversely, low-dose exposure seems to activate genes involved with the elimination of this toxicant.[29] Therefore, we need not deny ourselves the enjoyment of occasionally consuming browned foods. Searing is one of the best methods for cooking red meat with minimal browning.

Soups and stews also make wonderful meals. In the upcoming recipe chapter, you will learn how to make delicious puréed vegetable soups, coconut curries, and slow-cooked stews. A slow cooker is an excellent kitchen machine for simple, one-pot meals. A good-quality blender is essential for smoothies, soups, and sauces. Salads are quick, easy, and highly nutritious. On special occasions, of course, it's nice to spend some hours in the kitchen creating divine meals for family and friends. This book, however, focuses squarely on practical, simple, delicious, and nutritious recipes for modern, busy people.

Meal Planning

Preparing quick, delicious meals is much easier than you might suppose. One hour per day is generally enough time to prepare breakfast, lunch, and dinner for four people. If cooking only for yourself, you need even less time. The recipes in this book are designed for busy people with busy lives. Many people maintain irregular and otherwise unhealthy eating habits, including sporadic snacking, eating sweets, and frequent eating. By eating two or three meals per day at regular times you gradually establish physiological balance, thus reducing your cravings for snacks and sweets.

Times between meals should be thought of as short-term fasting opportunities. Your body needs these times to digest, rest, and regenerate your cells. Every night after dinner, a fast commences, eventually ending with breakfast (literally breaking the fast). To obtain the benefits of this fasting opportunity, avoid eating late at night. Also, it's okay to skip breakfast. Intermittent fasting (IF) is a practice of regularly skipping one or two meals per day. Our hunter-gatherer ancestors didn't eat three square meals per day and we, too, can benefit from eating less frequently.[30] If you condense your daily eating into an eight hour-window, you receive the benefits of IF, which include enhanced cardiovascular health and brain function.[31]

Breakfast and Snack Possibilities – Figure 8.2

Breakfast	Snacks
Buckwheat Pancakes (pg. 252)	Full-Fat Greek Yogurt
Steamed Anything (pg. 258)	Avocado with Lemon
Coconut Smoothie (pg. 272)	Goat Cheese
Almond Smoothie (pg. 272)	Goat Yogurt
Kefir Smoothie (pg. 272)	Soaked Nuts
Smoked Salmon	Miso Soup
Steamed Fish	Prosciutto
Miso Soup	Sardines
Bacon	Chorizo
Kefir	Olives
Fruit	Kefir
Eggs	Fruit

Breakfast

If you eat three meals per day, one meal should be relatively small. The other two should be more substantial. Some people prefer a light dinner with a more substantial breakfast and lunch. Others prefer a light lunch with a more substantial breakfast and dinner. By trying different approaches, you will see what gives you the best energy and what works best for your daily schedule. Personally, I skip breakfast entirely or eat a very light breakfast, followed by a more substantial lunch and dinner.

A protein-rich smoothie containing germinated almonds and antioxidant-rich fruits makes for a healthy breakfast. Having a couple pieces of fruit is also great. Eggs and other protein-rich foods are also excellent for breakfast. Additionally, you can eat vegetables, steamed fish, and fermented pancakes with your breakfast. Figure 8.2 shows breakfast and snack ideas. Figure 8.3 is a two-week menu plan offering many lunch and dinner suggestions. If breakfast is one of your more substantial meals, you can prepare the lunch menus for breakfast.

Lunch and Dinner

When planning lunch or dinner, first you should decide which protein-dense food you will center your meal around. This could be fish, eggs, beef, lamb, pork, chicken, lentils, beans, tempeh, or many others. Next think about which vegetables you want. Vegetables can be roots, ground vegetables, cruciferous vegetables, salad greens, and many others. The vegetables can be steamed, roasted, made into soups, or eaten raw in salads. After protein and vegetables, the third most important consideration is fat. Each meal should have some high-quality fat, primarily coconut oil, butter, olive oil, or avocado. If your meal involves some light pan-frying, use coconut oil or butter. For steamed vegetables, drizzle them with coconut oil, butter, or olive oil. For salads, make an olive oil- or avocado-based dressing. You can also eat guacamole regularly.

Generally we should be decreasing (or eliminating) our consumption of cereal grains. If you are accustomed to eating cereals, however, you might want to include one cereal dish with some meals. Fermented cereals are best, but simply soaking and cooking them is also acceptable. Buckwheat, quinoa, amaranth, and white rice are the best choices. These grains cook relatively quickly. They can also be cooked, chilled, and added to salads. For quick and easy cooking, you can also use gluten-free noodles. Always read the ingredients on the packaging. You will sometimes see, for example, "buckwheat noodles," which upon closer inspection are actually 90 percent wheat and

Two-Week Menu Plan – Figure 8.3

Week 1	Lunch	Pg.	Dinner	Pg.
Mon				
Main	Basic eggs, any style	n/a	Miso Beef Mushroom Stew	228
Sides	Broiled Herbed Zucchini	261	Mashed Sweet Potatoes	255
	Anything Salad	262	Anything Salad	262
Tue				
Main	Tuna Ceviche	241	Roasted Chicken w. Lemon	236
Sides	Guacamole	267	Curried Cauliflower Soup	255
	Steamed Anything	258	Anything Salad	262
Wed				
Main	Shiitake Omelet	239	Sage Rosemary Lamb	232
Sides	Vegetable Miso Soup	261	Roasted Parsnips	257
	Steamed Anything	258	Anything Salad	262
Thu				
Main	Basic Grilled Sardines	246	Slow-Roasted Steak	231
Sides	Gazpacho	265	Steamed Anything	258
	Steamed Anything	258	Anything Salad	262
Fri				
Main	Basic eggs, any style	n/a	Grilled Salmon	243
Sides	Garlicky Artichokes	260	Garlic Roasted Mushrooms	266
	Anything Salad	262	Steamed Anything	258
Sat				
Main	Cilantro Chili con Carne	231	Thai Chicken Curry	238
Sides	Coconut Sautéed Plantains	260	Roasted Kabocha Squash	260
	Anything Salad	262	Anything Salad	262
Sun				
Main	Stuffed Mackerel	244	Hungarian Pork Goulash	235
Sides	Broccoli Soup	256	Steamed Anything	258
	Anything Salad	262	Anything Salad	262

Two-Week Menu Plan – Figure 8.3 (continued)

Week 2	Lunch	Pg.	Dinner	Pg.
Mon				
Main	Basic eggs, any style	n/a	Ginger Seared Beef	228
Sides	Guacamole	267	Roasted Eggplant Spread	270
	Anything Salad	262	Anything Salad	262
Tue				
Main	Red Snapper Ceviche	241	Chicken Tagine	237
Sides	Sweet Potato Fries	256	Better Ratatouille	253
	Anything Salad	262	Steamed Anything	258
Wed				
Main	Spanish Parsnip Tortilla	240	Persian Lamb Stew	232
Sides	Steamed Anything	258	Roasted Beetroot with Feta	266
	Anything Salad	262	Anything Salad	262
Thu				
Main	Easy Steamed Halibut	244	Balsamic Glazed Steak	230
Sides	Roasted Celeriac Fries	266	Miso Vegetable Soup	261
	Anything Salad	262	Steamed Anything	258
Fri				
Main	Basic eggs, any style	n/a	Thai Vegetable Fish Curry	242
Sides	Mashed Sweet Potatoes	255	Steamed Anything	258
	Steamed Anything	258	Anything Salad	262
Sat				
Main	Sage Feta Meatballs	230	Peruvian Chicken Soup	236
Sides	Mashed Cauliflower	254	Broiled Herbed Zucchini	261
	Anything Salad	262	Steamed Anything	258
Sun				
Main	Simple Fish Cakes	243	Slow-Roasted Pork	234
Sides	Zucchini Leek Soup	254	Broccoli Soup	256
	Anything Salad	262	Steamed Anything	258

only 10 percent buckwheat. The best gluten-free noodles are 100 percent buckwheat or Asian-style noodles (usually made from 100 percent mung beans). 100 percent rice noodles are also okay. Avoid products sold in gluten-free sections of supermarkets. Typically, these products are based on corn (which is usually GMO) and also contain nasty, pseudo-food fillers and binders including guar gum, lecithin, and xanthan gum. Potato starch and tapioca starch are other binders with poor nutritional value, which are commonly added to gluten-free foods. A good strategy for cutting back on cereal grains is replacing them with starchy vegetables, including sweet potato, parsnip, pumpkin, and squash.

A balanced meal generally has two or three dishes. This means one protein-rich dish and at least one vegetable dish. The third dish could be another vegetable dish or an approved-carbohydrate dish. Figure 8.3 is a 14-day sample menu. The idea is not necessarily to follow this plan formulaically. Feel free to pick and choose from the different menus that appeal to you. Also, you should realize that by cutting back on carbs and eating more protein and fat, you will probably begin feeling more satisfied with lower quantities of food. For some meals, you might feel inclined to eat very lightly. Other times, you might want to replace a meal with a healthy snack. In other words, eat when you are hungry and don't presume that every meal must have three courses. Also, as a time-saving strategy, you might want to prepare larger portions of certain recipes to eat with subsequent meals. Once you feel comfortable creating meals, you can assemble them by using other recipes from this book, or even better, by developing your own recipes.

Notes

[1] Gnowfglins.com/2010/03/12/how-to-season-cast-iron/

[2] J Kuligowski et al., "Stainless steel cookware as a significant source of nickel, chromium, and iron," *Archives of Environmental Contamination and Toxicology*, August 1992, vol. 23, no. 2, pg. 211–215

[3] Ibid.

[4] Essam Zubaidy et al., "Effect of pH, Salinity and Temperature on Aluminum Cookware Leaching During Food Preparation," *International Journal of Electrochemical Science*, December 2011, vol. 6, pg. 6424–6441

[5] Anoop Shankar et al., "Perfluoroalkyl Chemicals and Chronic Kidney Disease in US Adults," *American Journal of Epidemiology*, August 2011, vol. 174, no. 8, pg. 893–900; Ryan Seals et al., "Accumulation and Clearance of Perfluorooctanoic Acid (PFOA) in Current and Former Residents of an Exposed Community," *Environmental Health Perspectives*, January 2011, vol. 119, no. 1, pg. 119–124

[6] Begley TH et al., "Perfluorochemicals: Potential sources of and migration from food packaging, Food Additives and Contaminants," *Food Additives and Contaminants*, 2005, vol. 22, no. 10, pg. 1023–1031; Zhishi Guo et al., "Perfluorocarboxylic Acid Content in 116 Articles of Commerce," US Environmental Protection Agency, March 2009

[7] "Teflon firm faces fresh lawsuit," *BBC News*, July 19, 2005

[8] Michael Hawthorne, "DuPont hit with $10 million fine," *Chicago Tribune*, Dec 15, 2005

[9] Anoop Shankar et al., "Perfluoroalkyl Chemicals and Chronic Kidney Disease in US Adults," *American Journal of Epidemiology*, August 26, 2011, vol. 174, no. 8

[10] EPA website, Epa.gov/oppt/pfoa/pubs/pfoarisk.html

[11] Press Release, "UCLA researchers report that exposure to perfluorinated chemicals (PFCs) may reduce women's fertility," January 28, 2009

[12] Christopher Lau et al., "Perfluoroalkyl Acids: A Review of Monitoring and Toxicological Findings," *Toxicological Sciences*, May 2007, vol. 99, no. 2

[13] Ibid.

[14] Sally White et al., "Effects of perfluorooctanoic acid on mouse mammary gland development and differentiation resulting from cross-foster and restricted gestational exposures," *Reproductive Toxicology*, June 2009, vol. 27, no. 3, pg. 289–298

[15] David Ellis et al., "Thermolysis of fluoropolymers as a potential source of halogenated organic acids in the environment," *Nature*, July 19, 2001, vol. 412, pg. 321–324

[16] Shusterman DJ, "Polymer fume fever and other fluorocarbon pyrolysis-related syndromes," *Occupational Medicine*, Jul–Sep 1993, vol. 8, no. 3, pg. 519–531

[17] Wells RE et al., "Acute toxicosis of budgerigars (Melopsittacus undulatus) caused by pyrolysis products from heated polytetrafluoroethylene: clinical study," *American Journal of Veterinary Research*, July 1982, vol. 43, no. 7

[18] Adam Bernstein and Walter Willett, "Trends in 24-h urinary sodium excretion in the United States, 1957–2003: a systematic review," *American Journal of Clinical Nutrition*, November 2010, vol. 92, no. 5, pg. 1172–1180

[19] American Heart Association, Sodium (Salt or Sodium Chloride), Heart.org

[20] Melinda Moyer, "It's Time to End the War on Salt," *Scientific American*, July 8, 2011

[21] Cohen HW et al., "Sodium intake and mortality follow-up in the Third National Health and Nutrition Examination Survey (NHANES III)," *Journal of General Internal Medicine*, September 2008, vol. 23, no. 9, pg. 1297–1302

[22] Garg R, "Low-salt diet increases insulin resistance in healthy subjects," Metabolism: Clinical and Experimental, July 2011, vol. 60, no. 7, pg. 965–968

[23] K Stolarz-Skrzypek et al., "Fatal and Nonfatal Outcomes, Incidence of Hypertension, and Blood Pressure Changes in Relation to Urinary Sodium Excretion," *Journal of the American Medical Association*, May 4, 2011, vol. 305, no. 17, pg. 1777–1785

[24] A Logan, "Dietary Sodium Intake and Its Relation to Human Health: A Summary of the Evidence," *Journal of the American College of Nutrition*, June 2006, vol. 25, no. 3, pg. 165–169

[25] Ibid.

[26] SL Drake et al., "Comparison of salty taste and time intensity of sea and land salts from around the world," *Journal of Sensory Studies*, February 2011, vol. 26, no. 1, pg. 25–34; Real Salt, "Are your facts real?" March 14, 2011, Blog.realsalt.com/2011/03/are-your-facts-real/

[27] N Kazerouni et al., "Analysis of 200 food items for benzo[a]pyrene and estimation of its intake in an epidemiologic study," *Food and Chemical Toxicology*, May 2001, vol. 39, no. 5, pg. 423–436; Donald Mottram et al., "Food chemistry: Acrylamide is formed in the Maillard reaction," *Nature*, October 3, 2002, vol. 419, pg. 448–449

[28] World Health Organization, Who.int/topics/acrylamide/en/

[29] A Ehlers et al., "Dose dependent molecular effects of acrylamide and glycidamide in human cancer cell lines and human primary hepatocytes," *Toxicology Letters*, February 27, 2013, vol. 217, no. 2, pg. 111–120

[30] David Stipp, "How Intermittent Fasting Might Help You Live a Longer and Healthier Life," *Scientific American*, January 11, 2013

[31] Mattson MP et al., "Beneficial effects of intermittent fasting and caloric restriction on the cardiovascular and cerebrovascular systems," *Journal of Nutritional Biochemistry*, March 2005, vol. 16, no. 3, pg. 129–137

CHAPTER NINE

Recipes

The following recipes are specifically designed for busy people with limited available time for cooking. The techniques are simple, but the results are scrumptious. Cooking should be fun and enjoyable, but shouldn't require hours and hours of peeling, slicing, and stirring. The recipes, concepts, and techniques presented here encapsulate my approach to cooking. As a trained chef with more than a decade of experience, I have been exposed to plenty of complex and time-consuming recipes. In my day-to-day life, however, these recipes never cross my mind. Even if I had time to prepare them, I would still opt for basic, humble, simply prepared food. Give me some steamed broccoli slathered with butter, an avocado-tomato-arugula salad, and some oven-roasted fish with lemon and olive oil and I am perfectly content.

These recipes are characteristic of the foods I eat and enjoy every day. You don't need any specialized culinary knowledge to prepare them. They are practical and straightforward. None of them are formulas. They will teach you certain techniques, from which there are endless variations. You don't need to follow the measurements precisely. Focus instead on the concepts. Chefs never really create recipes, nor do they prepare food. Nature handles these tasks exclusively. The real "recipes" are the genetic codes of plants and animals—and the symbiosis enabling them to coexist and thrive together. These are the real recipes, which we should respect and never alter. Food preparation doesn't happen in the kitchen. It happens in the gardens, forests, and seas. By the time food arrives to your kitchen, it's almost ready. We never really "make food." We simply put on the finishing touches.

Beef

Ginger Seared Beef SERVES 2

¾ pound lean beef
1½ inches ginger, grated
1 clove garlic, pressed
1 tablespoon tamari
2 teaspoons mirin (optional)
1 tablespoon coconut oil or butter

Cut beef into 4 pieces and leave at room temperature for 2 hours. Gather the grated ginger and squeeze its juices into a bowl. Add the garlic, tamari, mirin, and beef. Toss well and marinate 30 min at room temperature. Bring a sauté pan to medium-high heat with coconut oil or butter. Cook beef 3 to 4 min per side.

Miso Beef Mushroom Stew SERVES 2 – 3

1 pound chuck roast beef
1½ inches ginger, finely chopped
2 cloves garlic, pressed
6 dried shiitake mushrooms
1 onion, chopped
2 carrots, peeled and chopped
2 tablespoons dark miso
¼ pound fresh enokitake mushrooms (optional)
¼ bunch cilantro, finely chopped

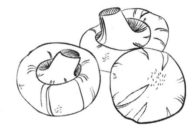

Put chuck roast (including bones), ginger, garlic, and shiitake in a casserole with enough water to cover. Bring to boiling, then reduce heat and simmer 3 hours. Remove the shiitakes, cut away the stems, and slice the caps finely. Add sliced caps back, along with onion and carrots. Simmer 1 to 2 more hours until meat is tender. Remove any bone material. Put miso in a bowl and add 2 ladles of broth. Stir until miso is dissolved. Pour back into stew and taste, adding more miso if necessary. Before serving, add the enokitake and cilantro. Recipe can be made using slow cooker.

Thai Coconut Beef with Lemongrass — SERVES 2

¾ pound lean beef
2 tablespoons coconut oil
1 clove garlic, pressed
1 inch ginger, finely chopped
1 piece lemongrass, finely chopped
¼ small red chili, finely chopped
½ cup homemade coconut milk (pg. 271)
1 Kaffir lime leaf or ¼ lime, juiced
Salt and pepper
¼ bunch cilantro, finely chopped

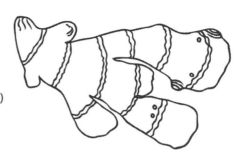

Cut the beef into 4 pieces. Create a marinade by sautéing the garlic, ginger, lemongrass, and chili in the coconut oil. Add the coconut milk, Kaffir lime, salt, and pepper and continue simmering until the mixture has reduced by half. If using lime juice instead of Kaffir lime, don't add now. Allow the marinade to cool, then toss with beef and marinate 30 min at room temperature. Bring a sauté pan to medium-high heat. Add beef along with marinade and sear several minutes on each side. Add chopped cilantro and lime juice. Stir and serve.

Chinese Beef with Ginger — SERVES 6

2 pounds beef shin or brisket, cut into large chunks
2 large tomatoes, peeled and chopped
2 onions, chopped roughly
1 inch ginger, finely chopped
3 cloves garlic, pressed
2 teaspoons Chinese five-spice
6 star anise, whole
1 teaspoon black peppercorns
1 tablespoon molasses (optional)
¼ cup tamari
Beef stock or water
½ bunch cilantro, chopped

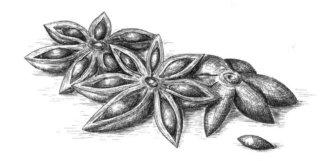

To peel the tomatoes, cut an "X" on the top and bottom of each and submerge in boiling water for 30 seconds, then put in cold water. The skins will peel away effortlessly. Chop peeled tomatoes and add to casserole with onions, ginger, garlic, Chinese five-spice, anise, peppercorns, molasses, and tamari. Add the beef plus enough beef stock (or water) to cover. Bring to boiling, reduce heat and simmer 5 hours or until beef is very tender. Adjust flavors, add cilantro, and serve.

Sage Feta Meatballs   SERVES 3

1 pound ground beef*
2 tablespoons full-fat yogurt
2 eggs, beaten
2 cloves garlic, pressed
Salt and pepper
2 spring onions, finely chopped
1 tablespoon sage, finely chopped
¼ cup parsley, finely chopped
¼ cup crumbled feta (optional)

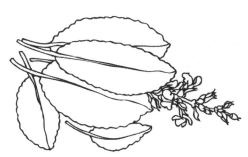

* Substitute ground lamb or turkey for beef.

Combine yogurt, eggs, garlic, a few pinches of salt, and some freshly milled pepper. Stir well and combine with beef. Stir in the spring onions, sage, parsley, and feta. Form into balls and place on a baking sheet lined with parchment paper. Bake the meatballs at 350°F for 10 to 15 min. Alternatively, you can cook them in a basic tomato sauce in a stove-top casserole or glass baking dish in the oven.

Balsamic Glazed Steak   SERVES 2

1 pound rib eye or tenderloin steak
¼ cup balsamic vinegar
¼ cup red wine
1 clove garlic, pressed
1 tablespoon coconut oil or butter
Salt and pepper

Allow beef to sit at room temperature 2 hours. To make the balsamic reduction, simmer the balsamic, wine, and garlic on the stovetop until the mixture reduces by half. Sprinkle the beef with salt and pepper. Bring a sauté pan to medium-high heat with the coconut oil or butter. Cook beef 3 to 4 min per side. Remove from heat and serve with the balsamic glaze.

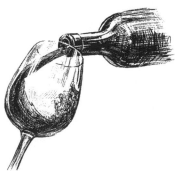

Cilantro Chili con Carne

SERVES 4

1 pound ground beef*
6 large tomatoes, peeled*
¾ cup precooked kidney beans*
2 cloves garlic, pressed
2 medium onions, chopped
½ red pepper, chopped
2 bay leaves
¼ teaspoon cayenne pepper
1 tablespoon oregano
1 tablespoon cumin
1 teaspoon coriander
Salt and pepper
¼ lime, juiced
1 bunch cilantro, chopped

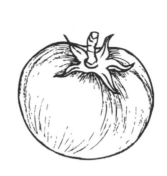
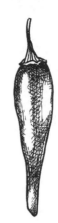

* Follow basic bean recipe on page 247 or use organic canned beans. Use bottled tomatoes as an alternative to fresh. Substitute beef for ground turkey or crumbled tempeh.

Chop 3 of the peeled tomatoes and set aside. Purée the other 3 in the blender. Put tomato purée and chopped tomatoes in a casserole and bring to boiling, adding slightly more water if necessary. Reduce heat to simmer. Add kidney beans, garlic, onion, red pepper, bay leaves, cayenne, oregano, cumin, coriander, salt, and pepper. Simmer 30 min. Add ground beef and cook another 10 min. Add lime, adjust seasoning, and serve with freshly chopped cilantro.

Slow-Roasted Cowboy Steak

SERVES 2

1 pound cowboy steak*
Salt and pepper

* Can also use other tender cuts of beef, as well as pork or lamb.

Sprinkle the steak with salt and pepper and your choice of herbs and spices. Allow steak to sit at room temperature 2 hours before cooking. Heat the oven to 250°F. Cook until the internal temperature reaches 130°F.

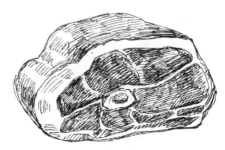

Lamb

Persian Lamb Stew SERVES 6

1½ pounds lamb stewing meat, cut into cubes*
2 dried lemons*
½ cup precooked kidney beans
2 cloves garlic, pressed
1 medium leek (white and green parts), chopped
3 spring onions, chopped
2 tablespoons fenugreek leaves*
2 teaspoons turmeric
Salt and pepper
1 bunch parsley, chopped
1 bunch cilantro, chopped
¼ pound spinach, coarsely chopped

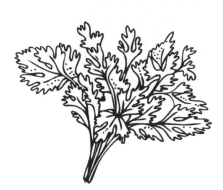

* If you wish, substitute beef for lamb. If you can't find dried lemons, use ½ fresh lemon, juiced. Omit fenugreek leaves if you can't find them.

Put lamb and dried lemons in a casserole (or use slow cooker). Add enough water to cover. Bring to boiling and reduce heat to lowest possible setting. Cover and simmer 2 hours. Add kidney beans, garlic, leek, spring onions, fenugreek leaves, turmeric, and a few pinches of salt and pepper. Continue simmering another hour. When lamb starts getting tender, add the parsley, cilantro, and spinach. When the greens are soft and lamb is very tender, adjust seasoning and serve.

Sage Rosemary Lamb Chops SERVES 2 – 3

1½ pounds lamb chops*
1 tablespoon sage, finely chopped
1 tablespoon rosemary, finely chopped
1 clove garlic, pressed
2 tablespoons coconut oil or melted butter
Salt and pepper

* Buy double chops if possible, single chops if not.

In a small bowl, mix sage, rosemary, garlic, and coconut oil. Rub this mixture into the chops. Sprinkle with salt and pepper and leave at room temperature for about 30 min. Heat a sauté pan to medium-high heat. Sear the chops 2 or 3 min on all sides. Remove pan from the heat, cover, and let stand for about 10 min.

Tandoori Lamb Chops

SERVES 6

2 pounds lamb chops*
Salt and pepper
½ cup full-fat yogurt
½ lime, juiced
1 clove garlic, pressed
1 inch ginger, finely chopped
½ teaspoon coriander
1 teaspoon cumin
Pinch cinnamon
1 teaspoon turmeric
1 teaspoon paprika

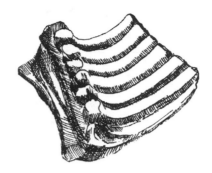

* Try the same recipe with beef or chicken (thighs and legs work best). You can also substitute the spices for a premade Tandoori spice mix.

Sprinkle chops with salt and pepper and set aside. In a bowl, combine yogurt, lime, garlic, ginger, and all spices. Mix with chops and marinate 2 to 4 hours. Preheat oven to 375°F. Cook for about 30 min or until internal temperature reaches 140°F. Alternatively, you can cook these on the grill.

Lamb Burgers

SERVES 6

1½ pounds ground lamb
2 cloves garlic, pressed
¼ cup full-fat yogurt (optional)
2 eggs*
2 teaspoons cumin
1 teaspoon coriander
½ teaspoon turmeric
Salt and pepper
1 spring onion, finely chopped
1 bunch parsley, finely chopped
1 bunch mint, finely chopped

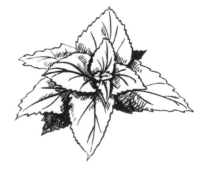

* If omitting the yogurt, also omit the eggs.

Combine pressed garlic with yogurt, egg, cumin, coriander, turmeric, a few pinches of salt, and some freshly milled black pepper. Stir well. Put lamb into mixing bowl along with egg mixture, spring onion, parsley, and mint. Mix well and form into burgers. Place on a baking sheet lined with parchment paper and bake at 350°F for 10 to 15 min.

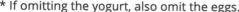

Pork

Ginger Pork Stir-fry   SERVES 6

¾ pound pork tenderloin, cut into bite-size pieces
Salt and pepper
1 teaspoon cumin
2 tablespoons coconut oil, divided
2 cloves garlic, pressed
½ inch ginger, finely chopped
1 onion, chopped
½ red bell pepper, chopped
Tamari
½ bunch parsley, finely chopped

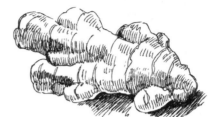

Sprinkle pork with salt, pepper, and cumin. Add 1 tablespoon of coconut oil to a sauté pan and bring to medium heat. Cook pork 10 to 15 min, stirring frequently, until cooked thoroughly. Remove from pan and set aside. Allow pan to cool slightly before adding the other 1 tablespoon of coconut oil. Add garlic, ginger, onion, and bell pepper, cooking over medium heat for about 5 min. Add pork and continue cooking another 2 min. Sprinkle with tamari, stir in parsley, and serve.

Slow-Roasted Rosemary Pork   SERVES 6

2 pounds pork loin, scored and tied
3 tablespoons butter
1 tablespoon mustard
2 tablespoons rosemary, finely chopped
Salt and pepper

Set oven to 325°F. Score the top of the loin, making several 1-inch deep cuts. Melt the butter and mix with the mustard and rosemary. Rub this butter mixture all over the loin, including between the cuts. Sprinkle with salt and pepper, wrap loin in aluminum paper, and place in a baking dish. Roast for 3 hours before removing from the aluminum paper and roasting an additional 30 min at 400°F.

Baked Bacon

15 to 20 pieces bacon

Preheat oven to 350°F. Place bacon strips on a baking sheet lined with parchment paper and bake for about 20 min or until the bacon looks crispy and delicious.

Hungarian Pork Goulash   SERVES 6

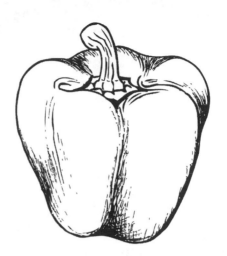

1¼ pounds pork tenderloin, cut into chunks
2 tablespoons coconut oil or butter, divided
2 cloves garlic, pressed
1 onion, chopped
¼ red chili pepper, finely chopped
1 green pepper, chopped
½ teaspoon paprika
½ teaspoon cumin
1 teaspoon caraway seeds, crushed
1 teaspoon oregano
1 teaspoon basil
3 tomatoes, peeled and chopped
1 cup chicken stock*
Salt and pepper
½ bunch parsley, finely chopped

* Can substitute for beef stock or water.

Heat a heavy casserole with coconut oil. Add garlic, onions, red chili pepper, and green pepper and cook 3 min. Add pork, paprika, cumin, caraway seeds, oregano, basil, tomatoes, and stock. Bring to boiling and reduce heat to low. Add 2 pinches salt plus some pepper. Cover and simmer 2 hours, adding more stock if necessary. When pork is very tender, adjust seasoning, stir in parsley, and serve.

Easy Marinated Pork Chops   SERVES 2 – 3

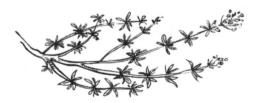

4 bone-in pork chops
2 cloves garlic, pressed
2 tablespoons tamari
1 tablespoon mixed Italian herbs
2 teaspoons cumin
Black pepper
2 tablespoons coconut oil or butter

Combine garlic, tamari, mixed herbs, cumin, and black pepper. Toss with pork chops and marinate for 20 min or longer. Bring a sauté pan to medium-high heat. Coat the chops with the coconut oil and sear 5 min per side. Then put in the oven at 350°F for 15 min or until thoroughly cooked.

Chicken

Roasted Chicken with Lemon and Rosemary   SERVES 4

1 whole chicken
2 tablespoons butter
3 cloves garlic, pressed
2 sprigs rosemary, finely chopped
1 lemon, juiced
Salt and pepper
Cavity stuffing (lemon and 2 more sprigs rosemary)

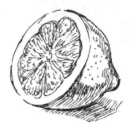

Preheat oven to 375°F. Melt butter in a small saucepan. Add garlic, rosemary, and lemon. Sprinkle chicken with salt and pepper, including inside the cavity. Put several slices of lemon plus 2 whole rosemary sprigs into the cavity. Brush the butter mixture over the chicken. Put chicken and shallow layer of water in baking dish and cook 60 min or until internal temperature reaches 170°F. If you don't have a meat thermometer, cook until chicken leg could easily be pulled away.

Peruvian Chicken Quinoa Soup   SERVES 4

1 pound of chicken pieces, bone in
1 clove garlic, pressed
1 onion, chopped
2 stalks celery, chopped
2 carrots, peeled and chopped
½ red bell pepper, chopped
1 cup kale or spinach, chopped
3 bay leaves
¼ cup quinoa, soaked overnight
Salt and pepper, to taste
1 bunch parsley, finely chopped
5 strands saffron, soaked in water
½ lemon, juiced

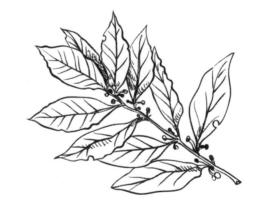

Make a flavorful chicken stock by boiling a whole chicken (cut in pieces) in a casserole with water to cover. Cook for 40 min before removing all chicken pieces. Set chicken aside and add all remaining ingredients to stock except parsley, saffron, kale, and lemon. Soaking water from quinoa should be discarded. Simmer for 30 min until vegetables are cooked. Meanwhile, pull chicken meat from bones and discard the bones. When vegetables and quinoa are fully cooked, add chicken meat, parsley, saffron water (remove strands), and lemon. Cook 5 more min. Adjust seasoning and serve.

Chicken Tagine with Lemon and Olive
SERVES 3 – 4

2½ pounds chicken, various pieces, skin removed
Salt and pepper
2 tablespoons coconut oil or butter
1 large onion, chopped
2 cloves garlic, pressed
¾ cup chicken broth (or water)
¾ cup green olives, pitted
1 teaspoon cinnamon
½ inch ginger, finely chopped
2 teaspoons grated lemon rind
1 lemon, juiced
¼ bunch cilantro, chopped
¼ bunch parsley, chopped

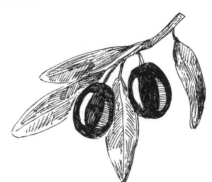

Sprinkle chicken with salt and pepper. Heat 1 tablespoon coconut oil in a large casserole over medium heat. Add chicken and cook 3 min per side or until lightly browned. Remove chicken from casserole. Add the other tablespoon of coconut oil and cook onion and garlic 2 min. Add chicken broth, chicken, olives, cinnamon, and ginger and bring to boiling. Cover, reduce heat, and simmer 45 min. Turn chicken over and cook, uncovered, another 15 min. Remove chicken from pan with a slotted spoon. Add lemon rind, lemon juice, cilantro, and parsley to broth and cook 30 seconds. Spoon the broth over the chicken and serve.

Basil Mint Pecan Chicken Salad
SERVES 2 – 3

1½ cups leftover cooked chicken, chopped*
½ cup pecans, soaked overnight and coarsely chopped
½ purple onion, chopped
3 radishes, chopped
1 stalk celery, chopped
¼ bunch basil leaves, torn
¼ bunch mint, chopped
½ bunch parsley, chopped
½ cup coconut mayonnaise (pg. 269)
Salt and pepper

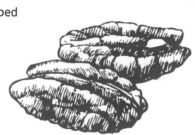

* Use chicken from Roasted Chicken with Lemon and Rosemary recipe (pg. 236).

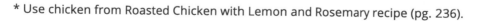

In a large bowl combine chicken, pecans, purple onion, radishes, celery, basil, mint, and parsley before stirring in the coconut mayonnaise. Taste and adjust seasoning, adding salt, pepper, lemon, and mustard according to your taste.

Thai Chicken Curry   SERVES 4

2¼ pounds chicken pieces
Salt and pepper
1 tablespoon coconut oil
2 pieces lemongrass, finely chopped
1 clove garlic, pressed
1 inch ginger, finely chopped
1 cup homemade coconut milk (pg. 271)
1 teaspoon red Thai curry paste*
1 Kaffir lime leaf (or ½ lime, juiced)
1 head broccoli, florets chopped
½ bunch cilantro, finely chopped

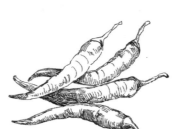

* Can use ¼ red chili, finely chopped, instead of curry paste.

Sprinkle chicken pieces with salt and pepper. Heat a casserole to medium heat and add coconut oil. Add lemongrass, garlic, ginger, and chicken pieces. Cook 5 min then add coconut milk, chili paste, and lime leaf. Bring to boiling then reduce heat, cover, and simmer 45 min. Add broccoli and continue cooking until tender. Adjust seasoning, add cilantro, and serve.

Greek Chicken Soup with Quinoa   SERVES 4

3 or 4 pieces of chicken, bone in
¼ cup quinoa, soaked overnight*
3 bay leaves
1 teaspoon cumin
1 teaspoon paprika
1 teaspoon turmeric
Salt and pepper
3 eggs, beaten
1 lemon, juiced
½ bunch parsley, finely chopped
½ bunch cilantro, finely chopped

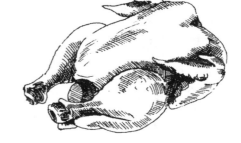

* This dish traditionally calls for rice. Use ¼ cup of white basmati rice instead if desired.

Put chicken in casserole with just enough water to cover. Bring to boiling, reduce heat to low and simmer 45 min. Remove chicken from casserole, cool, and remove meat from bones. Strain quinoa and discard soaking water. Cook quinoa in chicken broth 20 min along with cumin, paprika, turmeric, and salt and pepper to taste. Whisk eggs and lemon juice together in a mixing bowl. While whisking continuously, ladle some hot broth into egg mixture. Repeat several times until egg mixture is fully cooked. Pour egg mixture back into soup and stir to combine. Add shredded chicken and adjust flavors. Stir in parsley and cilantro and serve.

Eggs

Shiitake Omelet　SERVES 1

3 eggs, beaten
1 tablespoon butter or coconut oil
2 spring onions, finely chopped
4 fresh shiitake mushroom caps, sliced
Tamari
Salt and pepper
¼ bunch cilantro, chopped

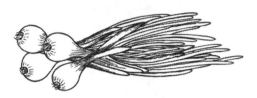

Mix eggs in a bowl with salt and pepper to taste. Bring a sauté pan to medium heat with butter. Cook the spring onion and shiitake 3 to 5 min. Sprinkle with tamari and stir. Pour in eggs and sprinkle with cilantro. Cover and reduce heat to very low. When eggs are solid, loosen them from the bottom of the pan and slide onto plate for serving.

Broccoli Smoked Salmon Mini Frittatas　SERVES 2

1 small head broccoli, florets chopped
1 tablespoon butter
4 eggs
2 teaspoons cumin
Salt and pepper
4 ounces smoked salmon, chopped*
1 spring onion, finely chopped

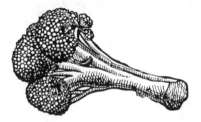

* You can substitute for prosciutto or cooked bacon.

Cut the broccoli florets into small pieces. Retain the rest of the broccoli for Broccoli Soup (pg. 256). Steam broccoli 15 min or until tender-firm. Preheat oven to 350°F. Rub butter on sides and bottoms of a 6-compartment muffin pan. Divide the steamed broccoli among the muffin compartments. In a bowl, stir the eggs, cumin, and salt and pepper. Spoon half the egg mixture into the muffin compartments. Distribute the smoked salmon and spring onion evenly among the compartments, followed by the remaining egg mixture. Bake for about 10 min or just until the eggs solidify.

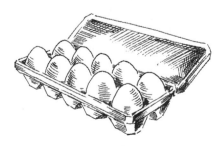

Spanish Parsnip Tortilla SERVES 2 – 3

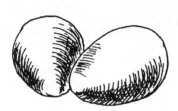

2 parsnips, cut as French fries
1 teaspoon cumin
Salt and pepper
2 tablespoon coconut oil or melted butter, divided
5 eggs, beaten
1 medium onion, chopped
½ bunch parsley, finely chopped

Preheat oven to 400°F. Toss parsnip slices with cumin, salt and pepper to taste, and 1 tablespoon coconut oil. Mix well using hands. Place on a baking sheet lined with parchment paper. Roast in the oven 30 min or until cooked thoroughly and lightly browned. Beat the eggs with salt and pepper to taste. Bring a sauté pan to medium heat with the other tablespoon of coconut oil and cook onion 3 to 5 min. Pour eggs into the pan and arrange parsnips and parsley evenly. Turn heat to very low and cover for 3 min or just until eggs are firm. Slide tortilla onto a plate. Place another plate, upside down, over the tortilla. Invert the entire 2-plate-tortilla sandwich so the browned side of the tortilla is now facing upwards on the second plate. Tortilla can be served warm or cold.

Green Eggs and Wham! SERVES 2

This is a great way to eat eggs for two reasons. First, your eggs will be green, thanks to plenty of delicious, aromatic herbs. Second, the experience will be enhanced by music from 1980s pop-culture sensation Wham!

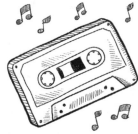

1 or more songs by Wham!
5 eggs
¼ bunch parsley, finely chopped
¼ bunch cilantro, finely chopped
2 tablespoons mint, finely chopped
1 spring onion, finely chopped
Salt and pepper
1 tablespoon butter

Play any music by Wham! For best results, put "Wake Me Up Before You Go-Go" on repeat. Crack the eggs and mix gently with a fork. Stir in the herbs, spring onion, and salt and pepper to taste. Heat a small sauté pan to medium heat. Add butter and tilt to coat the pan's surface. Add the egg mixture, cover, and reduce heat. When the eggs are just solid, they are ready. Don't overcook. Slide onto a plate and serve. Don't stop the music.

Fish and Seafood

Tuna Ceviche
SERVES 2 – 3

1 pound tuna fillet
1 inch ginger, grated
2 limes, juiced
1 mild red chili pepper
½ bunch cilantro, chopped
Freshly milled black pepper
Olive oil

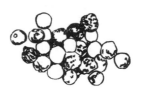

Cut tuna into bite-size chunks. Grate ginger, gather the pulp, and squeeze out the juice. Combine ginger juice with lime juice and toss with tuna. Marinate for 5 to 10 min. Deseed chili and slice thin. Toss tuna mixture with chili and cilantro and serve. Top with freshly milled black pepper. Drizzle with olive oil.

Simple Seared Tuna Steaks
SERVES 2 – 3

1 pound tuna steaks
1 inch ginger, grated
1 clove garlic, pressed
1 tablespoon tamari
1 tablespoon coconut oil

Grate ginger, gather pulp, and squeeze out the juice. Combine ginger juice with garlic, tamari, and coconut oil. Rub this mixture all over the tuna steaks and marinate 30 min at room temperature. Bring a sauté pan to medium-high heat. Sear tuna 2 min per side.

Red Snapper Ceviche
SERVES 2 – 3

1 pound red snapper fillets, cut into ½-inch pieces
2 limes, juiced
¼ orange, juiced (optional)
Salt and pepper
½ purple onion, finely chopped
1 tomato, chopped
¼ bunch cilantro, finely chopped
½ avocado, sliced

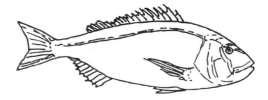

In a ceramic or glass dish, combine fish, lime, and orange juice. Marinate 10 to 15 min. Strain, retaining the marinade. Sprinkle fish with salt and pepper to taste. Toss with onion, tomato, cilantro, and avocado. Divide fish mixture into individual serving bowls. Pour the remaining marinade over each bowl.

Thai Coconut Fish Soup   SERVES 2 – 3

¾ pound white fish fillet, cut into chunks*
2 cups homemade coconut milk (pg. 271)
1 piece lemongrass, finely chopped
1 clove garlic, pressed
½ inch ginger, finely chopped
½ red pepper, chopped
6 fresh shiitake mushroom caps, sliced
2 Kaffir lime leaves or ¼ lime, juiced
½ head broccoli, florets only, chopped
Salt and pepper
¼ bunch cilantro, chopped

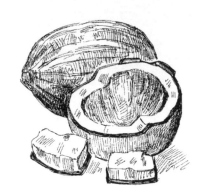

* Haddock, sole, cod, halibut, and monkfish all work well.

Bring coconut milk to boiling with lemongrass, garlic, ginger, red pepper, shiitake caps, and Kaffir leaves. Reduce heat to low and simmer 10 min. Add broccoli, cooking just until tender. Add salt and pepper to taste. If not using Kaffir leaves, add lime juice at this point. Adjust seasoning. Add fish and simmer for 5 min or just until tender-firm. Stir in cilantro and serve.

Thai Vegetable Fish Curry   SERVES 3 – 4

1 pound white fish fillet
1 tablespoon coconut oil
1 piece lemongrass, finely chopped
1 clove garlic, pressed
½ inch ginger, finely chopped
¾ cup homemade coconut milk (pg. 271)
2 teaspoons Thai curry paste*
2 Kaffir lime leaves or ¼ lime, juiced
Salt and pepper
1 carrot, peeled and sliced julienne
6 pieces baby corn
1 baby bok choy, leaves cut lengthwise
¼ pound baby asparagus, chopped roughly
½ bunch cilantro, finely chopped

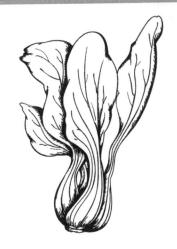

* Can use ¼ red chili, finely chopped, instead of curry paste.

Bring a sauté pan to medium heat with coconut oil. Add lemongrass, garlic, and ginger and cook 3 min. Add the coconut milk, curry paste, and Kaffir leaves. Add salt and pepper to taste. Reduce mixture by half. Stir in carrots and baby corn and simmer 5 min. Stir baby Bok Choy, asparagus, and fish and cook until fish is flaky. Stir in cilantro and serve.

Simple Fish Cakes   SERVES 2

¾ pound boneless white fish fillet
1 parsnip, chopped*
1 small onion, chopped
1 egg
¼ bunch parsley, chopped
¼ bunch dill, chopped
1 teaspoon turmeric
1 teaspoon cumin
Salt and pepper
1 tablespoon coconut oil
Tamari

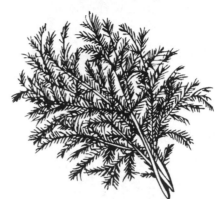

* You can substitute with celeriac or sweet potato.

Steam parsnip and onion until tender. Remove from steamer. Steam fish until tender. Allow parsnip, onion, and fish to cool down significantly. Beat the egg in a bowl. Put parsnip, onion, fish, parsley, dill, turmeric, cumin, and egg in food processor. Add a few pinches salt and pepper. Use the pulse function to process coarsely. Do not over-process. Remove and form into cakes. Refrigerate at least ½ hour. Bring sauté pan to medium heat. Heat coconut oil and lightly fry fishcakes 3 to 5 min per side. Sprinkle with tamari and serve.

Grilled Salmon with Salsa Verde   SERVES 2 – 3

1 pound wild salmon
2 tablespoons hazelnuts nuts, soaked overnight
¼ bunch mint, chopped
¼ bunch parsley, chopped
¼ bunch cilantro, chopped
2 spring onions, chopped
2 tablespoons capers
2 ounces canned sardines
½ lemon, juiced
2 tablespoons olive oil
¼ cup green olives, pitted and chopped
Salt and pepper

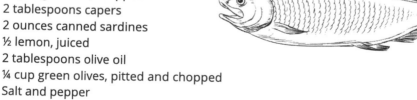

Preheat oven to 350°F. To make salsa, strain hazelnut soaking water and combine hazelnuts with herbs, spring onions, capers, sardines, lemon juice, olive oil, olives, and salt and pepper to taste. Process the mixture in a food processor, adding water if necessary. Put salmon fillets on baking sheet lined with parchment paper. Squeeze some lemon juice on the salmon and sprinkle with salt and pepper. Cook 10 to 12 min until tender and flaky. Serve with salsa.

Easy Steamed Seasoned Halibut   SERVES 2

1 pound halibut or other white fish fillet
2 pinches turmeric
1 pinch cumin
1 pinch coriander
Salt and pepper
1 tablespoon butter
½ lemon, cut into wedges

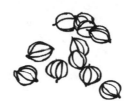

Toss fish fillets with spices, and salt and pepper to taste. Steam 10 min or until flaky and tender. Slather with butter and serve with lemon wedges.

Tamarind Mint Sole   SERVES 2 – 3

1 pound sole fillets or other white fish
1 tablespoon tamarind paste
1 tablespoon molasses
¼ cup water
2 tablespoons fish sauce (optional)
1 clove garlic, pressed
1 inch ginger, grated
¼ bunch mint, finely chopped

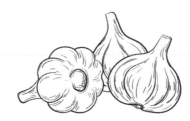

Make a sauce by combining tamarind paste, molasses, water, fish sauce, garlic, and grated ginger juice (squeeze juice from grated ginger). Adjust flavors, adding salt if necessary. Toss fish with sauce and mint, reserving some sauce for dipping. Either steam the fish or bake at 400°F for 10 to 15 min or until tender and flaky.

Stuffed Mackerel   SERVES 2

2 whole fresh mackerel
2 spring onions, finely chopped
1 clove garlic, pressed
½ bunch parsley
½ bunch cilantro
1 tablespoon butter, melted
½ lemon, juiced
Salt and pepper

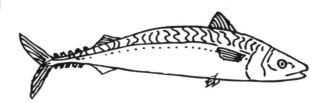

Cut the underbelly of each fish and remove the innards. Rinse under cold water. Either finely chop the spring onion, garlic, parsley, and cilantro, or process these ingredients in a small food processor. Add the butter, lemon, and salt and pepper to taste. Stuff each fish with this herb mixture. Place under the broiler of your oven for 5 to 10 min or until the fish starts to lightly brown. Turn off oven or turn to very low until fish is tender yet flaky.

Mackerel Cauliflower Caper Salad SERVES 2 – 3

1 large mackerel (or 2 small)
½ cauliflower, cut into florets
2 tablespoons capers
2 tablespoons olive oil
1 small clove garlic, pressed
¼ lemon, juiced
2 teaspoons cumin
Salt and pepper
¼ bunch parsley, finely chopped
¼ bunch mint, finely chopped

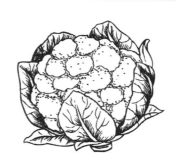

Cut the underbelly of each fish and remove the innards. Rinse under cold water. Place under oven broiler 5 to 10 min or until fish starts to brown. Turn off oven or turn to very low until fish is tender yet flaky. Steam cauliflower just until tender. Separate the mackerel meat from the bones. Make a dressing by mixing olive oil, garlic, lemon juice, cumin, and salt and pepper to taste. Combine cauliflower with capers, parsley, mint, and mackerel meat. Toss with dressing and serve.

Kerala Prawn Curry SERVES 2 – 3

1 pound jumbo prawns
1 tablespoon coconut oil
1 mild red chili, deseeded and sliced thin
1 small purple onion, chopped
½ inch ginger, finely chopped
1 teaspoon mustard seeds
1 teaspoon cumin seeds
1 teaspoon fenugreek seeds
¾ cup homemade coconut milk (pg. 271)
1 tablespoon curry powder
½ lime, juiced
Salt and pepper
½ bunch cilantro, chopped

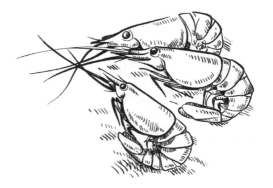

Bring a sauté pan to medium heat with coconut oil. Add the chili, onion, ginger, mustard seeds, cumin seeds, and fenugreek seeds and cook 3 min. Add the coconut milk and curry powder. Add salt and pepper to taste. Simmer until mixture reduces by half. Add the prawns. Stir and cook 5 min until prawns are tender, but firm. Stir in cilantro and serve.

Scallops with Capers and Tomatoes   SERVES 1 – 2

6 large scallops
1 tablespoon butter
1 clove garlic, pressed
1 tomato, grated*
2 teaspoons oregano
2 tablespoons capers, drained
Salt and pepper
¼ bunch basil, leaves torn into small pieces

* Cut tomato in half and grate on large holes of box grater until only skins remain.

Bring a sauté pan to medium heat with butter. Add the garlic and cook 2 min. Add tomatoes, oregano, capers, and salt and pepper to taste. Cook 3 additional min. Remove tomato mixture from pan. Sear scallops 1 min per side. Toss with tomato sauce and basil leaves. Cover 5 min before serving.

Basic Grilled Sardines   SERVES 2 – 3

1 pound fresh sardines
½ lemon, juiced
½ teaspoon oregano
½ teaspoon tarragon
Salt and pepper
Olive oil

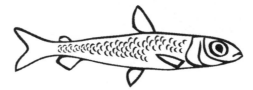

Cut undersides of sardines with a small, sharp knife. Remove innards and rinse fish under cold water. Leave heads and tails intact. Preheat oven to 400°F or turn on your oven's broiler. Arrange the sardines on a baking sheet lined with parchment paper. Squeeze some lemon juice over sardines. Sprinkle with oregano, salt, and pepper. Put sardines in oven. If using broiler, place baking sheet higher in the oven. If baking, place at mid-level. Cook 5 to 10 min or until sardines are tender and you can pierce them easily with a fork. If they start to brown, turn off the oven and keep closed inside until they are tender. Arrange on a serving plate, squeeze more lemon, and drizzle with olive oil.

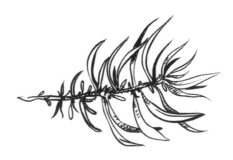

Cereals and Legumes

Basic Beans
SERVES 4

1 cup dried beans
2 bay leaves
Salt

Beans must soak at least 12 to 24 hours before cooking. Always discard the soaking water and bring the beans to boiling with fresh water. Foam will typically start to rise. Pour off all the foamy water while straining the beans. Return to casserole and replenish with fresh water. Again bring to boiling, reduce heat, add bay leaves, cover, and simmer 40 min or until beans are soft. To test doneness, position 1 bean between your thumb and index finger. It should squeeze with little resistance. Adding salt during the last 15 min of cooking helps soften them. Always add salt progressively. Taste and add more if necessary. You can cook beans in any heavy casserole with a lid. Another option is using a pressure cooker.

Canned beans are also okay, but always read the ingredients and only purchase beans with basic ingredients and no additives or preservatives. Look for beans with just sea salt. Eden makes excellent canned beans, sold in BPA-free cans.

Basic Buckwheat
SERVES 2

¾ cup buckwheat, soaked overnight (or at least 1 hour)
5 cups water
2 pinches salt

Pour off soaking water from buckwheat. Bring casserole of salted water to boiling. Add buckwheat. Reduce heat and simmer until buckwheat is tender-firm (about 10 to 15 min). Strain off cooking water and serve immediately. If you wish to use the buckwheat for salads, rinse with cold water to stop the cooking process.

Basic Quinoa
SERVES 2

1 cup quinoa, soaked overnight
1 cup water
1 pinch salt

Pour off the soaking water from the quinoa. Bring a casserole of salted water to boiling. Add the quinoa. Cover and reduce heat as low as possible. Simmer until quinoa is tender yet firm (about 15 to 20 min). Fluff with a fork. Serve warm or chill and combine with cold salads.

Red Lentil Coconut Curry   SERVES 4 – 5

1 medium eggplant, peeled and cubed
1 cup red lentils, soaked overnight
2 to 3 cups homemade coconut milk (pg. 271)
1 clove garlic, pressed
½ inch ginger, finely chopped
1 onion, finely chopped
½ red bell pepper, chopped
2 tablespoons curry powder
Salt and pepper
2 tablespoons coconut oil
½ lime, juiced

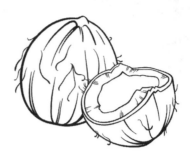

Toss eggplant with 2 pinches salt and set aside. Strain lentils and discard soaking water. Put lentils in a casserole with fresh water and bring to boiling. When foam starts to rise, strain again. Return lentils to casserole with coconut milk to cover. Bring to boiling. Reduce heat to very low. Rinse eggplant and squeeze to remove excess water. Add garlic, ginger, onion, red pepper, and eggplant to lentils. Simmer 30 min. Add curry powder and salt and pepper to taste and cook 10 additional min. Lentils should be very soft. Remove 1 cup of lentils and purée in the blender with the coconut oil, adding a little water if necessary. Pour lentil purée back into the casserole. Add lime, adjust flavors, and serve.

Lentil Herring Salad   SERVES 4 – 5

¾ cup lentils, soaked overnight*
2 bay leaves
4 ounces smoked herring or mackerel, chopped
Salt and pepper
1 carrot, peeled and chopped
4 radishes, sliced
2 spring onions, chopped
½ bunch parsley, chopped
½ bunch cilantro, chopped
½ lime, juiced
¼ cup olive oil

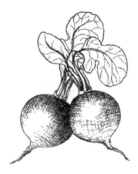

* Beluga or French green lentils are best because they retain their shape once cooked.

Strain lentils and discard soaking water. Put in casserole with fresh water and bring to boiling. Strain again and return lentils to casserole with enough fresh water to cover. Add bay leaves and smoked fish. Bring to boiling. Reduce heat, cover, and simmer 30 min or until tender. Strain and discard cooking water. Stir in salt and pepper to taste. When lentils cool down, toss with remaining ingredients.

Mediterranean Chickpea Salad

SERVES 4

¾ cup dried chickpeas, soaked overnight
1 lemon, juiced
1 clove garlic, pressed
¼ cup tahini
Salt and pepper
2 handfuls arugula, washed and spun dry
4 marinated sundried tomatoes, sliced
1 small cucumber, peeled and sliced
2 tablespoons olive oil

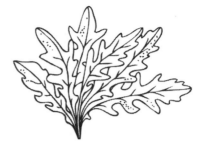

Prepare chickpeas according to Basic Beans recipe (pg. 247), reserving some of the chickpea cooking water. To make dressing, add lemon, garlic and tahini to a bowl and begin stirring. Tahini will start thickening. Slowly add some chickpea cooking water until tahini is light and fluffy. Stir in salt and pepper to taste and adjust seasoning. Add the cooked chickpeas (fully cooled). Toss with arugula, sundried tomatoes, and cucumber. Drizzle with olive oil and serve.

Greek Lentil Soup

SERVES 4

1 cup brown lentils, soaked overnight
2 large tomatoes, grated and skins discarded
1 leg of lamb with bone (about 1 pound)*
2 bay leaves
1 onion, chopped
1 clove garlic, pressed
2 tablespoons oregano
Salt and pepper
1 carrot, finely grated
1 stalk celery, chopped
½ lemon, juiced

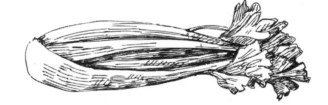

* Lamb is optional. Can also substitute beef or pork.

Strain soaking water and put lentils in a casserole with fresh water to cover. Bring to boiling. When foam starts to rise, pour off water and again add fresh water to cover. Add tomatoes, lamb, bay leaves, onion, garlic, and oregano. Simmer for 3 hours or until lamb is tender. Add salt and pepper to taste, carrots, and celery. Simmer 30 min more. Add lemon and adjust seasoning.

Buckwheat Mushroom Mint Falafels   SERVES 2 – 3

¾ cup buckwheat, soaked overnight
½ pound fresh mushrooms, chopped
Tamari
1 clove garlic, pressed
½ bunch mint, chopped
½ bunch cilantro, chopped
2 spring onions, chopped
2 tablespoons mild mustard
1 tablespoon cumin powder
Salt and pepper
1 tablespoon coconut oil

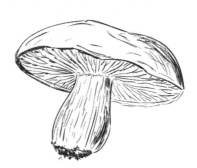

Cook buckwheat according to Basic Buckwheat recipe (pg. 247). Toss chopped mushrooms with tamari and garlic. Place on a baking sheet lined with parchment paper and bake 15 min at 400°F. In a food processor, combine buckwheat, mushrooms, mint, cilantro, spring onions, mustard, cumin and salt and pepper to taste. Process roughly until mixture holds together, working in batches if necessary. Form into falafel balls. Bring sauté pan to medium-high heat with coconut oil. Add falafels and cook several minutes, turning occasionally. Sprinkle with tamari and serve.

Caraway Cabbage Buckwheat Salad   SERVES 3 – 4

½ cup buckwheat, soaked overnight
¼ small green cabbage, finely chopped*
½ bunch parsley, finely chopped
½ bunch cilantro, finely chopped
1 handful cherry tomatoes, sliced
1 carrot, peeled and grated
½ lemon, juiced
¼ cup olive oil
Pinch caraway seeds
Salt and pepper, to taste

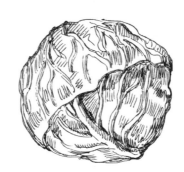

* Cabbage can also be finely grated.

Prepare buckwheat according to Basic Buckwheat recipe (pg. 247). Rinse with cold water to stop cooking. Put cooked buckwheat in a colander to completely dry. Next toss buckwheat with the remaining ingredients. Adjust seasoning and serve.

Fermented Pancakes – The Technique

As discussed in previous chapters, cereal grains have many nutritious attributes, but also contain anti-nutrients. Soaking and fermenting are traditional methods for minimizing anti-nutrients while increasing digestibility. Fermenting cereals, however, can be daunting, and requires perhaps more effort than most people care to make. Nevertheless, there is a very simple method, which involves making pancakes. Several recipes using this technique are below.

This technique works with cereal grains and cereal flours. If using whole cereal grains, you can remove more anti-nutrients than with flour by soaking the grains to begin the process. Commercial flour is generally processed from dry, non-soaked grains. The following simple, effective fermentation technique greatly improves the nutritional composition of cereals. Choose any non-gluten grains, especially quinoa, buckwheat, amaranth, rice, or teff. Even red lentils will work, as per the dosa recipe below.

This method involves puréeing soaked grains. You must strain and discard the soaking water, then add minimal amounts of fresh water, just enough to get the mixture spinning inside your blender. Pour this puréed mixture into a nonreactive bowl and stir in some yogurt and, optionally, a sweetener, like molasses. The yogurt introduces probiotic microorganisms, which are happy to feed on the cereals. Sweeteners are not necessary, but can enhance the fermentation by providing additional sugars for the culture. Fermentation can occur on the counter at room temperature or inside your oven with only the pilot light on. After 8 to 24 hours of fermentation, add the remaining ingredients and cook like pancakes.

Red Lentil Dosas   SERVES 3 – 4

¾ cup red lentils
¾ cup white basmati rice
2 tablespoons fenugreek seeds
2 tablespoons full-fat yogurt
2 tablespoons curry powder
Salt and pepper

Soak red lentils, rice, and fenugreek seeds all together 12 to 24 hours. Rice can be white or brown basmati, though white lends a nicer texture. Strain and discard the soaking water. In batches, process the soaked grains in your blender, adding just enough water to make a thick yet homogenous purée. Pour this purée into a nonreactive bowl and add yogurt. Cover and ferment 8 to 24 hours. Stir in curry powder and season with salt and pepper. Bring a nonstick sauté pan to medium-low heat. Ladle ½ cup batter onto the pan and cook 2 min per side.

Basic Buckwheat Pancakes   SERVES 2 – 3

1¼ cups buckwheat, soaked overnight*
2 tablespoons full-fat yogurt
1 tablespoon molasses or barley syrup (optional)
1 teaspoon baking powder (optional)
2 eggs
Salt
Butter

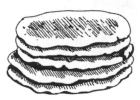

* Also try quinoa-buckwheat pancakes using 1 cup soaked buckwheat and ¼ cup soaked quinoa, or amaranth-buckwheat pancakes using 1 cup soaked buckwheat and ¼ cup soaked amaranth. The ratios are flexible as are the starting ingredients.

Strain buckwheat and discard the soaking water. Put buckwheat into the blender. Add just enough water to make a thick, yet homogenous purée. Pour this purée into a nonreactive bowl and stir in yogurt and sweetener. Cover and ferment 8 to 24 hours. Stir in all remaining ingredients. Bring a nonstick pan to medium-low heat with a little butter. Ladle ½ cup batter onto the pan and cook 2 min per side.

Quinoa Tabouleh   SERVES 2 – 3

1 recipe Basic Quinoa, cooled (pg. 247)
½ lemon, juiced
¼ cup olive oil
2 teaspoons cumin
Salt and pepper
½ bunch cilantro, finely chopped
½ bunch parsley, finely chopped
¼ purple onion, chopped
½ beefsteak tomato, chopped
4 marinated artichoke hearts, sliced
¼ cup feta, crumbled

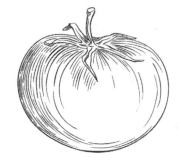

Make dressing by whisking together lemon, olive oil, cumin, and salt and pepper to taste. Mix all other ingredients. Toss with dressing.

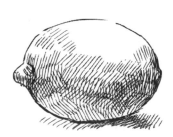

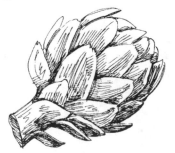

Vegetables

A Better Ratatouille

SERVES 3 – 4

Most ratatouille recipes use too much cooked olive oil. Here is a better, fat-conscious way to prepare this classic.

2 small eggplants, cut into large-bite pieces
2 tablespoons butter (or coconut oil)
1 clove garlic, pressed
1 onion, cut into large-bite pieces
1 tablespoon sage, chopped
1 tablespoon marjoram, chopped
1 red bell pepper, cut into large-bite pieces
1 zucchini, cut into large-bite pieces
Salt and pepper
¼ cup feta, crumbled

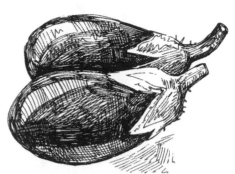

Sprinkle eggplant pieces with salt and set aside for 15 min. Rinse and squeeze out the excess water. In a large casserole (with lid), heat the butter and add garlic, onions, sage, and marjoram. Cook several minutes before adding bell pepper, zucchini, eggplant, and salt and pepper to taste. Stir well, then cover and reduce heat to low. Cook for about 30 min, stirring occasionally and adding water as necessary until vegetables have softened. Place the vegetables onto a baking sheet lined with parchment paper and bake at 350°F for 15 min or until slightly roasted. Serve with crumbled feta.

Creamy Sage Carrot Soup

SERVES 3 – 4

5 medium carrots, chopped
1 onion, chopped
1 clove garlic, pressed
2 bay leaves
Pinch of cumin
1 tablespoon sage, finely chopped
3 tablespoons coconut oil or butter
Salt and pepper

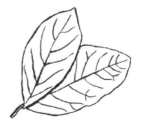

Put the chopped carrots, onion, garlic, bay leaves, cumin, and sage in a casserole. Add just enough water to cover and bring to boiling. Cook for about 25 min before testing the vegetables with a fork. Everything should be soft but not overcooked. Turn off the heat and add the coconut oil. Purée the mixture progressively in the blender. Return to casserole. Add salt and pepper. Adjust seasoning and serve.

Zucchini Leek Soup   SERVES 2 – 3

1 leek, green and white parts
4 medium zucchinis
1 small potato (optional)
1 clove garlic, pressed
2 bay leaves
1 teaspoon basil
1 teaspoon oregano
Salt and pepper
2 tablespoons butter
¼ lemon, juiced

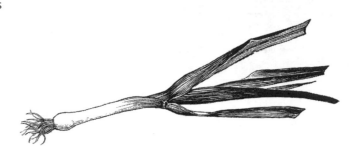

Pull away the outer layers of the leek and rinse with water, ensuring no dirt is inside. Chop both the white and green portions and put in a casserole with the zucchini, potato, garlic, bay leaves, basil, oregano, and salt and pepper to taste. Add just enough water to cover, bring to boiling, reduce heat, and simmer 20 min or until all vegetables are fully cooked. Add the butter and purée the soup in the blender. Add the lemon, adjust seasoning, and serve.

Mashed Cauliflower   SERVES 2 – 3

1 cauliflower, chopped roughly
1 clove garlic, pressed
2 tablespoons butter
1 tablespoon mixed Italian herbs
Salt and pepper
Homemade almond milk (pg. 271) or water

Steam cauliflower 20 min or until tender. Put all ingredients in food processor and process, adding just enough almond milk to achieve the desired consistency. Alternatively, you can mash everything with a potato masher.

Curry Roasted Cauliflower   SERVES 2 – 3

½ cauliflower, chopped into bite-size pieces
1 tablespoon coconut oil
2 teaspoons curry powder
Salt and pepper

Chop cauliflower and combine with coconut oil, curry powder, and salt and pepper to taste. Toss well with hands, ensuring the oil is evenly distributed. Arrange as a single layer on a baking sheet lined with parchment paper. Bake at 350°F for 20 min or until cauliflower is tender and lightly browned.

Curried Cauliflower Soup   SERVES 3 – 4

1 cauliflower, chopped
2 onions, chopped
1 clove garlic, pressed
2 bay leaves
2 tablespoons mild curry powder
2 cups homemade coconut milk (pg. 271)
Salt and pepper
3 tablespoons coconut oil

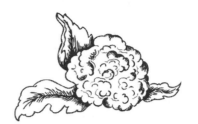

Put all ingredients except coconut oil in a casserole and add just enough coconut milk (or water) to cover. Bring to boiling, reduce heat, and simmer 25 min or until cauliflower is tender. Turn off heat and add coconut oil. Next, purée the mixture progressively in the blender. Adjust seasoning and serve.

Tarragon Mashed Sweet Potatoes   SERVES 4

2 medium sweet potatoes, cut into chunks
2 tablespoons butter
2 teaspoons tarragon
½ bunch parsley, chopped
Salt and pepper

Steam the sweet potatoes 20 min or until tender. Remove from steamer and place in a bowl with the remaining ingredients. Use a fork or potato masher and mash until you achieve the desired consistency.

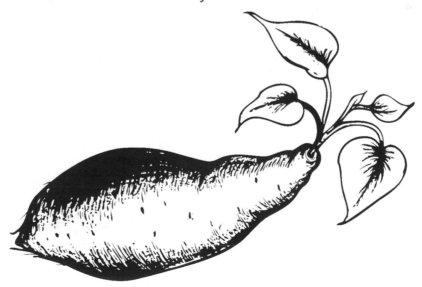

Baked Sweet Potato Fries   SERVES 4

2 medium sweet potatoes
Salt and pepper
1 tablespoon coconut oil or melted butter

Cut sweet potatoes as French fries. Place in a bowl and sprinkle with salt and pepper. Add coconut oil and toss well with hands, ensuring oil is evenly distributed. Arrange as a single layer on baking sheet lined with parchment paper. Bake at 350°F for 30 min until sweet potatoes are tender and lightly browned.

Broccoli Stalker Soup   SERVES 3 – 4

This soup is great for using up broccoli stalks that remain after the choice florets have been used in other recipes.

1 small head broccoli
3 or 4 broccoli stalks
1 whole leek, chopped
1 zucchini, chopped
1 onion, chopped
1 clove garlic, pressed
2 bay leaves
Salt and pepper
3 tablespoons coconut oil or butter
Small squeeze of lemon

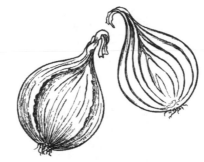

Clean the broccoli, cut the florets, and set aside. Cut away the tough outer layers of the stalks. Clean the leek, retaining the green and white parts. Add the stalks, zucchini, leek, onion, garlic, bay leaves, salt, and pepper to a casserole. Add just enough water to cover and bring to boiling. Reduce heat and simmer 15 min. Add broccoli florets and cook another 10 min until everything is tender. Turn off the heat and add the coconut oil. Purée the mixture progressively in the blender. Squeeze a small amount of lemon juice into the soup. Adjust seasoning and serve.

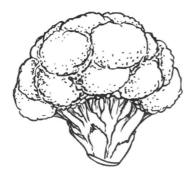

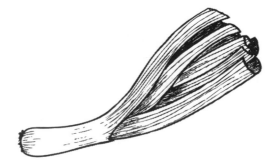

Borscht

SERVES 4 – 5

2 tablespoons butter
2 cloves garlic, pressed
1 onion, chopped
3 tomatoes, peeled and chopped
6 cups homemade pork stock (or beef stock)
3 medium beets, peeled and grated
1 leek, sliced into thin rings
1 carrot, peeled and chopped
1 stick celery, chopped
2 medium potatoes, chopped
½ teaspoon allspice
¼ teaspoon nutmeg
3 bay leaves
Salt and pepper
1 tablespoon molasses (optional)
½ lemon, juiced
¼ bunch parsley, chopped
¼ bunch dill, chopped

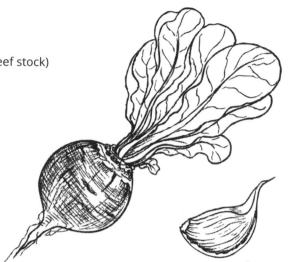

Bring a large casserole to medium heat. Add butter and cook garlic and onions. Put peeled tomatoes in the blender with 1 cup of stock. Add to casserole with all remaining vegetables, remaining stock, allspice, nutmeg, bay leaves, and salt and pepper to taste. Bring to boiling, reduce to low heat, cover, and simmer 30 min or until vegetables are tender. Add molasses and lemon. Adjust seasoning, add fresh parsley and dill, simmer a few more minutes, and serve.

Variation: If making homemade beef or pork stock, add some meat to the borscht as well. Secondly, this recipe can be made in slow cooker. Upon bringing mixture to boiling, transfer to slow cooker for 6 to 8 hours on low or 3 to 5 hours on high.

Roasted Parsnips

SERVES 2

3 parsnips
1 tablespoon coconut oil or butter
Salt and pepper

Cut parsnips as wedges or French fries. Put in a bowl and sprinkle with salt and pepper. Add coconut oil and toss well with hands, ensuring that oil is evenly distributed. Arrange as a single layer on baking sheet lined with parchment paper. Bake at 350°F for 25 min or until parsnips are tender and lightly browned.

Steamed Anything

Steaming is my favorite cooking method. Simple, quick, and healthy—steamed vegetables are delicious and very flavorful. After steaming, I typically slather vegetables with butter and/or drizzle them with olive oil. A little squeeze of lemon is also a nice touch. You can also toss your pre-steamed vegetables with various spices or dried herbs. Steaming time is generally 10 to 20 min, depending on the vegetables and how you cut them. You can also steam a medley of different vegetables. Cut them appropriately so they finish at the same time. For example, carrots require more time than equal-sized pieces of broccoli. Therefore, when steaming carrots and broccoli together, cut the carrots smaller. Alternatively, you could put the carrots in the steamer first, then add the broccoli after 5 to 10 min. With a little practice, you will quickly become a master steamer.

Favorite Vegetables for Steaming

Asparagus	Cauliflower	Snow peas
Bell peppers	Fennel	Squash
Broccoli	Kale	Tomatoes
Carrots	Parsnips	Turnips
Celeriac	Pumpkin	Zucchini

The Nicest Spices

Chop vegetables and toss with several pinches of one or several of the following spices before steaming.

Ancho chili powder	Cumin seeds	Paprika
Caraway seeds	Coriander powder	Ras el hanout
Cumin powder	Curry powder	Turmeric

Tasty Healing Herbs

Chop vegetables and toss with several pinches of one or more of the following dry herbs before steaming.

Basil	Oregano	Tarragon
Marjoram	Sage	Thyme

Fresh Herbs

Add fresh chopped herbs after steaming. Turn off heat and put them in the steamer with the vegetables. Close the lid for about 30 seconds, then transfer to a mixing bowl and stir.

Basil	*Dill*	*Parsley*
Cilantro	*Mint*	*Tarragon*

Post-Steaming Enhancements

Toss your steamed vegetables with one or more of the following.

Balsamic vinegar	*Coconut oil*	*Sea salt*
Black pepper	*Lemon*	*Sumac*
Butter	*Olive oil*	*Tamari*

Favorite Fruits for Steaming

Steamed fruits make a nice snack or dessert.

Apple	*Banana*	*Peach*
Apricot	*Mango*	*Pear*

The Nicest Spices for Fruits

Chop fruits and toss with several pinches of one or more of the following spices before steaming.

Anise	*Cinnamon*	*Coriander powder*
Cardamom	*Cloves*	*Ground ginger*

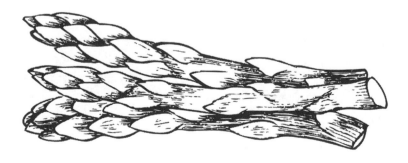

Roasted Kabocha Squash SERVES 3 – 4

½ kabocha squash
1 tablespoon coconut oil
1 tablespoon tamari

Cut the squash in half and remove the seeds. Cut into large, bite-size chunks. Place in bowl with coconut oil and tamari. Toss well with hands, ensuring the oil is evenly distributed. Arrange as a single layer on a baking sheet lined with parchment paper. Bake at 350°F for 20 min or until squash is tender.

Coconut Sautéed Plantains SERVES 2 – 3

3 ripe, yellow plantains
2 tablespoons coconut oil
Tamari

Peel the plantains and slice into ½ inch rounds. Bring a sauté pan to medium heat. Add the coconut oil and the plantains. Reduce heat slightly and cover. Cook about 5 min per side, adding water whenever the pan becomes too dry. Sprinkle with tamari and serve.

Garlicky Herbed Artichokes SERVES 2

5 artichokes
1 lemon, juiced
2 cloves garlic, pressed
¼ cup olive oil
1 tablespoon mixed Italian herbs
Salt and pepper

Prepare a bowl with lemon juice and 1 cup of water. Slice off the tops of the artichokes and peel away the outer leaves. Retain the inner leaves. Use a small spoon to scrape away the fuzzy-hairy part above the heart. Also retain the first inch or so of the stems near the heart. Use a peeler to remove the outer skin of the stems. Slice the prepared chokes in quarters and put in the lemon water.

Put the chokes into a small saucepan along with the lemon water and the garlic. Bring to boiling, reduce heat, cover, and simmer for 10 min or until chokes are tender-firm. Add more water while cooking if necessary. Remove from saucepan and strain away any excess water. Toss with olive oil, herbs, salt, pepper, and slightly more lemon juice.

Miso Vegetable Soup
SERVES 2

½ inch ginger, finely chopped
4 dried shiitake mushrooms
1 carrot, cut into matchstick pieces
1 stalk celery, chopped
½ head broccoli, florets chopped
3 tablespoons dark miso

Bring 2½ cups water to boiling with the ginger and shiitakes. Cover and simmer for 5 min. Remove shiitakes. Cut and discard the stems. Slice the caps thinly. Return the sliced caps to the water along with the carrots and celery. Cook 5 to 10 min. Add broccoli and cook until all vegetables are tender-firm. Remove from heat. In a separate bowl, combine the miso with ¼-cup broth, stirring well. Add this miso mixture back to the soup. Taste and add more miso if necessary. Do not boil miso.

Broiled Herbed Zucchini
SERVES 3

6 medium zucchinis
1 tablespoon coconut oil or melted butter
1 tablespoon mixed Italian herbs
1 tablespoon tamari
¼ bunch parsley, finely chopped
¼ lemon, juiced
2 tablespoons olive oil

Slice zucchini into ½-inch rounds. Put in a bowl with coconut oil, mixed herbs, and tamari. Toss well, ensuring the oil is evenly distributed. Arrange as a single layer on a baking sheet lined with parchment paper. Bake at 350°F for 15 to 20 min or until slightly browned and tender-firm. Remove from oven and toss with parsley, lemon, and olive oil.

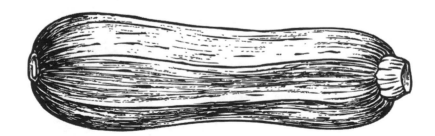

Anything Salad

Vegetables are an essential component of every meal. Salads are one of the best ways to consume vegetables. A salad can even be an entire meal. If you have some leftover beef or chicken, for example, slice it into small pieces and combine with your salad. Try to include a variety of vegetables, especially greens and herbs. You can also add root vegetables, steamed vegetables, nuts, and what I call "rich tastes." A little fruit is okay, but don't add too much since fruits digest differently from other foods. As for dressings, the standard is lemon (or lime) with olive oil. Sometimes, however, you might want to swap the citrus for some high-quality balsamic vinegar. Starting on page 267, there are several sauces and dressings suitable for salads. Every salad is unique. Try combining different foods from each of the following categories. Be creative.

Greens and Fresh Herbs

Arugula	*Mâche*	*Parsley*
Baby spinach	*Mint*	*Purslane*
Cilantro	*Mixed Baby Greens*	*Romaine*

Raw Vegetables

Beetroot, cabbage, and carrot are all great for salads when grated using the small holes on your box grater. You can use a mandoline or peeler to make thin slices of fennel.

Beetroot	*Cucumber*	*Radish*
Cabbage	*Fennel*	*Spring onion*
Carrot	*Purple onion*	*Tomato*

Cooked Vegetables

The following vegetables are great steamed or roasted and added to your salads.

Beetroot	*Cauliflower*	*Red bell pepper*
Broccoli	*Fennel*	*Squash*
Cabbage	*Parsnip*	*Sweet potato*

Rich Tastes

Rich tastes are the little flavor bursts that bring salads to another level. All nuts should be soaked beforehand. Depending on where you live, you might also be able to find presoaked, dehydrated nuts, which would be an excellent choice.

Almonds	*Goji berries*	*Other cheeses*
Apple	*Hazelnuts*	*Parmesan*
Avocado	*Hulled hempseeds*	*Pomegranate*
Dried figs	*Macadamias*	*Raw sauerkraut*
Feta	*Marinated artichokes*	*Sundried tomatoes*
Goat cheese	*Olives*	*Walnuts*

High Protein

Adding protein-rich foods turns your salad into a complete meal. Fish could be smoked, canned, or freshly steamed. Soft-boiled eggs are excellent with salads.

Anchovy	*Chickpeas*	*Pork*
Bacon	*Cured meats*	*Salmon*
Beef	*Eggs*	*Sardines*
Cannelloni beans	*Kidney beans*	*Shrimp*
Chicken	*Mackerel*	*Tuna*

Marinated Sundried Tomatoes

½ pound sundried tomatoes
1 clove garlic, pressed
½ lemon, juiced
¼ cup olive oil
1 tablespoon mixed Italian herbs
Salt and pepper

Put sundried tomatoes in a bowl and add boiling water to cover. After 10 min, pour off water, allow to cool, and squeeze tomatoes to remove all excess water. Combine tomatoes with all other ingredients. Store in refrigerator up to 10 days.

Arugula Salad with Pomegranate SERVES 2

2 handfuls arugula, chopped
1 handful sprouts (alfalfa or others)
¼ bunch coriander, chopped
1 carrot, peeled and finely grated
1 small cucumber, peeled and chopped
¼ pomegranate, seeded
¼ cup walnuts, soaked overnight
½ avocado, sliced
½ lemon, juiced
3 tablespoons olive oil

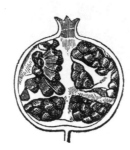

Toss all salad ingredients and drizzle with olive oil and lemon juice.

Purslane Salad SERVES 1

I first became aware of purslane during my years in Greece. Though typically known as a weed in the US, purslane is highly regarded in many parts of the world. Its tangy taste and crunchy texture make it perfect for salads. Purslane is rich in omega-3, primarily ALA but also EPA, which is rare for plants.

2 handfuls purslane, chopped
2 tomatoes, chopped
1 small cucumber, chopped
¼ cup feta, crumbled
½ lemon, juiced
2 tablespoons olive oil

Toss purslane, tomatoes, cucumbers, and feta. Drizzle with olive oil and lemon.

Grated Cabbage and Carrot Salad SERVES 2

¼ small cabbage (purple or green)
1 large or 2 small carrots
¼ bunch parsley, finely chopped
1 tablespoon caraway seeds
¼ cup feta, crumbled
½ lemon, juiced
3 tablespoons olive oil

Grate cabbage with box grater (large holes). Grate carrots with box grater (small holes). Toss cabbage and carrots with feta, caraway, parsley, lemon, and olive oil.

Italian Green Salad
SERVES 2 – 3

2 handfuls baby field greens
4 ounces marinated artichokes
1 large tomato, seeded and chopped
1 carrot, peeled and finely grated
1 cucumber, peeled and chopped
1 spring onion, chopped
½ lemon, juiced
3 tablespoons olive oil
Grated Parmesan

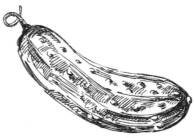

Toss all ingredients and serve immediately.

Cold Cucumber Avocado Soup
SERVES 2 – 3

6 small cucumbers, peeled and chopped
½ lemon, juiced
3 tablespoons olive oil
½ avocado
Salt and pepper
¼ bunch cilantro, leaves only

Put all ingredients in the blender except cilantro. Start blending, adding just enough water to achieve the desired consistency. Add the cilantro leaves and pulse-blend to gently disperse them. Chill and serve cold.

Gazpacho
SERVES 3 – 4

1½ pounds ripe tomatoes, chopped
¼ red bell pepper, chopped
1 clove garlic, pressed
¼ cup olive oil
½ lemon, juiced
½ avocado
Pinch of cayenne or ancho powder
Salt and pepper, to taste
¼ bunch parsley, chopped
¼ bunch cilantro, chopped
1 celery stalk, chopped
1 spring onion, chopped
¼ piece fennel, finely chopped or mandoline sliced

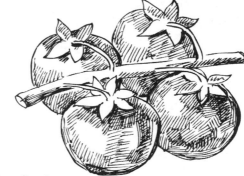

Put tomatoes, red bell pepper, garlic, olive oil, lemon, avocado, cayenne, salt, and pepper into blender. Add just enough water to achieve creamy soup consistency. Stir in remaining ingredients and chill soup in refrigerator. Serve cold.

Garlic Roasted Mushrooms

SERVES 2

¾ pound button mushrooms
½ pound fresh shiitake or other mushrooms
1 tablespoon coconut oil or butter
1 clove garlic, pressed
1 tablespoon mixed Italian herbs
1 tablespoon tamari

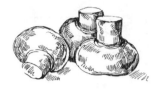

Button, shiitake, chanterelle, oyster, and portobello all work well for this recipe. Preheat oven to 350°F. Clean the mushrooms and put in a bowl with the coconut oil, garlic, Italian herbs, and tamari. Toss well with hands, ensuring the oil is evenly distributed. Arrange on a baking sheet lined with parchment paper. Cook 10 to 12 min or until mushrooms are tender.

Roasted Celeriac Fries

SERVES 3 – 4

1 celeriac (celery root), cleaned and peeled
2 tablespoons coconut oil or melted butter
1 tablespoon mixed Italian herbs
Salt and pepper

Clean the celeriac and cut as you would French fries. Toss with coconut oil, herbs, salt, and pepper. Line a baking sheet with parchment paper and arrange celeriac as a single layer. Bake at 350°F for 40 min or until celeriac is browned and tender.

Roasted Beetroot with Feta and Mint

SERVES 3 – 4

8 medium beetroots
2 tablespoons coconut oil
1 tablespoon cumin
Salt and pepper
½ cup feta, crumbled
½ bunch mint, leaves torn
½ lime, juiced
2 tablespoons olive oil

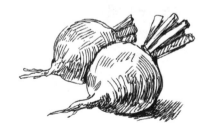

Wash and peel beetroots. Cut into irregular wedge-shaped pieces, around ½-inch thick. Preheat oven to 350°F. Put beetroot pieces in a bowl with coconut oil, cumin, and salt and pepper to taste. Toss well with hands, ensuring the oil is evenly distributed. Arrange as a single layer on a baking sheet lined with parchment paper. Cook 20 to 30 min, until tender. Remove from oven and cool for 5 min before tossing with feta and mint. Drizzle with lime and olive oil.

Sauces and Spreads

Guacamole

SERVES 2 – 3

2 ripe avocados
3 tablespoons olive oil
1 small clove garlic, pressed
1 lime, juiced
1 bunch cilantro, chopped
1 teaspoon cumin (optional)
Pinch of cayenne or ancho chili powder
Salt and pepper

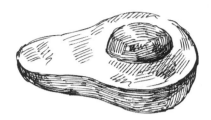

Mix olive oil, garlic, and lime juice in a bowl. Remove pits from avocados and scrape the flesh into the bowl. Add cumin, cayenne, salt, and pepper. Use a fork to mash the avocado. Stir in the cilantro and serve.

Cashew Zucchini Hummus

SERVES 2 – 3

2 tablespoons white tahini
½ lemon, juiced
3 cups zucchini, peeled and chopped
¼ cup cashews, soaked 2 hours
3 tablespoons olive oil
1 small clove garlic, pressed
1 teaspoon cumin
Salt and pepper

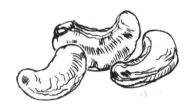

Put tahini and lemon juice in a bowl and stir with a fork. Add a little water, stirring until the mixture becomes fluffy. Put zucchini, olive oil, garlic, cumin, salt, pepper, and lemon-tahini mixture into the blender. Blend well, adding a little water if necessary to achieve the desired consistency. Adjust seasoning and serve.

Caper Gremolata

SERVES 2

1 bunch parsley, chopped
3 tablespoons olive oil
½ clove garlic, pressed
Zest of 1 lemon
½ lemon, juiced
¼ cup capers, chopped
Salt and pepper

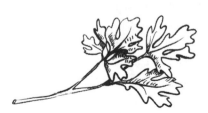

Combine all ingredients using a mortar and pestle or use food processor with pulse action. Adjust flavors and serve with steamed fish.

Green Cashew Ginger Sauce   SERVES 3 – 4

½ cup cashews, soaked 2 hours
½ bunch cilantro
½ bunch parsley
¼ bunch mint
1 spring onion
½ inch ginger, finely chopped
3 tablespoons olive oil
1 lime, juiced
Salt and pepper

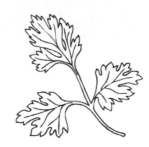

Discard cashew soaking water and put all ingredients into the blender. Blend until smooth and creamy, progressively adding small amounts of water as necessary. Adjust for salt and lime. Serve with salads, steamed vegetables, meat, or fish.

Homemade Ketchup   SERVES 6 – 8

2 tablespoons coconut oil or butter
2 cloves garlic, pressed
1 purple onion, chopped
1 inch ginger, finely chopped
1 bunch basil
1 tablespoon coriander seeds
¼ teaspoon cloves
½ fennel bulb, chopped
1 stalk celery, chopped
Salt and pepper
3 pounds cherry or plum tomatoes
½ cup apple cider vinegar
¼ cup barley malt

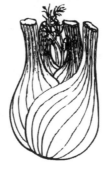
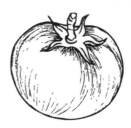

Warm the coconut oil in a casserole and add garlic, onion, ginger, basil stalks, coriander seeds, and cloves. Cook 3 min before adding fennel, celery, salt, and pepper. Cook for about 10 min over medium heat. Add the tomatoes and 1 cup water. Bring to boiling, then reduce heat and simmer gently until the sauce reduces by half. Put the sauce in a food processor or blender. Add the basil leaves and process. Pour the mixture into a fine sieve and push it through using the back of a spoon. Put the strained sauce in a saucepan and add vinegar and barley malt. Simmer until sauce reduces and thickens. You can add some tomato paste to thicken if necessary. Adjust seasoning.

Coconut Mayonnaise   SERVES 6 – 8

2 egg yolks
1 teaspoon mustard (optional)
1 tablespoon lemon juice
½ cup olive oil
½ cup coconut oil (warmed to be liquid)

Put the egg yolks, mustard, and 1 teaspoon lemon in a bowl or a blender with low-speed functionality. Start whisking vigorously (or turn the blender on low). Start adding the oil very slowly, drop by drop at the beginning. You are trying to create an emulsion. As the mixture starts to thicken, you can add the oil faster. Finally, add the remaining lemon, salt, and pepper. Adjust seasoning. Store in refrigerator.

Creamy Avocado Red Pepper Sauce   SERVES 2

2 roasted red peppers*
1 ripe avocado
2 tablespoons olive oil
1 lime, juiced
Salt and pepper

* Prepare according to Roasted Eggplant and Red Pepper Spread recipe on page 270.

Add all ingredients to blender and blend while slowing adding just enough water to achieve the desired consistency. Adjust for salt and lemon, and serve.

Silky Green Avocado Herb Sauce   SERVES 4

½ clove garlic, pressed
¼ cup olive oil
½ ripe avocado
½ lime, juiced
½ bunch cilantro*
½ bunch parsley
Salt and pepper

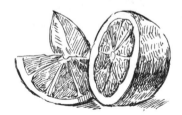

* Any mix of fresh herbs will work, giving preference to cilantro, basil, parsley and mint.

Combine garlic and olive oil in a small bowl. Put avocado in blender with garlic-oil mix, lime, and half the fresh herbs. Blend well, adding just enough water to achieve the desired consistency. Add salt and pepper to taste. Adjust seasoning, then add remaining herbs and pulse-blend so little pieces of the herbs remain.

Roasted Eggplant and Red Pepper Spread   SERVES 4 – 5

3 eggplants
1 red pepper*
1 small clove garlic, pressed
3 tablespoons olive oil
½ lemon, juiced
2 teaspoons cumin
1 teaspoon paprika
Pinch cayenne (optional)
Salt and pepper
¼ bunch mint, chopped
½ bunch parsley, chopped

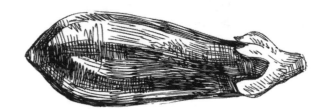

* Red pepper can be omitted.

Preheat oven to 425°F. Poke a few holes in each eggplant. Roast red pepper and eggplants 40 min or until skins have darkened and vegetables are soft. Remove from oven and cover with a kitchen towel 5 to 10 min. Remove the peels and discard them. Chop the soft flesh of the red pepper and eggplants. In a mixing bowl add garlic, olive oil, lemon, cumin, paprika, and cayenne. Stir in the red pepper and eggplants. Sprinkle with salt and pepper. Adjust seasoning. Stir in the mint and parsley.

Note: You can do many variations on this theme. The spices and fresh herbs are all optional, and all could be substituted for other tastes.

Roasted Red Pepper Sardine Spread   SERVES 2 – 3

1 tin sardines in olive oil, drained*
2 tablespoons capers, chopped
1 roasted red pepper, chopped
1 tablespoon dill, chopped
2 tablespoons parsley, chopped
1 spring onion, chopped
2 tablespoons lemon juice
¼ cup full fat Greek yogurt*
1 tablespoon oregano
Salt and pepper

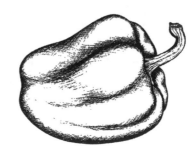

* Can also use homemade grilled sardines. Can substitute yogurt for homemade coconut mayonnaise (pg. 269).

Prepare peppers according to Roasted Eggplant and Red Pepper Spread recipe above. Remove sardine bones and mash sardines with a fork. Stir in all remaining ingredients. Adjust seasoning. Serve with salad or steamed vegetables.

Drinks

Homemade Coconut Milk

1 cup desiccated coconut
Water (roughly 3 cups)

Put the coconut in the blender. Pour just enough warm-hot water to cover. Blend on high for 2 min, gradually adding water until mixture is thick and creamy, yet still blends efficiently. Blend for a total of 2 to 3 min. Strain the contents through a fine cheesecloth, squeezing out all the coconut milk. You can use more or less water depending on the consistency you want.

Homemade Almond Milk

1 handful of soaked almonds*
3 cups water

* Hazelnuts can be used in combination with or instead of almonds.

Soak almonds for at least 12 hours in water. Remove soaking water and rinse. You can store soaked, strained almonds in the refrigerator for several days. This way you can make almond milk whenever needed. Take 1 handful of soaked almonds and put in the blender. Add just enough water to cover the almonds. Blend until smooth. Add the remaining water and blend 30 seconds. Strain contents through a fine cheesecloth. Squeeze out all the liquid and discard the pulp. You can use more or less water depending on how creamy you want the almond milk.

Almond Milk Iced Coffee   SERVES 1

1 single espresso or small cup of coffee, chilled*
1 cup homemade almond or hazelnut milk

* You can also use 2 teaspoons quality instant coffee, like the one manufactured by Clipper.

Add coffee and almond milk to blender. Blend and serve over ice.

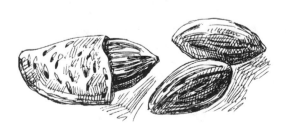
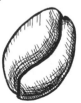

Basic Almond Smoothie   SERVES 1 – 2

1 handful almonds, soaked overnight (soaking water discarded)
1 handful frozen berries (blueberries, raspberries, etc.)
1 banana
5 ice cubes

Put almonds, berries, banana, and ice in blender. Add small amount of water and begin blending, adding more water until smoothie reaches desired consistency.

Basic Coconut Smoothie   SERVES 1 – 2

1 cup homemade coconut milk (pg. 271)
1 handful frozen berries (blueberries, raspberries, etc.)
1 banana
5 ice cubes

Put berries, banana, and ice in the blender. Add a small amount of coconut milk and begin blending, adding more until smoothie reaches desired consistency.

Basic Kefir Smoothie   SERVES 1 – 2

½ cup kefir
1 handful frozen berries (blueberries, raspberries, etc.)
1 banana
5 ice cubes

Put kefir, berries, banana, and ice in blender. Add a small amount of water and begin blending, adding more water until smoothie reaches desired consistency.

Smoothie Boosts

Add one of more of the following to your smoothies.

Acai powder	Chia seeds	Lemon
Avocado	Chlorella	Maca
Basil, fresh	Cilantro, fresh	Macadamia
Cacao nibs	Cinnamon	Matcha
Cacao powder	Coconut oil	Spinach
Camu powder	Ginger	Spirulina
Cardamom	Goji berries	Vanilla
Carob	Hemp protein	Whey protein

Desserts

Chocolate Avocado Mousse   SERVES 4 – 6

1 cup coconut milk, almond milk, or water (pg. 271)
1 cup dates, pits removed
1½ cups avocado
½ cup coconut oil
2 tablespoons maple syrup or honey
10 drops steviol glycosides
½ cup raw cacao powder
Pinch vanilla powder

Soak the dates in the coconut milk until soft. Put all ingredients in the blender and blend until smooth and fluffy. Chill and serve.

Homemade Ice Cream   SERVES 4

1 cup dates, pits removed
¾ cup homemade coconut milk (pg. 271)
¾ cup cashews, soaked 2 hours
2 tablespoons maple syrup or honey (optional)
10 drops steviol glycosides
1 or more flavor addition*

Soak the dates in the coconut milk 15 to 30 min. Add cashews (soaking water discarded), maple syrup, stevia, and one or more flavor additions. Blend well, working in batches. Taste and adjust sweetness if necessary. Pour into a plastic storage container and freeze, stirring roughly every hour. The ice cream needs about 8 to 10 hours to freeze. You can also freeze using an ice cream machine, which will speed up the process. Once the ice cream has become completely solid, simply remove from refrigerator 10 min before serving so it becomes less hard.

Ice Cream Flavors*

Add one or more to your ice cream. For chocolate, chop into small pieces and stir in (don't blend). For pistachios, remove the cashews. For essential oils, only use edible grade.

Cacao powder	Lavender essential oil	Raspberries
Cardamom powder	Lemon essential oil	Rose water
Chocolate, 85%	Mint essential oil	Strawberries
Cinnamon	Pistachios (unsalted)	Vanilla

Creamy Macadamia Sauce
SERVES 4

¾ cup macadamia nuts, soaked 2 hours
¼ cup maple syrup or honey
10 drops steviol glycosides
Pinch vanilla powder
¾ cup water
1 pomegranate, seeds removed
4 handfuls fresh berries

Put macadamias in the blender with maple syrup, stevia, vanilla, and water. Blend well, progressively adding more water to achieve the desired consistency. Serve over fresh berries and pomegranate.

Easy Apple Crumble
SERVES 2

½ cup soaked almonds
½ cup dates, pits removed
¼ cup desiccated coconut
4 tablespoons butter or coconut oil, divided
2 teaspoons cinnamon, divided
4 apples, cored and chopped into large chunks

Medjool and other soft dates don't require soaking. If your dates are not soft, chop them in small pieces and put them in water 10 to 15 min. Dates should be soft but not soggy. Discard the soaking water. Put the almonds, coconut, and 1 teaspoon cinnamon in food processor and process well. Add 2 tablespoons butter and process coarsely. Add dates and again process coarsely. Mixture should just be holding together. Crumble onto a baking sheet lined with parchment paper and bake at 200°F for 45 min. Toss apples with remaining 2 tablespoons of butter and remaining cinnamon. Bake in a separate dish while baking the crumble. When crumble has lightly browned, remove from oven and raise temperature to 350°F until apples are soft and browned. Remove from oven and toss with crumble.

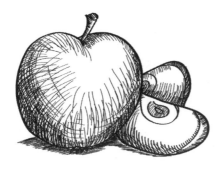

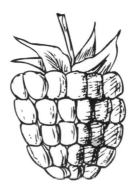

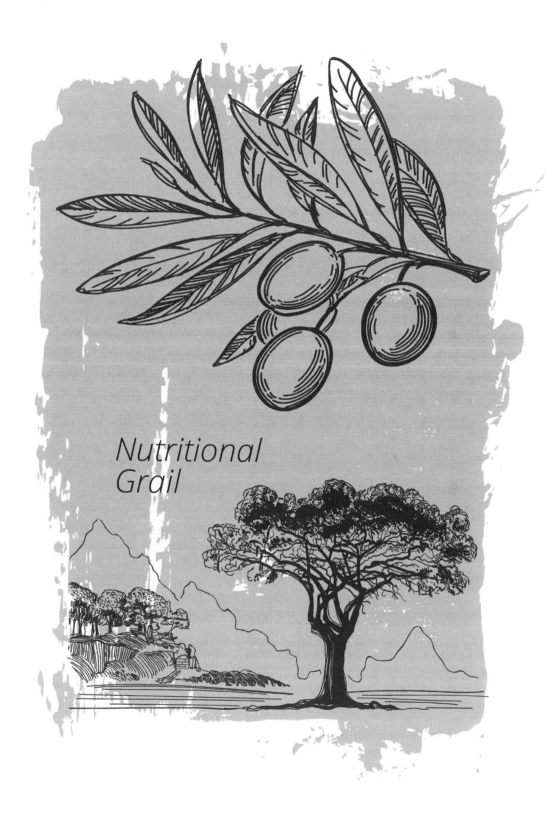

Nutritional Grail

Conclusion

What happened to health? For centuries, death by infectious disease was all too common. Today, infectious diseases are much more contained and manageable, but chronic, degenerative diseases have become the leading causes of death. Is this progress? What changed? The twentieth century was the Dark Ages of nutrition, a time when wholesome, traditional foods were considerably displaced by synthetic, highly processed, and otherwise nontraditional foods. A combination of decadence, naiveté, and greed catalyzed the most radical dietary misdirection in human history. The results speak for themselves.

In 2011, in only its second-ever general assembly regarding health (the first was for AIDS), the UN met to discuss non-communicable diseases, including cancer, heart disease, diabetes, stroke, and lung diseases. These so-called lifestyle diseases are primarily caused by unhealthy diets, physical inactivity, smoking, and alcohol abuse. They currently account for more than 63 percent of deaths worldwide.[1] During the past thousand years, life expectancy has slowly and steadily increased, but lifestyle diseases have decelerated this historical trend and now threaten its reverse.

In 2005, the *New England Journal of Medicine* published a report on the possibility that during the twenty-first century, life expectancy could decline in the US. Absent effective, population-level interventions to reduce obesity, the youth of today could "live less healthy and possibly even shorter lives than their parents."[2] According to the WHO,[3] obesity and being overweight currently account for:

- 44 percent of the diabetes burden
- 23 percent of the heart disease burden
- 7 to 41 percent of various cancer burdens

Two-thirds of US adults are now overweight, while 20 percent are obese. Obesity has doubled since 1980, and by 2015 the WHO predicts that 2.3 billion people will be overweight, of which 700 million will be obese.[4] While obesity does predict certain degenerative diseases, the relationship is more complex than simple causality.

Obesity is technically not a disease. Obesity is a condition characterized by excess body weight, generally caused by lifestyle, genetics, and diet. According to Dr. Robert Lustig, an endocrinologist and obesity expert, there are roughly sixty different obesity diagnoses.[5] Those who are obese, however, are not necessarily sick, and those who carry "normal" body weight are not necessarily healthy. The standard definition of obesity is based on body mass index (BMI) and calculated as body weight divided by height squared (kg/m^2). Being overweight is defined as BMI greater than 25, whereas being obese is defined as BMI greater than 30.

These calculations sometimes fail to accurately indicate who is metabolically healthy and who is not. BMI cannot distinguish, for example, between lean body mass and body fat. Most importantly, BMI cannot distinguish between subcutaneous fat (under the skin) and visceral fat (inside and around the organs). Visceral fat, not subcutaneous fat, drives degenerative disease. Upwards of 20 percent of those who are obese by BMI calculations are actually completely metabolically healthy.[6] On the other hand, up to 40 percent of those with normal BMI scores are actually "obese" and unhealthy in terms of visceral fat.[7]

During the summer of 2013, the American Medical Association voted to declare obesity a disease, reasoning that disease-status recognition would make diagnosing and treating obesity the professional obligation of physicians.[8] Although diagnosing obesity is surely important, BMI should be replaced by more-accurate measurements of visceral fat, especially as obesity is now becoming a matter of public policy. After all, obesity is a predictor of disease, but not a disease itself. So the question remains, are we getting healthier or sicker? Is health declining, and if so, can we reverse the trend through dietary changes?

Heart disease is the number one cause of death in the US and has been since around 1910.[9] Heart disease claimed 158.9 lives per 100,000 in 1910, compared to 193.6 today. During the 1960s, heart disease mortality peaked at 369 deaths per 100,000 and has been declining ever since. Is this cause for celebration? Has the $1.2 billion spent annually by the US on heart disease research been money well spent?[10] Have we turned the corner on the Dark Ages of nutrition?

Top 10 Causes Of Death By Year In USA – Figure 10.1

Year	Cause of Death	Deaths	Rate
2010	Heart disease	597,689	193.6
	Cancer	574,743	186.2
	Lung disease	138,080	44.7
	Stroke	129,476	41.9
	Accidents	120,859	39.1
	Alzheimer's disease	83,494	27.0
	Diabetes	69,071	22.4
	Kidney disease	50,476	16.3
	Influenza and Pneumonia	50,097	16.2
	Intentional self-harm	38,364	12.4
	All causes	2,468,435	799.5
1960	Heart disease	661,712	369.0
	Cancer	267,627	149.2
	Stroke	193,588	108.0
	Accidents	93,806	52.3
	Diseases of early infancy	67,094	37.4
	Influenza and Pneumonia	66,803	37.3
	Arteriosclerosis	35,876	20.0
	Diabetes	29,971	16.7
	Congenital malformations	21,860	12.2
	Cirrhosis of the liver	20,296	11.3
	All causes	1,711,982	954.7
1910	Heart disease	75,429	158.9
	Influenza and Pneumonia	73,983	155.9
	Tuberculosis	73,028	153.8
	Diarrhea and Enteritis	54,795	115.4
	Stroke	45,461	95.8
	Kidney disease	45,008	94.8
	Accidents	39,281	82.7
	Cancer	36,193	76.2
	Premature birth	17,904	37.7
	Senility	12,119	25.5
	All causes	696,856	1468.0

Rate equals deaths per 100,000.

Unfortunately, this downward trend in heart disease mortality can be accredited mostly to treatment, as opposed to risk-factor reductions.[11] The prevalence of heart disease remains very high. In other words, people are still getting heart disease, but modern medicine is keeping them alive longer. Instead of disease prevention, we have disease management. This is better than nothing, but far below our potential, especially considering the effectiveness of simple, proactive, relatively inexpensive (compared to paying for disease management) dietary adjustments.

Calculating disease prevalence largely depends on self-reporting and is limited by numerous other factors.[12] Nevertheless, there is abundant evidence that heart disease prevalence remains high. In the US, for example, inpatient cardiovascular operations and procedures increased 38 percent from 1997 to 2009.[13] Total direct medical costs of heart disease in 2010 amounted to $273 billion. The AHA expects this number to nearly triple, to $818 billion, by 2030.[14] Heart disease mortality has decreased since the 1960s, but heart disease has not gone away. To the contrary, it remains highly prevalent and highly profitable. Figure 10.1 shows the leading causes of US deaths and associated mortality rates for the years 2010, 1960, and 1910.[15]

Of today's top ten causes of death, at least seven are diet-related. And while heart disease mortality has decreased since the 1960s, cancer is an entirely different story. Cancer mortality has steadily increased, having claimed 76.2 lives per 100,000 in 1910, 149.2 in 1960, and 186.2 today. The WHO's International Agency for Research on Cancer first acknowledged in 2004 that obesity, diabetes, and metabolic syndrome all strongly predict cancer.[16] Each of these predictors, of course, is directly related to diet and lifestyle. Cancer is extremely rare in populations eating traditional diets.

By now, most of the world has adopted modern, westernized diets. Observational data regarding the Inuit people from the Arctic regions of Greenland, Canada, the US, and Russia dramatically shows the effects of this westernization. A 2011 study published in the *Canadian Medical Association Journal* demonstrated that 35 percent of Inuit living in Canadian territories are obese. Diabetes, previously nonexistent among Inuit, now afflicts them nearly as much as the larger Canadian population.[17] Likewise, cancer rates have also exploded, now accounting for 20 percent of all deaths in the Northwest Territories, second only to accidental deaths (38 percent).[18] A 2012 study published by the *International Journal of Circumpolar Health* concluded that Inuit cancer rates are increasing "due to changes to diet and lifestyle in recent decades."[19] The connections between diet and disease are now very well established. Of course there are certain genetic predispositions, but being healthy—attaining the nutritional grail—largely comes down to awareness and choice.

The quest for the nutritional grail begins by asking questions. Ask yourself, "Whom does my food serve?" Does it serve my higher Self? Does my food benefit me physically, mentally, and spiritually? Asking these questions begins the process of learning which foods are best for you, why they are best, and how to prepare them. Knowledge combined with action—this is the nutritional grail. By seeking nutritional knowledge, then implementing this knowledge, you serve your inner Perceval, your inner Fisher King, and your inner Grail Kingdom.

After many decades of darkness, a nutritional renaissance finally now is dawning. Accordingly, knowledge about healthy food and lifestyles is becoming increasingly relevant and important. If you are seeking the nutritional grail, you can serve others by sharing your knowledge and your experiences, and of course, by sharing meals.

The grail quest is certainly about asking questions and serving others, but it's also about responsibility and self-sufficiency. To be healthy, you cannot be dependent. You cannot always depend, for example, on others to cook for you. Inevitably, there will be times when your choices are: a) cooking for yourself, or b) eating substandard restaurant food. Learning to cook basic, healthy food can dramatically improve your quality of life. You don't need to study gourmet cooking. The simple recipes from this book provide a very strong foundation. But learning to cook and learning *what* to cook go hand in hand. And just as you shouldn't depend on others to prepare your meals, you also shouldn't depend on others to decide what is and isn't healthy for you.

This might seem like an unusual concluding statement for a book of nutritional advice. This book, however, is simply a reference point, showing you what has and hasn't worked for others. This book shows you the results of scientific experiments, clinical research, and epidemiological studies, as well as the dirty laundry of many industries, corporations, and special interest groups. But this book cannot prove what will actually work for you. Only you can do that, through careful experimentation and observation. This book can guide you, but your success depends squarely on you and your active participation in your own health.

Make your health your business and be the sole shareholder. Own your health. Be the CEO as well. To run a good business, you must understand how your business functions. You must make informed and intelligent decisions. You cannot outsource managerial decisions to other parties. Perhaps your company will need professional advice in certain areas. In this case, you would hire a consultant. A consultant gives you advice and information, but consultants do not make decisions for you. Doctors and other health professionals should be your health consultants.

As a human being, you must attain enough basic information about how your human organism functions so as to make your own informed decisions. Of course you can consult with doctors, dieticians, nutritionists, and other health professionals, but by all means, maintain control of your company. Every business owner must be cognizant of individuals selling products and services not in the best interest of the business. You, too, should be aware of such attempted sales. You must be your own CEO and decide what you need. Let your personal experience guide your decision-making. Try different foods and different food combinations and observe the results. Be scientific. Be intuitive. Create yourself.

Notes

[1] UN News Centre, "Battle against deadly lifestyle diseases figures high on UN agenda next week," September 15, 2011

[2] SJ Olshansky et al., "A Potential Decline in Life Expectancy in the United States in the 21st Century," *New England Journal of Medicine*, March 17, 2005, vol. 352, no. 11, pg. 1138–1145

[3] World Health Organization, "Obesity and overweight," Fact Sheet Number 311, March 2013

[4] World Health Organization, "Unhealthy Diets and Physical Inactivity," NMH Fact Sheet, June 2009; World Health Organization, "Obesity and overweight," Fact Sheet Number 311, March 2013

[5] Clare Leschin-Hoar, "Should Obesity Be Defined as a Disease? The AMA Thinks So," *Take Part*, June 27, 2013

[6] Robert H. Lustig, *Fat Chance: Beating the Odds Against Sugar, Processed Food, Obesity, and Disease*, published by Hudson Street Press, December 2012, pg. 109

[7] Nirav Shah and Eric Braverman, "Measuring Adiposity in Patients: The Utility of Body Mass Index (BMI), Percent Body Fat, and Leptin," *PLoS One*, 2012

[8] Melissa Healy and Anna Gorman, "AMA declares obesity a disease," *Los Angeles Times*, June 18, 2003

[9] Valentín Fuster et al., Promoting Cardiovascular Health in the Developing World: A Critical Challenge to Achieve Global Health, published by the National Academies Press, 2010, pg. 58

[10] National Institutes of Health, "Estimates of Funding for Various Research, Condition, and Disease Categories (RCDC)," April 10, 2013; Shelly Wood, "Part 2: Money—Is cancer beating cardiovascular disease?" *Heart Wire*, August 6, 2011

[11] Ibid., pg. 62

[12] Centers for Disease Control, "Prevalence of Coronary Heart Disease, United States, 2006–2010," *Morbidity and Mortality Weekly Report*, October 14, 2011, vol. 60, no. 40, pg. 1377–1381

[13] Véronique Roger et al., "Heart Disease and Stroke Statistics—2011 Update: A Report From the American Heart Association," *Circulation*, February 1, 2011, vol. 123, pg. e18–e209; Véronique Roger et al., "Heart Disease and Stroke Statistics—2012 Update: A Report From the American Heart Association," *Circulation*, January 3, 2012, vol. 125, pg. e2–e220

[14] Paul Heidenreich et al., "AHA Policy Statement: Forecasting the Future of Cardiovascular Disease in the United States," *Circulation*, March 1, 2011, vol. 123, pg. 933–944

[15] SL Murphy et al., Division of Vital Statistics, "Deaths: Final Data for 2010," *National Vital Statistics Reports*, May 8, 2013, vol. 61, no. 4; Centers for Disease Control, "Leading Causes of Death, 1900–1998," Cdc.gov/nchs/data/dvs/lead1900_98.pdf; David Jones et al., "The Burden of Disease and the Changing Task of Medicine," *New England Journal of Medicine*, June 21, 2012, vol. 366, no. 25, pg. 2333–2338

[16] Gary Taubes, "Is Sugar Toxic?" *New York Times*, April 13, 2011

[17] Grace Egeland et al., "Hypertriglyceridemic-waist phenotype and glucose intolerance among Canadian Inuit: the International Polar Year Inuit Health Survey for Adults 2007–2008," *Canadian Medical Association Journal*, June 14, 2011, vol. 183, no. 9, pg. E553–E558

[18] Inuit Tapiriit Kanatami, "Inuit & Cancer: Fact Sheets," Inuit Tapiriit Kanatami, February 2009, Itk.ca/

[19] Gisèle Carrière et al., "Cancer patterns in Inuit Nunangat: 1998–2007," *International Journal of Circumpolar Health*, 2012, vol. 71: 18581

Index

ABOUT THE AUTHOR

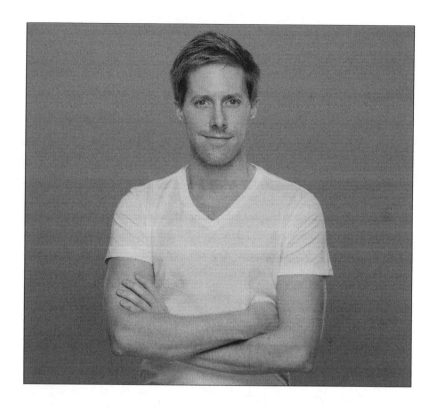

Christopher James Clark is an independent writer, researcher, consultant, and chef with specialized knowledge in nutritional science and healing cuisine. He has a Bachelors of Business Administration degree from the University of Michigan at Ann Arbor and formerly worked as a business analyst for a Fortune 100 company. For the past decade-plus, Christopher's work has focused on health and nutrition, including designing menus, recipes, and food concepts for restaurants and spas, coaching private clients, teaching healthy cooking workshops worldwide, and managing the kitchen for a yoga resort in Greece. For more information, visit christopherjamesclark.com

24657150R00165

Made in the USA
Middletown, DE
07 October 2015